DENTAL MANAGEMENT
OF PATIENTS WITH HIV

DENTAL MANAGEMENT OF PATIENTS WITH HIV

Michael Glick, DMD

Director, Infectious Disease Program
Associate Professor
Department of Oral Medicine
University of Pennsylvania School of Dental Medicine
Philadelphia, Pennsylvania

Quintessence Publishing Co, Inc
Chicago, Berlin, London, Tokyo, São Paulo, Moscow, and Warsaw

Library of Congress Cataloging-In-Publication Data

Glick, Michael.
    Dental management of patients with HIV / Michael Glick.
        p. cm.
    Includes bibliographical references and index.
    ISBN 0-86715-288-5
    1. HIV infections—Patients—Dental care. 2. HIV infections.
 I. Title.
    [DNLM: 1. HIV Infections. 2. Acquired Immunodeficiency Syndrome.
3. Dental Care for Chronically Ill. 4. Infection Control. 5. Oral
Manifestations. WD 308 G559d 1994]
RK55.H58G56 1994
616.97'92'00246176—dc20
DNLM/DLC
for Library of Congress   94-30147
                                          CIP

quintessence
books

©1994 by Quintessence Publishing Co, Inc

Published by Quintessence Publishing Co, Inc
551 North Kimberly Drive
Carol Stream, IL 60188

Editor: *Patricia Bereck Weikersheimer*
Production Manager: *Timothy M. Robbins*
Designer: *Jennifer Ann Sabella*

Printing and binding: Everbest Printing Co, Ltd, Hong Kong
Printed in Hong Kong

CONTENTS

CONTRIBUTORS

Susan E. Beekmann, BSN, MPH
Infection Control Specialist
Hospital Epidemiology Service
Warren Magnuson Clinical Center
National Institute of Health
Bethesda, Maryland

Scott Burris, JD
Assistant Professor of Law
Temple Law School
Philadelphia, Pennsylvania

Mary E. Chamberland, MD, MPH
Chief, Epidemiologic Studies Activity
HIV Infections Branch
Hospital Infections Program
National Center for Infectious Diseases
Centers for Disease Control and Prevention
Atlanta, Georgia

Clay J. Cockerell, MD
Associate Professor of Dermatology
    and Pathology
Director for the Division
    of Dermatopathology
University of Texas,
    Southwestern Medical Center
Dallas, Texas

James W. Curran, MD, MPH
Assistant Surgeon General·
Associate Director for HIV/AIDS
Centers for Disease Control and Prevention
Atlanta, Georgia

Barbara F. Gooch, DMD, MPH
Dental Officer
National Center for Prevention Services
Centers for Disease Control and Prevention
Atlanta, Georgia

David K. Henderson, MD
Associate Director for Quality Assurance
    and Hospital Epidemiology
Warren Magnuson Clinical Center
National Institute of Health
Bethesda, Maryland

Howard M. Kassler, DMD, FACD
Director of Managed Care
Delta Dental Plan of Massachusetts
Boston, Massachusetts

William J. Kassler, MD, MPH
Medical Epidemiologist
Division of STD/HIV Prevention
Centers for Disease Control and Prevention
Clinical Instructor of Medicine
Emory University
Atlanta, Georgia

M. Ann Ricksecker, MPH
Program Director
Pennsylvania Educational Training Center
    for AIDS
Hahnemann University
Philadelphia, Pennsylvania

Milton E. Schaefer, DDS, MLA, FACD
Peoria, Arizona

Robert M. Swenson, MD
Professor of Medicine and Microbiology
Section of Infectious Diseases
Temple University Health Sciences Center
Philadelphia, Pennsylvania

Susan R. Thompson
Training Coordinator
Pennsylvania Educational Training Center
    for AIDS
Hahnemann University
Philadelphia, Pennsylvania

John W. Ward, MD
Chief, AIDS Surveillance Branch
Division of HIV/AIDS
National Center for Infectious Diseases
Centers for Disease Control and Prevention
Atlanta, Georgia

PREFACE

It has been the habit of humankind to wait until the eleventh hour to spiritually commit ourselves to those problems which we knew all along to be of the greatest urgency. All of us world citizens—Eastern and Western, developed and developing, regardless of ethnicity, nationality, or geographic origin—must see AIDS as our problem. Developing countries must do more, not only out of a moral sense of purpose but because it is in their own self economic interest to do so. Nevertheless, we must try and we must succeed or our children and grandchildren will one day rightfully ask us why in the face of such a calamity we did not give our best effort. What shall we tell them—and their mothers in particular—if we don't measure up? How shall I answer my six-year-old daughter and what do we say to the estimated ten million AIDS orphans by the year 2000? That their parents' generation was so racked with political and cultural and religious discord that it was willing to needlessly condone millions of medical refugees?

—Arthur Ashe, December 1, 1992
Address to the United Nations

If it is the habit of humankind to wait until the eleventh hour to address those problems of most pressing concern, then it is no surprise that the HIV epidemic is creating new agendas for all professions touched by the disease. For health-care professionals, perhaps more than others, the epidemic has called upon skills, knowledge, and experience to care for infected persons. Yet for dental providers their role in this epidemic has extended far beyond what has traditionally been the realm of dentistry. Infected patients and society at large expect dentists, hygienists, assistants, and other dental staff members to know how to treat patients infected with HIV. But dental health-care workers are also often sought out, as health-care professionals, for advice on various medical topics. This makes it imperative that the information given to patients about HIV infection and AIDS is balanced, accurate, and based on fact. Misconception will only generate further discrimination and myths surrounding this disease.

Dental providers need to continue to render dental care to all patients, regardless of their social or religious background or sexual orientation. New laws and ethical standards have been formulated to uniquely deal with the provision of health care for HIV-infected patients. The license to practice dentistry is a privilege granted to us based on our training and exper-

9

tise, and we must use this license to provide the best care possible to all individuals seeking our help.

I have often been asked why patients with HIV disease and AIDS continue to seek dental care. One of my patients, who was severely debilitated by HIV wasting syndrome and numerous opportunistic infections that made his every movement an effort, answered this question simply—"I want to feel like everybody else." The need for regular dental care does not diminish during HIV disease progression. On the contrary, many patients present with oral pathologies associated with their disease, and dental providers must be familiar with these manifestations. Treatment of these lesions, which are sometimes accompanied by severe pain, will enable patients to continue oral nutrition and oral medications. Furthermore, many lesions are early manifestations of immune suppression and disease progression. Recognition of the significance of the appearance of these lesions will ensure early medical intervention that may prolong the patient's life. Patients will soon realize that dental care is an integral part of their overall medical care, and that dental providers are part of their treatment team. Questions concerning their health, including medications, disease progression, and alternative treatment protocols, will sometimes be put forth to the dental provider. It is therefore critical that dental providers become knowledgeable about many facets of HIV and AIDS.

Treating patients with HIV disease does not require a major modification of generally accepted principles and standards of dental practice, but it still presents a challenge. This book is intended to alleviate some of the fear and reduce the stigma associated with this disease. This book aims to empower dental-care providers. With information about HIV and AIDS, dental professionals can provide safe and appropriate dental care and take an active part in the overall medical treatment of infected patients. Their involvement in the care of HIV-infected patients will prolong patients' survival and enhance their quality of life. The information contained in this book will also help dental providers become much-needed resources in their community for information about this disease. To provide dental care for HIV-infected patients, we need not dedicated clinics but knowledgeable and dedicated personnel.

I would like to acknowledge my patients, teachers, and Barbie, Noa, Jonathan, and Gideon for all their support in the preparation and writing of this book. With their help, and that of countless others, it is my hope that this generation will go beyond its own discord in addressing AIDS.

1

AIDS in
Historical Perspective

Robert M. Swenson

The plague bacillus never dies or disappears for good; it bides its time in bedrooms, cellars, trunks and bookshelves; and the day will come when, for the bane and enlightenment of men, it would rise up its rats again, and send them forth to die in a happy city.

Albert Camus, The Plague[1]

In December 1981, an article appeared in the *New England Journal of Medicine* describing a curious cluster of seven men who, for no apparent reason, had severe infections with microorganisms that had previously infected only profoundly immunologically compromised individuals. Soon this disease became known as the Acquired Immunodeficiency Syndrome (AIDS). Since then the number of cases has increased at a startling rate. By October 1993, over 340,000 cases had been reported in the United States.[2] It is now estimated that 10 to 20 million people throughout the world are infected with the human immunodeficiency virus (HIV), the cause of the disease we recognize as AIDS.[3] This worldwide outbreak of a devastating new infectious disease has engendered much fear and apprehension, resulting in comparisons to previous epidemics. Although there may be significant differences between the AIDS epidemic and previous epidemics, it is instructive to examine previous epidemics for similarities that may be relevant.

There are at least three general ways to examine these questions. One can consider previous epidemics and the ways they have affected nations, politics, and even the structure of society. Alternatively, one can describe the "sociological responses" to an epidemic, ie, the social and political responses that occur during the course of an epidemic. These reactions tend to be similar in all epidemics, and many have already occurred during the AIDS epidemic. Lastly, because AIDS is a sexually transmitted disease, it is illuminating to compare the response to AIDS with society's responses to other sexually transmitted diseases early in this century. Each of these approaches provides a different perspective on the AIDS epidemic.

Epidemics and Nations

Infectious diseases have had a major influence on Western history. Although epidemics have been frequent and devastating, one can easily categorize the ways in which epidemics have produced these effects. The first of these is through a widespread epidemic affecting the entire population relatively uniformly, resulting in the disruption of social structures and in long-term historical change. The most obvious, and perhaps only, example of this is the epidemic of bubonic plague that occurred in Europe in the fourteenth century.

Epidemics may have markedly different effects on different populations, resulting in significant shifts in the balance of power. The importation of smallpox into the Central American native population is a dramatic example of this effect. Many military battles, in which one military force is more severely affected than the other, are common examples. Frequently, one army suffers from disease more severely than the opposing force, dras-

tically altering the outcome of a battle. In general, since the defending forces tend to be more resistant to their own endemic diseases, this differential effect is most marked on the invading force. A dramatic example of this occurred during Napoleon's invasion of Russia. In June 1812, Napoleon assembled a force of 500,000 men to invade Russia. By the time they reached Moscow, only 80,000 able-bodied soldiers remained. Most of the others were dead or disabled from typhus and dysentery. These catastrophic losses continued, and by June 1813 only 3,000 soldiers were alive to complete the retreat. The vast majority of deaths were due to infectious diseases rather than battle injuries or exposure to the severe Russian winter. Thus, the power of Napoleon in Europe was undermined more by diseases, especially typhus, than by military opposition.

In the last 150 years, smaller epidemics have produced social change through laws enacted and social structures developed in response to the epidemic. Many of our present-day public health laws were enacted during the recurrent cholera epidemics in the United States and England in the mid-nineteenth century. To begin to put AIDS in some historical perspective, it is useful to examine some of these epidemics in greater detail.[4]

Bubonic Plague

Bubonic plague struck Europe in 1347, but events of the previous two hundred years had set the stage for this great epidemic. The eleventh and twelfth centuries were politically stable and disease-free, and food production had increased dramatically. As a result, the population, which had numbered 25 million in 950 A.D., tripled to 75 million by 1250 A.D. Around 1300 A.D. a significant drop occurred in the mean temperatures of Europe, and widespread crop failures ensued. The resulting famine forced many peasants to move to the cities and towns, producing severe crowding and poverty. Under these conditions the black rat population thrived.

In urban areas, plague is a disease affecting rats; it is spread by the rat flea. In an epidemic among rats (an epizootic), large numbers of rats die. (In Camus's *The Plague,* the epidemic is heralded by large numbers of dead rats suddenly appearing on the streets.) Infected fleas leave the dead rats for a new host; if other rats are not available, they will attempt to feed on humans, thereby infecting them. Thus, it is easy to see how under the appropriate conditions of poverty, crowding, and poor sanitation an epidemic such as this could occur.

Plague was already established in several areas of Asia. However, it was not until the mid-fourteenth century that overland travel was efficient enough to carry plague westward to the Mediterranean Sea. The epidemic arrived in Marseilles in 1348, and by 1351 all of Europe was affected. The immediate effects of the epidemic were devastating. The most accurate estimate for total deaths during the first wave of the epidemic is 25 million, or one-third of the population of Europe. No segment of society was spared. Following this epidemic, recurrent waves of plague kept the population at this level for another 150 years.

The consequences of the epidemic were far-reaching. Since the population was devastated, real wages increased dramatically. As peasants' wages increased, they were able to demand a commutation of their services. The population decreased more rapidly than the fall in food supplies, and the resultant drop in food prices made it impossible for landowners to support their large manors. These changes led directly to the end of the manorial system.

The effects of the plague on clergy and the Catholic Church were tremendous. The mortality among clerics was greater than 50%. Yet the epidemic had even more profound effects on the church itself and religious thinking. People turned away from traditional religion, which was perceived as having failed during the epidemic. Many turned to superstitious religion (for example, the flagellants), and, for generations after, much religious thinking focused on the apocalypse. This dissatisfaction with the church contributed significantly to the Reformation.

The plague also affected medicine profoundly. Many cleric-physicians died. These physicians were viewed as having failed, which resulted in a tremendous rise in the number and popularity of surgeons. New medical texts were developed, and the rudiments of scientific inquiry began. The initial theories of contagion were developed, and the concept of quarantine was first recognized. This resulted in the first primitive hospitals and the development of early public health measures.

Two additional points are important. Plague could not occur where it did, when it did, or take the form it did until a variety of conditions had occurred to make it possible. For example, the urban population had to reach a certain density, and living conditions had to decline to a certain level. The rat population also had to reach a certain density and reside in close proximity to humans. And, lastly, travel from Asia had to be sufficiently rapid and frequent to bring the plague bacillus to the European continent. If any one of these had not occurred, the plague epidemic would not have happened. Furthermore, the devastating effects of plague continued because there were recurrent epidemics for the next 150 years. If there had been only a single initial epidemic, however catastrophic, the effects would not have been as great and certainly not as long lasting. Before AIDS the most recent worldwide epidemic was the influenza pandemic of 1918–19. Despite being the largest epidemic in history, it had little long-term effect because the epidemic was relatively short-lived and the population losses were rapidly replaced.

Smallpox

Epidemics have a major effect when the disease has a different impact on two populations. The most dramatic example of this was the importation of smallpox into Central America by the Spanish in 1520. Humans are the only reservoir for the smallpox virus, and transmission is only from human to human. Smallpox had been widespread in Europe for thousands of years so that those who had survived smallpox now had life-long immunity. It appears that when Asians migrated across the Bering Strait sometime before 10,000 B.C., they did not bring smallpox with them. Thus, the native populations of the western hemisphere had never been exposed to smallpox and remained susceptible to infection.

In 1520 a small expedition led by Pánfilo de Narváez left Cuba and sailed for Central America. When the expedition landed in Mexico, one crewman had active smallpox, and infection was established among the susceptible Indian population. From there smallpox spread rapidly throughout Central and South America. Epidemics occurred frequently throughout the sixteenth century, eventually complicated by measles epidemics. It has been estimated that of the native population of 25 million, 18 million eventually died of smallpox. Thus, a major factor, if not the major factor, in the Spanish conquest of the Americas was the importation of smallpox into the susceptible native population.

Cholera

From the mid-nineteenth century to the present, as government bureaucracies became larger and took control of public health functions, much smaller epidemics produced change through legislation and public health measures in response to the epidemics. The cholera epidemics in the United States in 1832, 1849, and 1866 provide excellent examples of these changes.

The largest cholera epidemic began in 1832. The city of New Orleans was hardest hit with 5,000 cases. By historical standards, this was a very small epidemic, but it engendered the clear beginnings of public health policy. In early 1832, the New York state legislature passed laws enabling communities to establish local boards of health, and in the summer of 1832 the New York City Board of Health was created. Quarantine regulations were passed and enforced. Cholera hospitals were established. Housing and care for the destitute were set up. Slum clearance was begun, and early efforts of food and drug control were undertaken. As the epidemic subsided, however, the government felt the measures were no longer necessary, and the New York Board of Health was disbanded.

By the time of the 1866 epidemic, few physicians doubted that cholera was a transmissible disease. With the threat of a third cholera epidemic, New York State passed the law creating the permanent Metropolitan Sanitary District and Board of Health in New York City. This first strong, permanent board of health in the United States exists to this day. The sanitary and public health measures were similar to those employed in 1832, but were more extensive and rigorously enforced. They were also much more

effective as only 591 cases of cholera occurred in New York City during this epidemic. Many of these regulations remain in effect and form the basis of present-day public health policy.

The Social Anatomy of Epidemics

The impact of epidemic diseases can also be analyzed by examining the societal responses to the epidemic, what may be called the "social anatomy" of an epidemic. This means the array of responses of individuals, groups, and society as a whole to a given epidemic. There are certain attitudes and behaviors that occur during all epidemics.

The first is denial of the disease. In 1832, when the New York Medical Society stated publicly that nine cases of cholera had been diagnosed in New York City, the announcement was immediately attacked by New Yorkers who felt that it was premature or totally unwarranted. Business leaders were particularly upset, realizing that the fear of cholera and a possible quarantine of the city would be disastrous for business. Not until six weeks later, when the evidence was overwhelming, was the outbreak officially recognized by the New York Board of Health. Denial also occurs at the national level. The initial outbreak of influenza in 1918 was at Camp Funston, Kansas. Major epidemics occurred two months later in England, France, and Spain. Initially, each country attempted to deny the presence of influenza within its borders (noting, of course, that influenza was present somewhere else.)

Once an epidemic is recognized, someone, or something, is quickly blamed. As bubonic plague swept through Europe in 1348, it was widely claimed that it had been caused by the Jews, who were believed to have poisoned the wells. As a result, thousands of Jews were burned at the stake. The cholera epidemics in the United States affected the poor disproportionately. At that time, poverty was viewed as a consequence of idleness, slothfulness, and intemperance. The latter was also clearly believed to make one more susceptible to cholera. Since new immigrants were often the poorest, they were blamed for their susceptibility to cholera, as well as for bringing the disease into the country. Prostitutes were also blamed for the epidemic, even though cholera was not thought to be a venereal disease. Many believed that their "moral corruption" caused cholera in them, as well as in their clients.

Blame could also be placed at a national level. After the initial outbreak of influenza in the United States, epidemics occurred in Spain, England, and France. In addition to attempting to deny their own epidemics, the countries blamed one another. The French referred to the epidemic as the Plague of the Spanish Lady, and the English called it the French Disease. Even today we refer to the Asian Flu.

An epidemic represents the recurrence of an old, dreaded disease or the appearance of a new and terrifying one. In either case, once an epidemic is recognized and acknowledged, fear ensues. Ironically, those most at risk tend to be least afraid, and those least at risk are most afraid. Thus, public policy and responses to the epidemic tend to be driven by a fearful middle-class majority that wants to protect itself from the infected and dangerous poor. These fears frequently distort policy and produce the call for unnecessary and restrictive measures.

Epidemics represent old diseases that are not yet understood, and thus controlled, or new diseases. In either case, physicians do not have the knowledge either to prevent the epidemic or treat its victims effectively. As a result, society views the physicians and the medicine of the time as having failed. A corollary of the failure of the existing methods of medicine is the rise of alternative therapies during an epidemic. During the plague epidemic, innumerable new preventatives and therapies arose. This is hardly surprising since existing texts and measures provided no effective treatment. During the cholera epidemics in the United States, allopathic physicians employed a variety of "heroic therapies," including bleeding and the administration of mercury and opiate treatments. These measures failed to treat cholera and had numerous harmful side effects. Given the failure and hazards of traditional medicine, it is no surprise that it was surpassed in popularity by botanical medicine during the early cholera epidemics.

Epidemics of Sexually Transmitted Diseases

To understand the public response to the AIDS epidemic, it is helpful to review the syphilis and gonorrhea epidemics in the early part of this century. At that time the organisms causing syphilis and gonorrhea had been identified, and it was clear that the diseases were sexually transmitted. It was also known that these were not trivial infections, but diseases with grave consequences, such as infertility and death. As a result, it was concluded that there was a great need for sex education. Despite this there were tremendous obstacles to what became known as the social hygiene movement. First, the remaining tenets of Victorian respectability made it virtually impossible to discuss venereal diseases. The basic assumptions of the time were that men were driven by lust and that discussing sex with them would only make them lose their last vestiges of control. The major question became: How can sex education be presented to men without their recognizing the subject? The answer was to veil the discussion in talk about plants, birds, and bees. Given these subterfuges, there could be little effective sex education.

At that time, large numbers of middle-class wives were being infected by their husbands, who had contracted their infections from prostitutes. With the recognition that gonorrhea was a common cause of infertility, some feared that the middle class was committing "race suicide." In response to the epidemic of venereal diseases among the middle class, physicians actively promulgated the idea of casual, nonsexual transmission (sine coitu) of syphilis and gonorrhea. It was apparently more important to protect the reputation of middle-class men than to provide a proper understanding of these diseases. The idea of casual transmission remained firmly entrenched well into the AIDS epidemic, even though there has been no evidence to support it.

As might be expected, prostitutes were blamed for the spread of venereal diseases early in the century. They were viewed as not only a moral threat, but as a health threat to the family as well. Because of this concern, the United States embarked on an effort to eradicate prostitution. Suggestions that prostitution could be regulated, as in France, were unacceptable. These ideas have persisted in one form or another throughout the twentieth century, with profound effects on our efforts to control sexually transmitted diseases, including AIDS.

Epidemiology—AIDS and Hepatitis B

AIDS

Before discussing the AIDS epidemic specifically, it is useful to examine why new infectious diseases occur. The answers are complex but may be summarized briefly.[5] The appearance of truly new organisms is extremely rare. New infectious agents do not arise in a vacuum but evolve from preexisting ones, usually among animal populations. We do not know the origins of HIV, but a primate origin is suggested and appears likely, particularly for HIV-2. The origin of HIV-1 is more problematic. The existence of animal lentiviruses with a predilection for the CD4+ T lymphocytes strongly suggests an animal origin for this virus also. However, it has been proposed that the nonpathogenic precursor of HIV-1 has infected humans for a long period, and that relatively recently it mutated to become the pathogenic virus that causes AIDS.[6]

Although we may know how HIV-1 evolved, we do not know exactly where it evolved. The precise area of the world where this occurred will probably remain unknown. Nevertheless, it seems clear that the oldest part of the epidemic began in Subsaharan Africa, where some of the earliest AIDS cases can be traced to the 1960s. By the mid-1970s, changes in modern air travel brought HIV to the rest of the world. Rapid urbanization around the world, the development of jumbo jets, and relatively low airfares produced dramatic increases in international travel to and from Central Africa, distributing HIV widely. As fourteenth-century travel had to become rapid and frequent enough to bring plague from Asia, modern jet travel had to expand greatly to spread HIV throughout the world.[7]

In the United States, HIV was introduced first into the population of homosexual males. Once there, HIV was carried to those areas with the largest concentration of homosexual men—New York, San Francisco, and Los Angeles. Additional factors account for the rapid spread among homosexual males. First, anal intercourse is the most effective sexual means of transmitting HIV. Second, homosexual males are a small, relatively sexually closed community, concentrated in major urban areas. Finally, with the Gay Liberation Movement promiscuity among some homosexual males increased dramatically, producing rapid and widespread dissemination of the virus among homosexual men. However, because of the long latency period between HIV infection and the development of AIDS, the first cases did not appear in the United States until 1978.

The next group infected with HIV were injection drug users. Homosexual drug users, already infected with HIV, infected other injection drug users through the sharing of needles. This second wave of the epidemic occurred in the early 1980s, three or four years after the first wave of the epidemic. Drug users now account for 35% of the AIDS cases.[8] The third wave of the epidemic, which began in the late 1980s, is the development of AIDS among the sexual partners of bisexual males and injection drug users. The final wave of the epidemic, which is now beginning, will be when AIDS cases occur in greater numbers among the remainder of the population.

AIDS, the final stage of HIV infection, occurs, on average, ten years after initial infection with HIV. In diagnosing a case of AIDS in 1994, we are literally recognizing an infection transmitted around 1984. It is more pertinent to ask: What is the extent of the spread of HIV infection in 1993? There are no complete answers to this question, but some insight can be gained from examining hepatitis B infection.

Hepatitis B

Hepatitis B is similar to HIV and is frequently used as the epidemiologic model for HIV. However, there are two major differences. First, hepatitis B is far more transmissible, that is, more infectious. Second, the hepatitis B epidemic is twenty years ahead of the HIV epidemic. Thus, it is possible to use information on the epidemiology of hepatitis B now to predict the epidemiology of HIV twenty years from now. In the United States, hepatitis B infection is spread throughout the population at an endemic level of 3% to 5%, that is, this percentage of healthy blood donors anywhere in the United States has had hepatitis B infection.[9] In all likelihood the spread of HIV will be similar. By the year 2010, HIV infection will be spread through the entire population of the United States, although because it is significantly less transmissible the level will be closer to 0.2% to 0.5% of the population. HIV infection will continue to be concentrated among certain populations: gay men, injection drug users, the urban poor, and those with other sexually transmitted diseases. As the HIV epidemic evolves in the United States, the pattern of transmission will become increasingly that of heterosexual transmission (resem-

bling increasingly the pattern of transmission in Africa), as indeed it has already begun to.

AIDS in Perspective

Several assumptions are necessary to speculate on the ultimate impact of the AIDS epidemic. First, it seems certain that the number of persons infected with HIV will continue to grow. For now, the only methods for slowing the spread of the virus are abstinence from sexual intercourse, "safer sex," or, in the case of drug users, stopping injection drug use. We have never before successfully controlled a sexually transmitted disease (STD), and there is little to suggest that we can do so now. The threat of STDs may slow sexual activity somewhat, but in the past this has not had significant impact. In less-developed areas, with few birth control programs, it seems inconceivable that widespread condom use will occur. Similarly, drug abuse programs have been notoriously ineffective. Increased poverty and worsening social conditions in many countries, including the United States, will provide fertile ground for the spread of HIV among the poor.[10] These are but a few of the factors that will contribute to the increasing spread of HIV throughout the world and our inability to control this spread.

How does the AIDS epidemic compare to the epidemic of plague in the fourteenth century? During the first three years of the plague epidemic, one-third to one-half of the population of Europe died. Obviously, nothing comparable is happening in the AIDS epidemic. However, recurrent epidemics of plague kept the population at a reduced level for the next 150 years and had powerful impact on existing social structures. Over time AIDS may have a similar impact in undeveloped areas of the world, most notably Subsaharan Africa.

In Central Africa, HIV infection has continued to spread widely, particularly in urban areas. The prevalence of HIV infection in areas of Rwanda and Uganda ranges from 15% to 25% of the population.[11] The burden of infection falls on two groups: young men and women, and children born of infected women. Already, the prevalence of neonatal AIDS has eroded improvements in infant mortality rates attained over the past 20 years. The deaths of young men and women have begun to erode governmental and other societal structures. The economic drain has been immense and has extended far beyond the public health sector of these nations. The impact of AIDS in Africa is beginning to resemble the long-term impact of the plague epidemic of the fourteenth century. Since it is unlikely that effective medications and vaccines, even when available, can be supplied to these countries, the consequences of this continuing epidemic will be devastating.

Since HIV infection is not distributed evenly throughout the population of the United States, it is possible to look at the different effects on populations in this country. The most obvious group is the gay community, which has been hardest hit by the AIDS epidemic. For the gay community, AIDS has been the Great Plague. The events and emotions that now define their lives revolve around AIDS and its consequences, and the gay community is now organized around the fight against the disease. The attention focused on AIDS has brought more public attention to homosexuals. While this has engendered more public support for them, it has also resulted in a backlash as states and communities pass increasing numbers of "anti-homosexual laws."

AIDS is increasingly a disease of the poor; most drug users are in fact poor. Society views drug users as the conduit of HIV into the rest of society and a source of crime and violence. Faced with the choice of spending great sums of money either to attempt to alleviate poverty and rehabilitate drug users or separate them from the rest of society, we have so far made the latter choice. As in the cholera epidemics of the 1800s, the poor are blamed for their disease and feared as a threat to the "decent people" of society.

The sociologic responses to the AIDS epidemic have been strikingly similar to other epidemics in history. In the first years of the epidemic, it was common to hear that AIDS was not an epidemic—that is, it was common to deny its existence. When it was recognized that AIDS could be transmitted by blood products, some in the blood-banking industry vehemently denied this possibility, in part because of the economic consequences of the measures required to control such transmission. As the epidemic grew and it was recognized that homosexual males and drug users were primarily affected, people began to deny that AIDS would spread to the rest of the population. Although it is now incontrovertible that HIV is spreading, and will continue to spread, throughout all segments of society, there continues to be disbelief or denial that this will happen.

Once the AIDS epidemic was recognized, it engendered widespread fear. As in other epidemics, those least at risk—the middle-class majority—were most afraid. And those most at risk—the poor—seemed to be least afraid. Thus, the concerns of the media as well as public health policy were driven by the distorted fears of the middle class. For example, from early in the epidemic there was widespread panic over acquiring HIV from a blood transfusion. The risk, although real, was never of great magnitude, but it nevertheless engendered great fear because now *anyone* was in danger of being infected.

A more recent example of this sort of distorted fear has been the furor over the possibility of acquiring HIV infection from an infected health-care worker.[11] Despite the minute risk of such an occurrence, public fear drove the CDC to initially promulgate highly restrictive policies for the HIV-infected health-care worker. Clearly the fear of transmissibility of HIV infection is tremendously exaggerated in the public psyche. In fact, this fear is the single major stumbling block to instituting reasonable, rational public policies. In the fourteenth century Jews were burned at the stake because they were believed to have started the bubonic plague. Earlier in the AIDS epidemic, a home in Arcadia, Florida, was burned to the ground because it was feared that their HIV-infected hemophiliac boys were a threat to other children. There seems to have been little progress in 500 years.

The AIDS epidemic has provided ample opportunities to cast blame. Initially the world seemed to "blame" Africa for starting the epidemic. In response, Africans denied that AIDS even existed there, even though there was overwhelming evidence to the contrary. Americans blame homosexuals for starting the epidemic and drug users for spreading it to the rest of society. For many it was clearly the moral failings of these groups that caused them to be infected. Some of America's fundamentalist evangelists cited AIDS as a sign of God's wrath on homosexuals and drug users. These sentiments are reminiscent of the nineteenth-century view of poverty as a moral failing and cholera as God's wrath on the poor and wicked.

As in other epidemics, medicine today has been criticized for its failures. Throughout the epidemic there have been claims that not enough resources are being devoted to finding a cure for AIDS. (Such statements usually imply, or even state, that part of the reason for this is that society really does not care about the groups most at risk for AIDS.) There has been an ongoing controversy between AIDS activists and researchers over the ways clinical trials should be conducted. In the United States this has essentially resulted in the abandonment of the placebo-controlled trial, premature termination of trials, and approval of drugs even before they have been completely evaluated.[13]

With no cure for AIDS available, innumerable alternative therapies have arisen. People have grasped at claims of the value of high doses of vitamins, a variety of nutritional remedies, and other alternative treatments. It is no surprise that people faced with an incurable illness have turned to these alternative therapies. Yet, despite a certain superficial sophistication, many of these alternative therapies seem strikingly similar to the claims of botanical medicine voiced 150 years ago during the cholera epidemics.

Early in the AIDS epidemic the approach to the control of its spread was remarkably similar to that proposed to control syphilis and gonorrhea in the early 1900s. Because AIDS is a sexually transmitted disease, the only way to control transmission today is to educate people, including children, about sex, sexually transmitted diseases, and AIDS. In 1910, the question was how to teach men about sex without their recognizing the subject. Earlier in the AIDS epidemic the question seemed only slightly different— how can we teach people about AIDS without talking about sex? Apparently most Americans still believe that talking to people about sex will cause them to have sex. These beliefs resulted in such confusing euphemisms as "exchange of body fluids." Although it is lessening, there remains widespread opposition to explicit and effective sex and AIDS education for American children.

Because many Americans believe that people with AIDS have become infected because of some kind of immoral, illegal, or otherwise unacceptable behavior, many continue to support a morality- or criminal-based approach to the control of the disease. This entwining of morality with public health makes it exceedingly difficult to implement appropriate, effective public health measures. Education about homosexuality is viewed as promoting homosexuality; needle exchange programs for drug users are believed to condone illicit drug use; measures to educate and protect prostitutes are thought to lend support to infidelity and extramarital sex; and measures to protect sexually active teenagers are seen as promoting early premarital sex. Until, and unless, we separate public health from private morality, our efforts to control this epidemic will remain ineffective.

There is one unique aspect to the AIDS epidemic. Most epidemics fall first, and disproportionately, on the poor. The AIDS epidemic, however, began among middle-class gay men. These men were well educated and highly motivated, and many were already organized and active in the Gay Liberation Movement. Thus, very early in the epidemic the images of the epidemic were created by gay men. To a gay man in urban America it appears that as many as 50% of his community is infected and will be dead in ten years, and much of the rest of society seems indifferent. To the rest of heterosexual society, the

AIDS epidemic appears as a "small epidemic" occurring somewhere else in society. The clash of these opposing images of the epidemic has been, and continues to be, a source of great conflict over the meaning and significance of AIDS.

As the epidemic has evolved, however, AIDS has increasingly become a disease of the poor. AIDS in America is becoming more and more like AIDS in a developing country. The reasons for this are many, but they are primarily the result of the socioeconomic conditions in America. The rates of infectious diseases, including AIDS, have always been determined more by social conditions than by biology, medicine, or public health.[14]

As scientific understanding has increased and superstitions subsided, much has changed about epidemics throughout history. In important ways, this has made the AIDS epidemic unlike any previous great epidemic. However, society's responses to the AIDS epidemic have been similar to society's responses to previous epidemics. Although our advanced biotechnology has allowed us to apply sophisticated techniques to the medical problems of AIDS, our human responses have changed little, hindering us from dealing effectively with many of the social problems integral to the AIDS epidemic.

References

1. Camus A. The Plague. Random House: New York, 1946.

2. Karon JM, Buehler JW, Byers RB, Farzio KM, Green TA, Hanson DL, Rosenblum LS. Projections of the number of persons diagnosed with AIDS and the number of immunosuppressed HIV-infected persons—United States, 1992–1994. MMWR 1992;41(RR-18):1–29.

3. Merson M. Slowing the spread of HIV: agenda for the 1990s. Science 1993;260:1266–1268.

4. Swenson RM. Plagues, history and AIDS. The American Scholar 1988:57(2):183–200.

5. Morse SM, Schluederberg A. Emerging viruses: the evolution of viruses and viral diseases. J Infect Dis 1990;162:1–7.

6. Smith TF. The phylogenetic history of immunodeficiency viruses. Nature 1988;333:573–575.

7. Grmek M. History of AIDS: emergence and origin of a modern pandemic. Princeton: Princeton University Press, 1990.

8. Schoenbaum E, Hartel D, Selwyn PA, et al. Risk factors for human immunodeficiency virus infection in intravenous drug users. N Engl J Med 1988;321:874–878.

9. Hadler SC, Margolis HS. Epidemiology of hepatitis B infection. In Ellis R (ed): Hepatitis vaccines in clinical practice. Marcel Dekker: New York, 1993:141–157.

10. Feinstein JS. The relationship between socioeconomic status and health: a review of the literature. Milbank Quart 1993;71:41–64.

11. N'Galy B, Ryder RW. Epidemiology of HIV infection in Africa. J Acquir Immune Defic Syndr 1988;1:551–558.

12. Chamberland M, Bell DM. HIV transmission from healthcare workers to patient: what is the risk? Ann Intern Med 1992;116:871–873.

13. Rothman DJ, Edgar H. Scientific rigor and medical realities: placebo trials in cancer and AIDS research. In Fee E, Fox D (eds): AIDS: the making of a chronic disease. Berkeley: University of California Press 1992:194–206.

14. Wilkinson RG. National mortality rates: the impact of inequality? Am J Pub Health 1992:1082–1084.

2

Law and Ethics and the Decision to Treat

Scott Burris

By the beginning of this century, the medical profession had adopted an approach to ethics, and to government regulation, that strongly favored professional autonomy and linked it to the proper exercise of the doctor's art.[1] Dentistry followed suit and, if anything, dentists in independent private practice became among the least-regulated health-care practitioners in the country. The HIV epidemic, however, has begun to change this. The specter of HIV transmission has led to mandated infection-control practices, and the reality of discrimination has led to new limits on the freedom of dentists to pick and choose their patients. The presence of HIV has also raised the stakes regarding the confidentiality of medical information and led to new laws that regulate how and when health-care providers can divulge it.

Case Study

J.B. had been receiving dental care from Dr Clausen since 1986. During that time, Dr Clausen had treated J.B. about 20 times, providing routine examinations, cleaning, fabrication of dentures, and extractions. In 1987, J.B. had tested positive for HIV but had remained asymptomatic and did not inform Dr Clausen of his condition.

In 1989, J.B. provided an updated dental history for Dr Clausen and disclosed that he had HIV. Dr Clausen continued to provide routine care to J.B., seeing him twice in 1989 and in March 1990. During the March visit, J.B. stated he was taking azidothymidine (AZT). J.B. made a September appointment for a cleaning, but Dr Clausen later had his receptionist cancel the appointment and refer J.B. to the dental clinic at a local university, a clinic known in the community as a place that would treat HIV-infected patients, and to which Clausen had referred two other patients with HIV. Dr Clausen made the decision to refer without consulting J.B., J.B.'s physician, or anyone knowledgeable about HIV. J.B., who declined to go to the university clinic, filed a complaint with the state human rights commission, which investigated the case and eventually brought J.B.'s complaint before a judge.

Dr Clausen told the judge that he believed he should refer any patients with HIV to protect their health, and because of his lack of knowledge about the disease. He insisted that his act should be treated as an appropriate referral and not a refusal to treat, and that he was simply exercising reasonable medical judgement in light of what is known about HIV. The judge, however, saw the evidence differently.

The judge did not accept Clausen's characterization of his actions as a referral. The routine cleaning for which J.B. was scheduled was not outside of Dr Clausen's area of expertise; in other words, Dr Clausen would not have made a similar referral for a person who did not have HIV. The American Dental Association and other experts were clear that this kind of care was safe and appropriate for a dentist to provide to a person with HIV. Although Dr Clausen claimed to be concerned about J.B.'s health, he did not discuss the matter with J.B. or his doctor. Finally, a patient who is referred to a specialist usually returns to his primary care provider. This was a terminal referral.

The judge was equally skeptical of Dr Clausen's medical judgment. Dr Clausen believed, and found another dentist to testify, that people with HIV should be treated in isolation rooms to protect them from exposure to aerosols from adjacent rooms. (Dr Clausen incorrectly believed that the university clinic used isolation rooms.) The judge, drawing on general public health guidelines and two experts put forward by J.B., found no reasonable probability of harm to either patient or dental staff under normal infection control conditions. The fact that Dr Clausen could find at least one dentist who saw a danger was not sufficient to insulate Dr Clausen's judgment from legal review.

Because Dr Clausen's proffered reasons for the referral had little or no medical basis, the judge found them unworthy of credence and merely a pretext for discrimination. The judge ordered Dr Clausen to pay damages of $10,000 to J.B. for mental anguish and suffering, and to pay a $5,000 civil penalty to the state. This is a true story—the judge's decision was affirmed on appeal[2]—and it illustrates the kind of limits that the law now places on the discretion of health-care providers to pick and choose their patients.

All dentists should be aware that they are ethically and legally required to treat patients with HIV as they would any other patient. Nevertheless, many dentists are not entirely sure where the obligation originates and have questions about the details of the obligation. Many dentists continue to deny care to people with HIV. After reviewing the basic legal and ethical framework governing the treatment of HIV-infected patients, I will discuss some of dentists' most common legal questions.

Ethics

The ethical position of the American Dental Association is summarized in a 1988 opinion of the Council on Ethics, Bylaws and Judicial Affairs[3]:

> A dentist has the general obligation to provide care to those in need. A decision not to provide treatment because the individual has AIDS or is HIV seropositive, based solely on that fact, is unethical. Decisions with regard to the type of dental treatment provided or referrals made or suggested, in such instances, should be made on the same basis as they are made with other patients, that is, whether the individual dentist believes he or she has need of another's skills, knowledge, equipment, or experience and whether the dentist believes, after consultation with the patient's physician if appropriate, the patient's health status would be significantly compromised by the provision of dental treatment.

This ethical position could well have been drafted by a lawyer—and not just because it is so wordy and larded with poorly punctuated qualifications. Like the law, the Code of Ethics takes it for granted that a dentist using universal precautions can treat a person with HIV without endangering the patient, other patients, or the dental team. There is an assumption that any procedures that can be provided to a patient without HIV can be provided to a patient who has HIV. Like the law, however, the Code of Ethics does not say that HIV status can never be a factor in the decision about what treatment, if any, a dentist should provide. In fact, dentists can play an important role in the diagnosis and treatment of HIV disease because of its tendency to express itself in oral symptoms.[4,5] When treatment would pose a real threat of harm to the patient, or when specific complications of HIV put treatment beyond the capacity of a nonspecialist, a denial of treatment or a referral may be justifiable. The suggestion that such a decision should be made after consultation with the patient's doctor, and the stipulation that the patient's health be significantly compromised both indicate that these situations will be unusual and based strictly on valid medical facts.

Throughout the first decade of the epidemic, persistent reports of discrimination indicated a failure by the profession to heed the call of ethics. Some have suggested that dentistry's obligation to relieve pain and suffering has never been taken seriously enough by dentists. "The pervasive attitude among dentists is that dental care is an optional health service with no particular right of access even for healthy patients," a defect attributed to flaws in dental education.[6] Surveys conducted during the 1980s indicated that a minority of dentists would refuse to treat an asymptomatic HIV-infected patient, and that a majority would prefer not to treat patients with more advanced HIV disease or AIDS.[7,8] Later surveys indicate some improvement in dentists' attitudes,[9] and at least two studies of patients' experiences have suggested that, for all their professed reluctance, most dentists do not actually refuse to treat when confronted with a real patient.[10,11] Few would dispute, however, that the profession has been ambivalent about treating HIV-infected patients, and that many dentists continue to decline to provide care. Even many of those who treat HIV-infected patients have done so quietly, almost shamefacedly, fearing to be known to other patients or the public as an "AIDS dentist." In many communities, special clinics have opened to meet the needs of patients with HIV who cannot get dental care elsewhere.[12]

Even if they are not always followed, ethical rules are important in the culture of dentistry. Ethics represent a profession's commitment to the community it serves. Dental ethics—like medical ethics—constitute an acceptance of the additional responsibility that comes with the training and privileged status of a healing profession. Ethics are also part of the structure of justification for professional self-regulation. The government is kept out of

the business of setting behavioral standards on the ground that the profession can and does police itself. A failure to live up to its own ethical standards invites the community to step in and set mandatory standards. In 1989, Michael Davis warned dentists that a "profession that seems to prefer its own safety even when that means turning the needy from its door resembles a trade association rather than a profession. The public is likely to treat dentists accordingly."[13] One could argue that Davis' warning came true in the passage of new laws directly prohibiting discrimination by dentists.

Perhaps the most important function of the ethical rule against discrimination is its potential use within a program of education. If the behavior of dentists is to be changed, both practitioners and those still in training need to accept the responsibility to learn about HIV and provide care. Norms of behavior—the collective values of the profession—are an important part of this social learning. The sense that one's peers and role models expect one to provide care, and do so themselves, is invaluable in changing behavior. Moreover, the problem of negative patient reaction to treating HIV-infected patients can only be overcome if the public understands that all dentists treat HIV-infected patients.[14]

Antidiscrimination Law

For decades, the legal analysis of a dentist's choice of patients began and ended with the contract. The dentist and the patient were free agents, agreeing to exchange services for money. Both dentist and patient could choose each other or not, for any reason. With some minor limits, to be discussed, each was free to end the relationship when it was no longer to his or her liking.[15] Unless a dentist agreed to surrender his right to choose patients, usually by accepting employment in a clinic or contracting to provide services to clients of a health maintenance organization, the law had little to say about the decision to treat. Antidiscrimination law and HIV have added a significant limitation: a dentist may not refuse to treat someone, or provide unequal services, based solely on a patient's disability or even perceived disability. The development of this legal rule has taken several years, a history worth reviewing.

The Rehabilitation Act of 1973

Perhaps the most important moment in the legal history of the HIV epidemic came when the Supreme Court ruled, in a 1987 case called *School Board of Nassau County v Arline*,[16] that a communicable disease could fit the legal definition of a handicap in the Rehabilitation Act of 1973, which was then the only national law prohibiting discrimination against people with physical disabilities. Although the ruling dealt with tuberculosis, it implicitly endorsed several lower court decisions treating HIV as a disability, and laid down a legal approach that made it inevitable that future cases would reach the same conclusion.[17,18]

Justice Brennan, writing for the Court, described the law's basic purpose as being "to ensure that handicapped individuals are not denied jobs or other benefits because of the prejudiced attitudes or the ignorance of others." In passing the law, Brennan explained:

> Congress acknowledged that society's accumulated myths and fears about disability and disease are as handicapping as are the physical limitations that flow from actual impairment. Few aspects of a handicap give rise to the same level of public fear and misapprehension as contagiousness. . . . The [Rehabilitation] Act is carefully structured to replace such reflexive reactions to actual or perceived handicaps with actions based on reasoned and medically sound judgments. . . . [16]

For the first time, people with serious communicable diseases were protected under the law against unnecessary discrimination.

The special problem posed by communicable diseases is, of course, the risk to others. No one has ever argued that the sick have a right to infect the healthy. Under the approach introduced in the *Arline* case, a person with a communicable disease is protected against discrimination only if he or she does not pose a "significant risk" of harm to another. Although there have been some exceptions, most cases applying this standard have found that the low risk of HIV transmission arising in the treatment of patients with HIV is not significant enough to justify discrimination.[2,15]

The protection of people with HIV under the Rehabilitation Act was a landmark legal development, but it actually had very little direct impact on dental patients. The Rehabilitation Act only forbids discrimination in programs or activities receiving federal funds, including business contractors and federal agencies. Only individuals and groups receiving such federal funding must abide by the antidiscrimination rules. Dental clinics in federally funded institutions are covered, as are all clinics that receive federal funding in the form of Medicare or Medicaid Part A reimbursements,[19,20] but a dentist working as an independent contractor in an institution that is covered by the Rehabilitation Act is not personally subjected to it unless the dentist is an actual recipient of federal funds in his or her own right.[21,22] Thus, the only private dentists potentially covered by the Rehabilitation Act are those who treat patients with Medicare and Medicaid under Part B of the program, but there is no case law yet that has said so.[23,24]

On the other hand, where the Rehabilitation Act does apply, its coverage is broad. The obligation to not discriminate applies to everyone the funding recipient deals with, not just the intended beneficiary of the program. So, for example, a hospital that receives Medicaid funding is barred not only from discriminating against patients with Medicaid, but also from discriminating against any patient or employee on the basis of disability.[25]

The Americans with Disabilities Act of 1990

When Congress passed the Americans with Disabilities Act (ADA) in 1990,[26] it adopted the basic rules and approach of the Rehabilitation Act, but made them applicable to a much broader class of businesses and activities. Its employment discrimination provisions apply to all businesses with 15 or more employees.[27] Far more important for dentists, however, is Title III of the ADA, which states that "[n]o individual shall be discriminated against on the basis of disability in the full and equal enjoyment of the goods, services, facilities, privileges, advantages or accommodations of any place of public accommodation."[28]

"Public accommodation" is legalese for a business, service, or activity open to the general public. Examples are hotels, restaurants, and trains. Traditionally, the definition of public accommodation was interpreted to exclude "purely private" facilities, like social clubs, and it was assumed that professional offices were well within this exception. When HIV discrimination by health professionals first became prevalent, there was no federal law regulating discrimination in places not receiving federal funds, but many states had disability discrimination laws that covered discrimination in public accommodations. Those alleging discrimination sought relief under these laws, with mixed results. In some, the term "public accommodation" was interpreted to include dental offices,[29,30] but other patients were unsuccessful in establishing this point.[31]

With the passage of the ADA, these laws have become much less important. The ADA not only provides a strong rule against discrimination that is independent of these state laws, but also leaves no doubt that a dental office is a public accommodation. The ADA provides a list of covered public accommodations, rather than a general definition, and prominent on the list is the "professional office of a health-care provider." Subsequent regulations issued by the Department of Justice (used by courts and lawyers to interpret the law) further define this term to mean "a location where a person or entity regulated by a State to provide professional services related to the physical or mental health of an individual makes such services available to the public," a definition broad enough to cover even home offices.[32] With the ADA in place, the focus of litigation will turn from whether dentists are covered to the precise nature of the obligation not to discriminate.

Sanctions

Both the Rehabilitation Act and the ADA are powerful tools for an aggrieved patient. Under both, the patient can seek an immediate order requiring the accused discriminator to treat, and under the Rehabilitation Act, the patient can seek monetary compensation for actual losses and any pain and suffering (including humiliation) the refusal to treat has inflicted. Damages are also available under many state and local antidiscrimination laws. (In one District of Columbia case, for example, a person with HIV was awarded damages of $60,000 against a dentist who had refused him treatment.)[30] The public accommodations portion of the ADA does not authorize any monetary damages, but like the Rehabilitation Act, it authorizes a court to make a losing defendant pay the plaintiff's attorneys' fees, and complainants may combine their federal claims with claims under state and local laws that do allow damages.

Licensure Laws

All states have laws and regulations governing the licensure of individuals to practice dentistry, and these rules include substantive requirements of professionalism, competence, and good conduct. A dentist who discriminates against a person with HIV could be accused under the applicable licensing law, and be ordered to treat the patient, or be disciplined. In Maryland and New Jersey, licensure rules explicitly prohibit a licensed provider from refusing to treat a patient he or she could otherwise care for based solely on HIV status.[20] In Pennsylvania, a violation of a state disability discrimination statute is automatically referred to the relevant licensing board for possible professional discipline.[33]

A more vigorous enforcement of nondiscrimination rules by professional licensing boards would certainly help spread the message that discrimination is illegal. It might even be more of a deterrent to dentists than antidiscrimination law, since the loss of one's license is a penalty far more intimidating than even an award of money damages and attorneys' fees. Nevertheless, for several reasons, individual litigants are not likely to pursue license sanctions as a main avenue of relief. Lay people (and their lawyers) may be skeptical of the willingness of licensing boards to consider their claims seriously and to impose serious penalties on offenders. Lay people, even lawyers, may also be unaware that there is a complaint procedure. The process is slow, and it ultimately offers only the most abstract satisfaction for the complainant, who gets no recompense for injuries.

Tort Law and Malpractice

Dentists have always been subject to suit if they fail to provide care that meets the standards of the profession. A dentist who fails to treat a patient thoroughly or competently will not be able to defend this carelessness on the ground that the patient had HIV. Indeed, if a dentist takes the position that a patient's HIV status was the ground for quick or incomplete work, the dentist could well face greater tort liability than that which would arise out of ordinary malpractice. A health-care provider who mistreats a patient in a way that a reasonable person would consider outrageous may be liable for intentional infliction of emotional distress, with attendant damages for the victim's emotional pain.[34]

Confidentiality

Health-care providers are generally aware of an obligation to maintain the privacy of patient's medical information, although in practice, information often flows quite freely. The HIV epidemic has led to the passage of confidentiality legislation in most states, protecting HIV test results or, in many states, any information that would reasonably identify a patient as having or being at risk of HIV. These statutes dictate how, and how carefully, a provider should maintain dental records including HIV-related information, and commonly control how such information may be passed on to other people, including other health-care providers.[35] Every dentist should know what the law is in his or her state.[35] Every dentist should carefully guard the confidentiality of a patient's medical information through thorough staff training and careful attention to the security of records. A record should never be released to a third party unless the dentist is certain that the recipient has the proper authorization. In one extreme case, a New York court ruled that a doctor could be liable for up to $50,000 in punitive damages for releasing HIV information to an attorney pursuant to a subpoena that was not, in fact, legally binding.[36]

Common Questions and Some Answers

Under the federal disability discrimination laws, and under many state laws, dentists do not have the right to deny treatment to an HIV-infected patient based solely on the patient's HIV status. Accepting that obligation, however, does not eliminate all questions.

Q. Can I test patients for HIV, or insist that they fill out a medical questionnaire?

A. Implementing the universal precautions required by the Occupational Safety and Health Administration (OSHA) eliminates any need to know a patient's HIV status for infection control purposes. On the other hand, an HIV test is, in medical terms, a diagnostic tool that may be of value to the patient, and any practitioner can be of more help if he or she is fully informed of the patient's medical history.

Testing for or asking about HIV to decide whether or not to treat is clearly illegal.[37] Testing patients with "suspected" HIV on an ad hoc basis would be difficult to justify as a medical practice and would therefore support an inference of improper purpose. Similarly, denying treatment to a patient who refuses to be tested or complete a history would also be questionable, because the provider is expected to treat the patient regardless of HIV status, and the sort of clinical symptoms that might indicate a referral would be apparent without an HIV test. A consistently applied policy of seeking complete medical histories from every patient, but not requiring any patient to disclose any information, is the most legally defensible approach. There have been no patient testing cases yet under the federal antidiscrimination laws.

The Justice Department's analysis of the ADA explains that the law prohibits attempts to unnecessarily identify the existence of a disability.[38] There has been a case under Hawaii state law in which a dentist was freed of any liability for refusing to treat a patient who refused to take an HIV test prior to treatment.[39] The court held that the refusal to treat was based on the patient's refusal to provide information, not on the patient's HIV status. The court assumed and the dentist claimed that he would have provided treatment even had the result been positive. However, in light of universal precautions, this is probably very weak ground to stand on in a future case outside Hawaii.

Dentists should also be aware that in most places, HIV testing is governed by detailed state laws. These commonly require the patient's informed, written consent for testing and for the release of any information, and also often require the tester to provide pre- and post-test HIV counseling to the patient.[35]

Assuming that a dentist is not seeking information with the intention of refusing treatment, HIV-related inquiries should never become a matter of dispute, legal or otherwise. If a dentist legitimately needs the information for the benefit of the patient, he or she should be able to explain this to the patient and win the patient's co-operation. The best prophylactic measure against litigation is a trusting, confidential relationship with the patient.

Q. Can I refuse to treat people because I know or suspect they are homosexual, or a present or former injection drug user?

A. Opinion surveys have found that many dentists object to homosexuals or drug users and are reluctant to treat them, for moral reasons supposedly unrelated to HIV.[7,8] Only a few states and cities prohibit discrimination based on sexual preference, and under the federal disability discrimination laws, current illegal drug use excludes an individual from protection.[40,41] However, regulations limit this exclusion when it comes to health and drug rehabilitation services.[42] The American Disability Act specifically prohibits discrimination against a disabled person who has undergone or is undergoing a supervised rehabilitation program or who is erroneously regarded as engaged in drug use.[40]

Even if discrimination based on sexual preference is strictly legal, the dentist who engages in it could well have serious legal trouble. Federal law protects not just the actually disabled, but also those who are perceived as disabled. In other words, it is just as illegal to discriminate against someone you believe to have HIV as someone you know has HIV. A homosexual or former injection drug user who is denied medical care may well believe, and will have a good chance of convincing a judge or jury, that the denial was really based on a fear of HIV rather than merely a more general prejudice.[21,36,39,40,43]

Q. What if I just don't feel competent to treat HIV-infected patients?

A. Get additional training. Subjective feelings of inadequacy will not be accepted as a justification for refusal to treat. All dentists will be expected to comply with universal precautions requirements and will be presumed to be able to provide the same services to patients with HIV as they supply to other patients.

Q. Is a referral discrimination?

A. Some dentists seem to think that a referral is different from a refusal to treat. From a legal point of view, however, it is not. A dentist's obligation under antidiscrimination law is not to treat a person differently merely because he or she has HIV. The law is broken whether the patient is thrown out of the chair or denied an appointment over the phone—or sent to a different practitioner. The emphasis here, unlike that in the area of abandonment, is not whether the patient's dental needs are ultimately met, but whether the dentist complied with the law.

On the other hand, all referrals are

not illegal. Department of Justice regulations for the ADA explain that patients with HIV are entitled generally to the same services as those made available to other patients. However, the law does not require a dentist to provide categories of care outside his or her area or specialty to a patient just because the patient has HIV.[44] For example, if a dentist ordinarily does not perform root canals, the dentist does not have to perform the procedure just because a patient has HIV. In such a case, a referral to a specialist would be perfectly appropriate.

On occasion, a patient with HIV may present the reasonable prospect of serious complications, even in a procedure the dentist customarily performs. In such a case, the issue is not the dentists' lack of dental expertise, but the need for greater expertise in the care of a seriously ill patient. It is not the government's intention to prevent the referral of a disabled patient if the disability itself creates specialized complications for the patient's health.[45] Such a patient is the exception rather than the rule, especially in the area of HIV, but when the exception presents itself a referral to a specialist is not illegal.

The touchstone for assessing a referral is the zone of one's ordinary practice and area of competency. If the service sought is within that zone, it must be provided. A dentist contemplating a referral of an HIV-infected patient should be sure he or she has clear answers to some basic questions: What, specifically, is the problem the patient has that you feel incapable of treating? Why? Have you made an effort to learn more about the problem before referring? Unusual is not the same as complex. What service does the dentist referred provide that you cannot with reasonable effort provide yourself? Have you consulted the patient's physician in assessing the need for the referral? Do the patient and the patient's physician agree with your assessment of the risks? In practical terms, the most important element is, once again, communication and trust between dentist and patient. Providers should particularly be aware that some patients may prefer less expert care by a provider they know and trust to the best efforts of a more qualified stranger. If the patient cannot be convinced that a referral is the best course, a provider should reassess the plan.

Q. What if I think that the patient would just be better off in a clinic, even though I could, in theory, provide the necessary treatment?

A. Questions of patient welfare present particularly difficult problems for law. No one wants the law to force dentists to go against their best professional judgment, or to interpose fear of litigation between the dentist and the patient. Yet patient welfare is also a common pretext for discrimination, and it is precisely the sort of rationalization for unnecessary discrimination that would delude a well-meaning but misguided dentist into thinking discrimination is kindness.

Cases raising this defense will be among the most difficult, as the courts will have to second-guess a delicate medical judgment, measuring the dentist's objective abilities and the exact condition of the patient. It is likely, however, that courts in such cases will side with the plaintiffs, not the dentists, because the statute's focus is on the risk the patient poses to others, rather than the risks to the patient himself, particularly if those risks are small. If it is for the patient's good, it should generally be the patient's choice. The fact that a lawsuit was brought in a case like this would suggest that the patient was not convinced of the need for a referral. One important indicator of the propriety of the referral in legal terms is whether it is terminal: even if a particular procedure requires a different dentist, there is no reason to stop providing all care to the patient.

Q. If a patient denies having HIV, but I find symptoms on examination, can I refuse further treatment?

A. This is probably not an uncommon situation. Many people who have HIV don't know it, and the first clue may be oral symptoms. The question assumes that the patient has deliberately deceived the dentist, but that could well not be the case. Even if a patient does know, there is generally no obligation to inform a health-care worker of one's condition (although a recent case in California found that a patient who had affirmatively denied having HIV after repeated direct questions had committed a fraud on the health-care worker who inquired,[46]

and many states authorize disclosure of a patient's HIV status after an exposure that could transmit the disease to a health-care provider.)[35]

Any decision to stop treating a patient is also limited by the tort of abandonment.[47] As long as services within a course of treatment are still needed, a dentist cannot unilaterally terminate the relationship with the patient without providing sufficient notice to allow the patient to make a smooth transition to another provider.[20]

Q. I understand the medical facts, but what if my staff will not treat?

A. You cannot use staff reluctance as a justification for discrimination. Your proper response is to educate your staff and, if necessary, discipline employees who refuse to perform their duties.[30] As the employer and the person ultimately providing the public accommodation, you are legally responsible for the discriminatory acts of your staff. If a person with HIV is turned away by a receptionist, you will be liable as if you had done it yourself.[34,36,21,48]

Q. What if my other patients will be upset and go elsewhere?

A. Many dentists voice concern that their practices could be hurt if other patients learn that people with HIV are being treated in the office. Depending on the community and the prevailing level of concern about dental transmission of HIV, this can be a real problem. Of course, it may also be no problem at all. The legal bottom line is, however, that "customer preference" is no defense.[30] Allowing the unjustified fear of other patients to justify discrimination would be contrary to the basic purposes of the antidiscrimination laws. As far as the law is concerned, the solution to this problem is for all dentists to accept their responsibilities, rather than let the irresponsibility of others justify more irresponsible behavior.

Q. Can I ask my HIV-infected patients to come at a special time, say the end of the day, to avoid their mixing in the waiting room with other patients?

A. This seems to be a common response to the concern about other patients' reactions. As with other points, much depends on how the problem is approached. You are not likely to be sued for asking the patient to do you this favor, provided it is truly a request and the patient appreciates your concerns. On the other hand, Department of Justice regulations specifically prohibit different or separate services for the disabled.[49] Forcing a patient to come at odd or inconvenient or special times would be an obvious violation of the law, and even asking the patient to consider it could lead to legal trouble.

Q. What if the person is in a wheelchair, and my office just isn't set up to accommodate that?

A. This is not a valid justification for discrimination. The ADA was passed to combat discrimination against *all* disabled people. Providers of public services, like dentists, are required to make their offices accessible to the handicapped, which would include access not just to the office itself but also to the waiting room, bathrooms, and examination and treatment areas.[41] The Department of Justice has issued detailed regulations governing accessibility, which should be consulted for details on the ADA's specific requirements in new and existing facilities.[50]

Q. Can I charge more for special services, like draping the work area?

A. Like referral, this is a question of medical necessity, although this one has an easy answer. Public health authorities advise specific universal precautions for all patients. Additional precautions, even if provided at no charge, are discriminatory because they are unnecessary. Even if they were necessary, Department of Justice regulations prohibit special charges for modifications and procedures that do not create unreasonable new costs or burdens.[21] Special fees for unnecessary services would also get you into trouble with the authorities under the Medicare and Medicaid programs.[48]

Q. Can I take additional precautions, like draping, as long as I don't charge the patient for them?

A. Precautions above and beyond those specified in OSHA and CDC universal precautions guidelines are legally risky even if the patient is not made to pay an additional charge. If the patient is humiliated, or if others can deduce the patient's HIV status from the extra measures, both discrimination and privacy laws could be implicated. There have, however, been two recent cases under New York law holding that free, additional draping of work surfaces for patients with HIV is not discriminatory, at least in the absence of evidence that the patient actually suffered humiliation.[51,52]

Conclusion

Health-care professionals commonly regard the legal system as a source of lightning bolts: unexpected, arbitrary, and terribly dangerous attacks can come at any time from nowhere. This view is partly based on inaccurate and politicized reporting of the so-called malpractice explosion. Careful studies actually show that only a small fraction of malpractice victims ever sue, and that those who sue do not actually receive disproportionate awards. The view is also based, however, on true cases in which professionals have been attacked for bad outcomes even the best exercise of one's training could not have prevented. Generally, however, the best way to avoid litigation is

to concentrate on meeting the dental needs of the people who entrust themselves to your care.

References

1. Starr P. The Social Transformation of American Medicine: The Rise of a Sovereign Profession and the Making of a Vast Industry. Basic Books, 1982.

2. *Beaulieu v Clausen*, 491 NW2d 662 (Minn 1992).

3. American Dental Association. Principles of ethics and code of professional conduct. J Am Dent Assoc 1988;117:657–661.

4. Glick M. General protocol for treating patients with HIV disease. Gen Dent 1990; Nov-Dec:418–425.

5. Gerbert B, Badner V, Maguire B. AIDS and dental practice. J Public Health Dent 1988; 48:68–73.

6. Rogers V. Dentistry and AIDS: ethical and legal obligations in the provision of care. Med Law 1988;7:57–63.

7. Moretti R, Ayer W, Derefinko A. Attitudes and practices of dentists regarding HIV patients and infection control. Gen Dent 1989;Mar-April:144–147.

8. Gerbert B. AIDS and infection control in dental practice: dentists' attitudes, knowledge, and behavior. J Am Dent Assoc 1987; 114:311–314.

9. Sadowski D, Kunzel C. Are you willing to treat AIDS patients? J Am Dent Assoc 1991; 122:29–32.

10. Hazelkorn H. The reaction of dentists to members of groups at risk of AIDS. J Am Dent Assoc 1989;119:611–619.

11. Gerbert B, Sumser J, Chamberlain K, Maguire BT, Greenblatt RM, McMaster JR. The dental care experience of HIV-positive patients. J Am Dent Assoc 1989;119: 601–603.

12. Goldstein M. A dentist who fills a gap. Newsday; June 8, 1992.

13. Davis M. Dentistry and AIDS: an ethical opinion. J Am Dent Assoc 1989;Supp:9–11.

14. Burris S. Education to reduce the spread of HIV. In Burris S, Dalton H, Miller J (eds): AIDS Law Today. New Haven, CT: Yale University Press; 1993:82–114.

15. Brennan TA. Patients and health care workers. In Burris S, Dalton H, Miller J (eds): AIDS Law Today. New Haven, CT: Yale University Press; 1993:377–403.

16. School Board of Nassau County v Arline, 480 US 273 (1987).

17. *Chalk v United States,* 840 F2d 701 (9th Cir 1988).

18. *Cain v Hyatt,* 734 F Supp 671 (EDPa 1990).

19. *United States v Baylor University Medical Center,* 736 F2d 1039 (5th Cir), *cert denied,* 469 US 1189 (1984).

20. Jackson M, Hunter N. The very fabric of health care: the duty of health care providers to treat people infected with HIV. In Hunter N, Rubenstein W (eds): AIDS Agenda: Emerging Issues in Civil Rights. New York: The New Press; 1992, 123–146.

21. 28 CFR §36.301(c) (1993).

22. *Glanz v Vernick,* 756 F Supp 632 (D Mass 1991).

23. 43 CFR App A, §2 (1987).

24. Parmet W. An anti-discrimination law: necessary but not sufficient. In Gostin (ed): AIDS and the Health Care System. New Haven, CT: Yale University Press; 1990, 85–97.

25. Tucker B, Goldstein B. Legal Rights of Persons with Disabilities; vol 3. Horsham, PA: LRP Publications; 1992:18–26.

26. 42 USC §§12101 et seq (Law Co-op 1993).

27. 42 USC §12111(5) (Law Co-op 1993).

28. 42 USC §12182(a) (Law Co-op 1993).

29. *Hurwitz v NY City Commission on Human Rights,* 535 NY2d 1007 (Sup 1988).(NY City Commission on Human Rights June 30, 1993) later proceeding Campanella v Hurwitz, no GA-0021-03/04/87 (final decision and order awarding complainant $7500 in damages).

30. In re Lewis v Runkle, no 92-254-PA[N] (DC Commission on Human Rights July 1, 1993), AIDS Litigation Reporter (Andrews) p 10641 (September 28, 1993).

31. *Sattler v NY City Commission on Human Rights,* 580 NY2d 35 (Sup Ct App Div 1990).

32. 28 CFR §36.401(d)(i) (1993).

33. Pennsylvania Human Relations Act. 43 Pa Cons Stat Ann §959(f)(3) (West Supp 1993).

34. *Miller v Spicer,* CA no 90-586 (D Del May 7, 1993) AIDS Litigation Reporter (Andrews), p 10274 (July 13, 1993).

35. Burris S. Testing, disclosure, and the right to privacy. In Burris S, Dalton H, Miller J (eds): AIDS Law Today. New Haven, CT: Yale University Press; 1993: 82–114.

36. *Doe v Roe,* no 0369 (App Div NY May 28, 1993) AIDS Litigation Reporter (Andrews), p 10294 (July 13, 1993).

37. Neugarten J. Note: The Americans with Disabilities Act: magic bullet or band-aid for patients and health care workers infected with the human immunodeficiency virus? Brooklyn Law Rev 1992; 57:1277.

38. 28 CFR App B §36.301(a) (1993).

39. *Doe v Kahala,* 808 P2d 1276 (Haw 1991).

40. 42 USC §12210 (Law Co-op 1993).

41. Mahoney J, Gibofsky A. The Americans with Disabilities Act of 1990: changes in existing protection and impact on the private health services provider. J Legal Med 1992;13:51–75.

42. 28 CFR §36.209(b) (1993).

43. *Leckelt v Board of Commissioners of Hospital District no 1,* 909 F2d 820 (5th Cir 1990).

44. 28 CFR §36.302(b) (1993).

45. 28 CFR App B §36.302(b) (1993).

46. *Boulais v Lustig,* no BCO38105 (Cal Super Ct June 6, 1993) 2 Health Law Reporter (BNA) p 857 (1993).

47. McIntyre L. The action of abandonment in medical malpractice litigation (Comment). 36 Tul L Rev 834 (1962).

48. 42 USCA §1320(a)-7(b) (1993).

49. 28 CFR §36.202(c) (1993).

50. 28 CFR App A §36.101 et seq (1993).

51. *North Shore University Hospital v Rose,* 600 NY 2d 90 (Sup Ct App Div 1993) (draping consistent with professional practice when acts occurred in 1985).

52. *Syracuse Community Health Center v Wendi AM,* 604 NYS 2d 406 (Sup Ct App Div 1993) ("[P]roof adduced at the factfinding hearing demonstrated that draping of surfaces that might become contaminated by blood or saliva is an acceptable precaution against the spread of HIV infection. It was also established that the treatment rooms are not visible from the waiting area, that the doors to the treatment rooms are kept closed except when staff members go in and out, and that no one but the patient and clinic staff members were aware that the precaution of draping had been utilized.")

3

Epidemiology and Prevention of HIV Infection and AIDS

Barbara F. Gooch, Mary E. Chamberland,
John W. Ward, and James W. Curran

Since the recognition of the first cases of AIDS in 1981,[1,2] infection with HIV has emerged as an immense and complex challenge to public health. The number of AIDS cases reported has increased each year (Fig 3-1). By December 1992, more than 250,000 AIDS cases, the most severe manifestation of infection with HIV, had been reported in the United States.[3] In 1992, 47,095 AIDS cases were reported to the Centers for Disease Control and Prevention (CDC), an increase of a few percent over the previous year. This number was almost 20% of all cases reported to the CDC since the beginning of the epidemic.[3] In late 1989, it was estimated that in the United States, approximately 1 million persons were infected with HIV, and 40,000 to 80,000 persons were being infected annually.[4]

HIV infection has become a leading cause of death, particularly among young adults.[5] The number of deaths attributable to AIDS in the United States has increased each year, from 125 deaths in 1981,[6] to more than 33,000 deaths in 1992.[7] By 1992, HIV infection was the most common cause of death among men aged 25 to 44 years, and the fourth leading cause of death among women of the same age.[8]

During the 1990s, it is expected that the number of AIDS cases reported annually in the United States will continue to increase, but at a slower rate than earlier in the epidemic.[9,10] How-

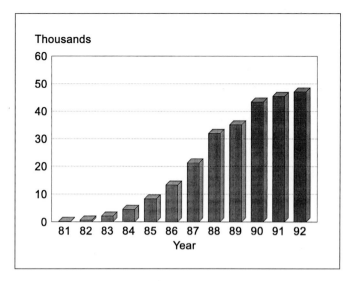

Fig 3-1. Annual AIDS cases by year of report, United States, 1981–92.

ever, the number of persons reported with AIDS each year will remain high, and these persons will be in need of prevention and treatment services within the health-care system.[9,10]

Approximately 50% of AIDS cases in the United States continue to be reported among homosexual/bisexual men; the burden of disease among these men will continue to be enormous. The nature of the epidemic, however, is changing. In 1992, the number of homosexual/bisexual men reported with AIDS decreased slightly from the previous year.[3] At the same time, women and men with AIDS who were infected through heterosexual contact accounted for the most rapid increase in any HIV-exposure group.[3] Most women diagnosed with AIDS in 1992 had been infected through heterosexual contact.[3] These changing trends reflect the multiple epidemics of HIV infection and AIDS among different population groups and different regions in the United States.

Globally, almost every country has been affected by HIV infection and AIDS. The World Health Organization (WHO) estimated in mid-1993 that worldwide, about 13 million adults and 1 million children had been infected with HIV.[11,12] Of these, more than 2.5 million persons had developed AIDS since the beginning of the pandemic, approximately 80% of those in developing countries.

Although nearly two thirds of the world's persons with HIV live in sub-Saharan Africa, transmission of HIV infection has been rapid in other regions, such as South and Southeast Asia. WHO estimates that 1.5 million infections have occurred there since the mid-1980s. The majority of the world's HIV infections have been acquired through heterosexual transmission, which will continue to account for an increasing proportion of all infections.[12] Five of every 11 new

HIV infections among adults occur in women.[13] It is expected that tens of millions of persons will be infected with HIV over the next decade and beyond with most of these persons residing in developing countries.[12]

Surveillance for HIV/AIDS in the United States

The CDC, in collaboration with state and local health departments, initiated a surveillance system in the United States for AIDS soon after the first cases were reported and well before the causative agent, HIV, had been identified. The national AIDS surveillance system is based on a standard case definition and has been an essential indicator of the course of the HIV epidemic in this country. AIDS is a reportable condition in all 50 states, the District of Columbia, and U.S. territories. Standardized reports of people who meet the surveillance case definition are sent without names from state and local health departments to the CDC. Although the completeness of reporting of AIDS cases can vary, recent studies indicate that at least 80% of AIDS cases are reported.[14]

Since 1982, the CDC's surveillance case definition for AIDS has been revised three times—in 1985, 1987 and, most recently, in 1993. These revisions resulted from an increased understanding of HIV infection, disease progression, and the availability of laboratory tests to confirm infection and monitor immune status.[15–17]

The original case definition included life-threatening opportunistic infections and cancers recognized to be most common among persons with cellular immunodeficiency.[6] For persons with laboratory-confirmed HIV infection, the 1987 revision incorporated HIV encephalopathy, wasting syndrome, and other indicator diseases such as *Pneumocystis carinii* pneumonia (PCP) and Kaposi's sarcoma that are diagnosed presumptively (ie, without laboratory evidence confirming the opportunistic disease or condition).[16] In addition to the 23 clinical conditions in the 1987 AIDS case definition, the 1993 expanded case definition included adults and adolescents with HIV and CD4+ T-lymphocyte counts of less than 200 cells/mm^3 or a percent of total lymphocytes of less than 14%, and persons with HIV diagnosed with pulmonary tuberculosis, recurrent pneumonia (more than two episodes in a 12-month period), and invasive cervical cancer.[17]

The 1993 surveillance case definition should more accurately monitor the number of persons diagnosed with severe HIV-related immunosuppression because the population of persons with HIV and CD4+ T-lymphocyte counts < 200/mm^3 is substantially larger than the population of persons with AIDS-defining conditions.[17] Also, since the surveillance case definition was last revised in 1987, the increasing use of prophylaxis against PCP and anti-retroviral therapy for persons with HIV has slowed the rate at which these persons develop AIDS-defining clinical conditions. Finally, the 1993 surveillance case definition is consistent with the classification system for HIV infection revised in 1993, which emphasizes the clinical importance of the CD4+ T-lymphocyte count in the categorization of HIV-related clinical conditions and medical management of persons with HIV.[17]

Because symptoms of AIDS can develop 10 years or longer after an initial infection with HIV, trends among persons reported to have AIDS result from earlier patterns of HIV transmission and may not reflect the current patterns of HIV infection in a community, population subgroup, or country. HIV serologic surveys are necessary to accurately monitor trends in the prevalence and incidence of HIV infection, to assist in targeting and evaluating prevention efforts, and to estimate current and future needs for prevention and treatment services.[18] In the United States, the CDC collaborates with state and local health departments and other institutions and agencies to conduct surveys of HIV seroprevalence among persons treated at selected clinics and hospitals in metropolitan areas, blood donors, applicants for military service, Job Corps entrants, and newborn infants.[18] Another source of information on HIV infection in the United States is the standardized HIV-infection reporting system also developed by the CDC in collaboration with state and local health departments. Since 1985, 26 states have implemented HIV infection reporting by patient name to state health departments.[19,20]

Changing Trends

Demographic Trends for AIDS

Since 1981, approximately 90% of AIDS cases in adults and adolescents have been reported in men; more than 40,000 reported cases were among men in 1992 alone (Table).[3,7] In 1992 the AIDS case rate among men (40 per 100,000 men) remained much higher than that among women (6 per 100,000 women)[7] and resulted primarily from large numbers of reported cases among homosexual/bisexual men. However, since at least 1989, the rate of increase of women with AIDS has been more rapid than the rate of increase of men with AIDS. From 1989 to 1992, the proportion of women among persons with AIDS increased from 11% to more than 13%.[21] Nearly three quarters of all AIDS cases among women are directly associated with the use of injection drugs (50%), or indirectly through sexual contact with a male who injected drugs (22%).[7] In 1992, for the first time, the number of women infected through heterosexual contact nearly equaled the number infected due to their own injection drug use.[3]

In 1992, 62% of all persons diagnosed with AIDS were between 20 and 39 years of age, as the epidemic continues to impact younger adults disproportionately. Of all cases reported among women with AIDS in 1992, 85% occurred among women of childbearing age—15 to 44 years, and about one quarter occurred among those who were between 20 and 29 years of age.[3] AIDS cases among those

Table. Characteristics of Reported Persons with AIDS in 1992

Category	Number	Percent	Rate*	% Change 1991–1992
Sex				
Male	40,453	85.9	32.6	2.5
Female	6,642	14.1	5.1	9.8
Age (years)				
0–4	624	1.3	3.2	16.6
5–12	146	0.3	0.5	−7.0
13–19	159	0.3	0.6	0
20–29	7,982	16.9	19.5	−1.4
30–39	21,212	45.0	49.1	2.2
40–49	11,963	25.4	36.7	8.5
50–59	3,515	7.5	16.0	4.7
60+	1,494	3.2	3.5	5.9
Race/ethnicity†				
White	22,328	47.4	11.8	0.6
Black	15,890	33.8	53.7	8.8
Hispanic	8,282	17.6	31.0	1.0
Asian/Pacific Islander	314	0.7	4.3	11.3
American Indian/Alaskan Native	113	0.2	6.1	37.8‡
Region				
Northeast	13,507	28.7	26.5	0.7
Midwest	5,296	11.2	8.9	17.9
South	15,788	33.5	18.3	0.3
West	10,881	23.1	20.2	8.3
US territories	1,623	3.5	45.6	−9.7
HIV exposure				
Homosexual/bisexual men	23,933	50.8	—	−1.1
History of IV drug use				
Women/heterosexual men	11,423	24.3	—	1.0
Homosexual/bisexual men	2,429	5.2	—	−4.7
Persons with hemophilia				
Adult/adolescent	316	0.7	—	0
Child (aged less than 13 yrs)	21	< 0.1	—	−16.0‡
Transfusion recipients				
Adult/adolescent	673	1.4	—	−3.2
Child (aged less than 13 yrs)	19	< 0.1	—	−51.3‡
Heterosexual contacts	4,111	8.7	—	17.1
Perinatal	696	1.5	—	13.4
No identified risk	3,474	7.3	—	
Total	47,095	100.0	18.5	3.5

*Per 100,000 population.
†Excludes persons with unspecified race/ethnicity.
‡Estimate of percentage change in cases may be less reliable due to small number of cases.
Source: CDC. Update: acquired immunodeficiency syndrome—United States, 1992. *MMWR* 1993;42:548.

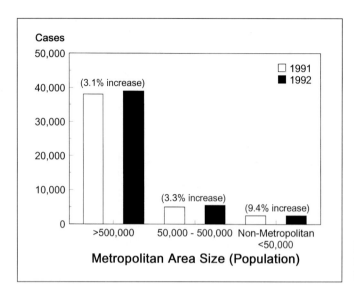

Fig 3-2. Increase in reported AIDS cases by metropolitan area size, United States, 1991–92.

in their twenties include many persons who were infected in their teenage years.

Of all AIDS cases reported through 1992, more than 4,000 have been reported in children less than 13 years of age.[7] Most of these children (86%) were born to mothers with or at risk of HIV infection.[7] About 12% of these cases can be related to blood transfusion or treatment of hemophilia. The 624 AIDS cases reported in 1992 among children aged 0 to 4 years represented an increase of 17% over 1991. Most of these infants and young children (96%) were infected perinatally, and this number reflects the increase in prevalence of AIDS and HIV infection among women in their childbearing years.[3]

Although most AIDS cases through 1992 were reported in non-Hispanic whites, racial and ethnic minorities have been disproportionately affected by the AIDS epidemic. In 1992, more than 50% of reported cases were among non-Hispanic blacks and Hispanics, while these two population groups represented about 20% of the total U.S. population. When compared to the 1992 case rate among non-Hispanic whites (12 per 100,000), rates were approximately 4.5 times greater for blacks (54 per 100,000) and three times greater for Hispanics (31 per 100,000).[3] Among women and children differences in AIDS case rates among ethnic and racial groups are even more striking. In 1992, rates among women were 17 times higher for black women (31.3 per 100,000) and 8 times higher for Hispanic women (14.6 per 100,000) than for white women (1.8 per 100,000).[3] More than 80% of children reported with AIDS in 1992 were black or Hispanic.[3] Racial differences probably reflect social, economic, behavioral, or other factors rather than race or ethnicity *per se*.[22]

AIDS cases have been reported in all 50 states, the District of Columbia, Puerto Rico, the Virgin Islands, and Guam, but the geographic distribution of these cases has remained uneven. Through 1992, about 60% of all reported cases were from 5 states: New York, California, New Jersey, Florida, and Texas. The incidence was highest in the most populous metropolitan areas of these states.[7] In 1992, annual AIDS incidence rates by state varied from approximately 1 per 100,000 persons in North Dakota, to 46 per 100,000 in New York State. The highest annual AIDS incidence rate (119 per 100,000) was in Washington, D.C.[7]

The geographic distribution of persons with AIDS has changed over time. The rate of AIDS cases per 100,000 persons has remained highest in the Northeast and in Puerto Rico. Beginning in 1989, however, the largest number of reported cases has been in the South. In 1992, 15,788 cases or 34% of the cases reported were in the South. In all regions, incidence rates remained highest in the largest urban centers, but in recent years the rate of increase in reported cases has been greater in smaller metropolitan and non-metropolitan areas (Fig 3-2).

Geographic distribution also varies by the reported mode of HIV transmission. From 1988 to 1991, the largest number of cases and largest increase in cases among homosexual/bisexual men occurred in the South (Fig 3-3a).[23] In contrast, in the Northeast, the annual number of diagnosed cases among homosexual/bisexual men remained stable or decreased. During this time, among women and heterosexual men who inject drugs the greatest rate of increase in cases occurred in the South (Fig 3-3b), although the absolute number of AIDS cases among persons who inject drugs remained highest in the Northeast. And finally, cases among persons exposed to HIV through heterosexual contact increased in all regions from 1988 to 1991 (Fig 3-3c), but the largest increase in cases occurred in persons in the South, where, in the past few years, the largest number of cases attributed to heterosexual contact have been diagnosed.[23]

Demographic Findings—HIV Infection

Findings of HIV serologic surveys are generally consistent with demographic patterns among reported AIDS cases.[18] In many settings, prevalence rates of HIV are higher in males than females, higher in blacks and Hispanics than non-Hispanic whites, and higher in urban than rural areas. The highest HIV prevalence rates are reported in persons at risk of infection such as homosexual/bisexual men and persons who inject drugs. The lowest rates of infection are found among groups from which persons at increased risk are excluded, such as blood donors and applicants for military service. Information available from states with confidential reporting of HIV infection suggests that, in comparison to persons reported with AIDS, persons

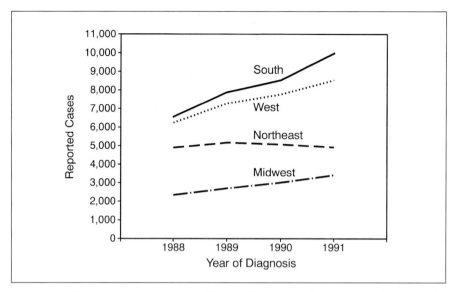

Fig 3-3a. AIDS cases among homosexual/bisexual men, excluding injection-drug users, by region and year of diagnosis, United States, 1988–91. South comprises the South Atlantic, East South Central, and West South Central regions; West comprises the Mountain and Pacific regions; Northeast comprises the New England and Middle Atlantic regions; and Midwest comprises the East North Central and West North Central regions.

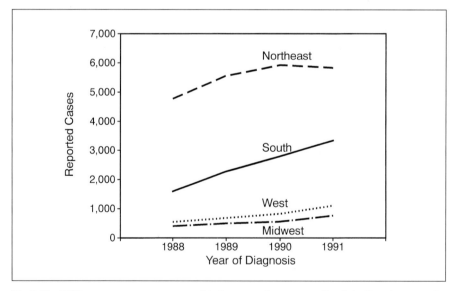

Fig 3-3b. AIDS cases among women and heterosexual men reporting injection-drug use, by region and year of diagnosis, United States, 1988–91. South comprises the South Atlantic, East South Central, and West South Central regions; West comprises the Mountain and Pacific regions; Northeast comprises the New England and Middle Atlantic regions; and Midwest comprises the East North Central and West North Central regions.

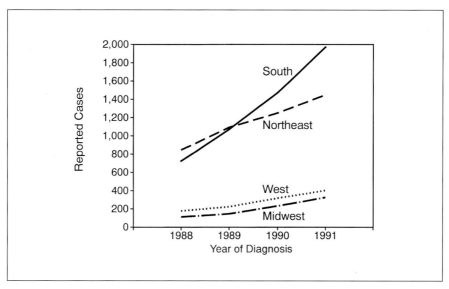

Fig 3-3c. AIDS cases among persons reporting heterosexual contact with persons with or at high risk for HIV infection, by region and year of diagnosis, United States, 1988–91. (Data adjusted for reporting delays.) South comprises the South Atlantic, East South Central, and West South Central regions; West comprises the Mountain and Pacific regions; Northeast comprises the New England and Middle Atlantic regions; and Midwest comprises the East North Central and West North Central regions. Each group analyzed includes a percentage of persons with no identified risk (NIR) who belong to the same geographic categories. The redistributions of cases diagnosed from 1984 through 1988 were initially assigned to NIR category but were subsequently reclassified.

reported with HIV are more likely to be young, black, and female.[24]

Among more than 3.7 million applicants for military service screened from October 1985 through December 1992, the overall HIV seroprevalence rate was 0.11% or 1.1 per 1,000 persons.[18,25] Infection rates among applicants decreased especially among men during this time. By 1991–1992, rates were only slightly higher among men (0.06%) than women (0.05%). Rates also decreased among the three largest racial and ethnic groups, but remained higher among blacks (0.22%) and Hispanics (0.10%) than among whites (0.02%).[18]

In 1992, the prevalence of HIV infection among U.S. blood donors was 0.012% or 1.2 per 10,000 donors.[26] Similar to trends among military applicants, infection rates among blood donors have declined over time. These declining rates are probably a result of the decreasing likelihood that persons who knew that they were infected or at high risk for infection applied for service or donated blood.

HIV seroprevalence data collected from U.S. Job Corps students, aged 16 to 21 years, suggest that disadvantaged youths who are not in school have an increased risk of infection with HIV.[27,28] From 1988 to 1992, the overall rate of HIV infection among these students was 0.30% or 3.0 per 1,000 students, a high infection rate for such a young population.[28] Since 1988, infection rates among males have steadily decreased while infection rates among females have increased. By 1992, the HIV prevalence rates of young black women exceeded those of young black men.[18,28] These findings suggest an increasing role for heterosexual transmission of HIV in this group. Because young women tend to have sex with men who are older, rates of other sexually transmitted diseases are generally higher among women than among men in the youngest age groups.[18,28]

Among applicants to military service and entrants to the Job Corps, infection rates among women were similar to or higher than those among men. These data suggest that in the 1990s HIV incidence among very young men and women may be more equal than in the 1980s when, according to the AIDS surveillance information, most infections occurred in men.[18]

The CDC has supported a population-based national survey to estimate rates of HIV infection among women giving birth in the United States.[29] The survey relies on the blinded testing for HIV antibody in residual blood specimens that are routinely collected from newborns for metabolic screening. Based on data from 35 states, there were approximately 7,000 annual births to HIV-infected women during 1991–1992 for an estimated annual national HIV prevalence of 1.7 per 1,000 childbearing women.[30] Assuming a perinatal transmission rate of 20% to 30%, an estimated 1,400 to 2,100 infants born in the United States in 1992 were infected with HIV. Infection rates were highest among black women and among women from large metropolitan areas. Women with HIV, however, were found in both urban and rural areas, especially in the South. Infection rates among childbearing women in the South rose from 1.7 to 2.1 per 1,000 women from 1989 to 1992, and an increase in the incidence of AIDS in women and children in this region is predicted.[30]

Modes of HIV Exposure

For surveillance purposes, AIDS cases are counted only once in a hierarchy of exposures to HIV (see Table). Persons with more than one reported mode of exposure to HIV are classified by the exposure risk listed first in the hierarchy, except for men with both a history of sexual contact with other men and injection drug use. Exposure categories are based on the three well-established modes of HIV transmission: sexual, exposure to blood through injection drug use and transfusion, and perinatal.

Male Homosexual/Bisexual Contact

Since the beginning of the epidemic, the largest number of persons with AIDS in the United States has been

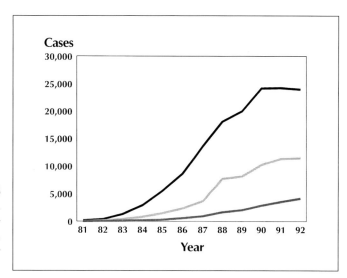

Fig 3-4. Trends in reported AIDS cases, United States, 1981–92. Exposure categories: black, homosexual/bisexual men; light gray, injection drug users; dark gray, heterosexuals.

homosexual/bisexual men. The number of AIDS cases among these men increased most rapidly in the early to mid-1980s.[9,10] In 1987, the rate of increase in case reports for this HIV-exposure group began to slow (Fig 3-4).[9,10] This was most apparent among homosexual/bisexual men in New York City, San Francisco, and Los Angeles.[10] Possible reasons include actual declines in the incidence of new HIV infections (due to the success of prevention efforts in decreasing risk behaviors); the effect of treatment strategies in delaying the onset of AIDS in infected persons; and declines in the completeness of case reporting.[4] As a result, the percentage of AIDS cases in adults and adolescents attributed to homosexual/bisexual contact alone decreased from 63% in 1988[31] to 51% in 1992.[3] In 1992, reported cases in this exposure category decreased slightly from the previous year (Table).

Some cohort studies of homosexual/bisexual men demonstrated a decrease in HIV seroconversion rates and risk behaviors.[32,33] Other studies, however, have documented that unsafe sexual behaviors continue among specific groups of gay men, particularly among those who are young and those in racial and ethnic minorities.[34,35]

Surveys of HIV seroprevalence have found high rates of infection among homosexual/bisexual men throughout the United States.[36] In 1991–1992, a study of unlinked serologic specimens collected from homosexual/bisexual men attending sexually transmitted disease clinics in 36 cities had a median seroprevalence rate of 26%, with a range of 4% to 47%.[18] Infection rates among homosexual/bisexual men had decreased since previous surveys in many of the same clinics. The median decrease was about 6%. These findings suggest that the incidence of new infections also may have decreased. However, seroprevalence remains high in this population and new infections continue to occur.

Use of Injection Drugs

One third of all AIDS cases reported to the CDC through December 1992 were associated with the injection of drugs and included cases among persons who inject drugs (23%), homosexual/bisexual men who inject drugs (6%), heterosexual persons whose sex partners injected drugs (3%) and children born to a mother who either injected drugs or had sex with an injection drug user (1%).[7] The rate of increase in case reports among persons who inject drugs began to slow in 1987 (Fig 3-4).[10] This slowing in case reporting occurred primarily in New York City and New Jersey with little slowing in the rest of the United States.[10] Most AIDS cases in persons who inject drugs are in the Northeast (see Fig 3-3b), but as previously noted, from 1988 to 1991 the greatest increase in cases in this exposure category was in the South.[23]

The use of injection drugs underlies the AIDS epidemic among women in the United States. Among women reported with AIDS through December 1992, 50% injected drugs,[7] 36% were the sex partners of men with or at risk of HIV infection, and 60% of these male sex partners injected drugs.[7] In most parts of the United States, the proportion of AIDS cases attributed to injection drug use is higher in blacks and Hispanics than in non-Hispanic whites.[37] In 1992, 38% of AIDS cases reported in blacks, 38% in Hispanics, and 11% in whites were among heterosexual men and women who injected drugs.

Results of seroprevalence surveys among intravenous drug users entering drug treatment in the United States indicate that transmission of HIV among persons who inject drugs remains an important public health problem. In 1991–1992, surveys in 35 cities found a median HIV seroprevalence rate of 7.5% (range of 1% to 53%) among injection drug users entering drug treatment programs.[18,38] Rates were similar for males and females at each treatment center, but varied by geographic area with highest rates observed along the Atlantic coast and in Puerto Rico. Rates were much higher among blacks than whites in all regions of the United States. Rates were higher among Hispanics than whites, but this difference primarily resulted from higher rates among Hispanics in the Northeast region.[18]

Receipt of Blood Transfusions or Blood Products

Since the late 1980s, the number of persons reported with AIDS who were infected through receipt of blood transfusion or blood products such as clotting-factor concentrates has remained stable or declined slightly for adults and adolescents and declined markedly in children (see Table).[39,40] The more gradual decline in AIDS cases in adults reflects the longer period between infection and disease in that age group and the large number of adults infected prior to 1985. In 1992, approximately 2% of all AIDS cases were reported among persons with hemophilia or recipients of blood transfusions.[3]

Donated blood has been screened for HIV antibodies in the United States since 1985. In addition, clotting-factor concentrates, derived from the plasma of hundreds or thousands of different individuals, has undergone heat treatment. Since the institution of these preventive measures, transmission of HIV to recipients of blood transfusions or clotting factors has been virtually eliminated in the United States. After 1985, transmission has been documented only in rare instances through the receipt of blood or blood products obtained from a donor originally testing negative but later confirmed to be infected with HIV.[41] A recent study by the CDC and the American Red Cross estimated that the risk of HIV transmission from screened blood in 1990 was 1 in 210,000 units.[42] Since AIDS can develop in infected persons up to ten years or more after initial infection with HIV, AIDS cases will continue to be reported among those individuals who received blood or blood products before the institution of screening practices and treatment processes.

Heterosexual Contacts

Cases attributed to heterosexual contact have been increasing steadily in the United States (see Fig 3-4). In 1992, heterosexual contact accounted for 9% of reported cases and for the fastest rate of increase (17%) in any exposure category (see Table).[3] Heterosexual contacts include persons reporting heterosexual contact with a person with or at risk of HIV infection and persons born in a country where heterosexual transmission predominates.

Since the beginning of the epidemic, women have accounted for most persons (60%) infected through heterosexual contact.[7] In 1992, 39% of reported AIDS cases in women were attributable to heterosexual contact.[7] In 1992, the number of women infected through heterosexual contact nearly equaled the number infected through injection drug use.[3] Among women 20 to 29 years, those diagnosed annually with heterosexually acquired AIDS has almost doubled from 1988 to 1992, with larger increases among non-Hispanic black women than among non-Hispanic white and Hispanic women. Most heterosexual transmission has occurred among women who were sex partners of injection drug users. Other factors that are associated with an increased risk of heterosexual transmission of HIV include the use of smokable "crack" cocaine, which may involve the exchange of sex for drugs or money,[43] and the presence of other sexually transmitted diseases.[44]

Surveillance of HIV infection in clinics for treatment of sexually transmitted diseases (STDs) can provide information on the sexual spread of HIV infection among heterosexuals, since those at greatest risk of heterosexual transmission of HIV are among those also at risk of acquiring other STDs. Available data from these clinics indicate that rates of HIV infection are higher among heterosexual persons who inject drugs than other heterosexual men and women.[18,36] In 1988–89, studies in STD clinics found a median seroprevalence rate of 2.3%, with a range of 0% to 14%, in heterosexual persons who did not report injection drug use but who either had a partner at risk of infection or were born in a country where heterosexual transmission is common. The median rate in heterosexual patients who did not report a risk of HIV infection was 1.0%, with a range of 0% to 11%.[36]

Perinatal Transmission

Increases in HIV infection and AIDS among women of childbearing age are reflected in reports of AIDS attributable to perinatal transmission among infants and young children. Since the beginning of the epidemic, most AIDS cases in children have been due to perinatal transmission. In 1992, perinatal transmission accounted for 96% of cases in infants and children less than 5 years and 90% of all AIDS cases in children. Cases attributed to perinatal transmission in 1992 represented an increase of more than 13% over the previous year, the second largest percentage increase among HIV exposure groups. An estimated 1,400–2,100 infants born in the United States in 1992 were infected with HIV.[30]

No Reported Risk for Infection

In 1992, 7% of AIDS cases had no reported history of exposure to HIV through any of the modes described in the Table. Most of these persons remain under investigation by local health department officials. When follow-up information has been available for persons initially reported with an undetermined risk, more than 90% have been reclassified into an appropriate exposure group.[7]

Transmission in Health-Care Settings

Most health-care workers with AIDS have nonoccupational risk factors for HIV infection.[45] Percutaneous, mucous membrane, and cutaneous exposure to blood or blood-contaminated body fluids, however, do occur in health-care settings[46–49] and have resulted in occupationally acquired HIV infection.[45,50,51] By 1993, the CDC had received reports of 39 health-care workers in the United States documented as having seroconverted following a specific occupational exposure to a known source with HIV.[52] Another 81 health-care workers were reported as possibly having acquired their infection occupationally. For each of these 81 workers, no other risk of infection, such as a behavioral or transfusion risk, could be identified; however, seroconversion as a result of a specific exposure was not documented for this group.[52]

Data from prospective studies among health-care workers indicate that the average risk of seroconversion after percutaneous exposure to HIV-infected blood is approximately 0.3%.[50,51] Transmission of HIV after mucous membrane and cutaneous exposure to HIV-infected blood has been reported, although there are inadequate data to quantify the risk precisely. This risk, however, is clearly much lower than the risk of transmission after percutaneous exposure. Data from 21 studies worldwide include one seroconversion (0.09%) among 1,107 mucous membrane exposures.[53]

Because health-care workers are more likely to experience blood contact than patients, the risk of HIV transmission from patient to health-care worker clearly exceeds that from health-care worker to patient.[54] Transmission of HIV from a health-care worker to patients has been documented in only one practice—a dental practice in Florida.[55,56] The investigation of the patients of a dentist with AIDS in Florida strongly suggests that HIV was transmitted during dental care to 6 of 1,100 patients tested. Although the precise mechanism of HIV transmission may never be identified, available evidence indicates that transmission occurred from the dentist to his patients. Each of these patients had no confirmed exposure to HIV other than receiving care from a dentist with AIDS. Each patient was infected with HIV strains that were very similar to the strain infecting the dentist, but distinct from other HIV strains found in HIV-infected persons in the local region. The very small risk of a health-care worker transmitting HIV to a patient probably depends on several factors, including the procedures performed, the technique, skill and medical status of the worker, and the titer of the circulating virus.[54,57]

Transmission of HIV from patient-to-patient through improper infection-control practices has been reported.[58] Available information strongly suggests that HIV was transmitted from one patient to four others in the office of an HIV-negative surgeon in Australia. All five patients underwent minor surgical procedures on the same day, including a man with known risk factors for HIV infection. The precise mechanism of transmission was not identified. Two patients undergoing nuclear medicine procedures were infected with HIV by the inadvertent, intravenous injection of blood or other material from HIV-infected patients.[59] Accidental intravenous or percutaneous exposure to HIV-infected blood was a likely cause of HIV transmission in home health-care settings.[60] In Romania and the Soviet Union, nosocomial outbreaks of HIV transmission resulted from improper sterilization or reuse of contaminated needles and syringes.[61,62]

Mortality Among Persons with HIV Infection and AIDS

During the 1980s, HIV infection (including AIDS) emerged as a leading cause of death in the United States; the greatest impact on mortality was among young adults.[5,8] During 1992, HIV infection accounted for 1.5% of all deaths and became the eighth leading cause of death among all persons in the United States and the second leading cause of death among persons aged 25 to 44 years.[8] Approximately three quarters of HIV-related deaths have occurred among persons in this age group. In 1992, HIV infection became the leading cause of death for men between 25 and 44 years and the fourth leading cause of death for women in this age group (Figs 3-5a and 3-5b).[8]

HIV infection has more severely affected mortality among blacks and Hispanics than other racial/ethnic groups. For example, the death rate from HIV infection in 1992 for persons aged 25 to 44 years was 3 times as high for black men (136.0 per 100,000) as for white men (42.1 per 100,000) and 12 times as high for black women (38.0 per 100,000) as for white women (3.3 per 100,000).[8] In addition, the impact of HIV infection on death patterns has been dramatic in many large U.S. cities.[5] In 1990, HIV infection was the leading cause of death for young men in 64 cities in 28 states; the proportion of deaths due to HIV ranged from 16% in Bridgeport, Connecticut, to 61% in San Francisco. Among young women, HIV infection was the leading cause of death in nine cities in five states on the East Coast, with the proportion of deaths due to HIV infection ranging from 15% in Baltimore to 43% in Newark, New Jersey.[5]

The Global Context

The estimated distribution of adult infections throughout the world in 1993 is shown in Fig 3-6.[11,12] Based on available data, WHO has estimated that during the 1990s, approximately 10 to 15 million adults and 5 to 10 million children worldwide will become infected with HIV. Cumulatively, 40 million adults and children may be infected by the year 2000, with more than 90% of these persons from developing countries. The cumulative number of HIV-related deaths among adults may rise to more than 8 million.[11,12]

The modes of HIV transmission throughout the world are similar, but the relative importance of different transmission modes varies by geographic area and, as previously discussed for the United States, may change over time. In North America, Australia, Western Europe, and some parts of South America, transmission among homosexual and bisexual men and persons who inject drugs has predominated since the beginning of the pandemic.[63] Overall, since the mid-1980s transmission of HIV among homosexual men has decreased in some of these regions. In many places, transmission of HIV among persons who inject drugs has increased. Heterosexual transmission, historically accounting for only a small percentage of infections in these regions, has increased since the mid-1980s.[12]

Increases in heterosexual transmission have occurred most frequently in urban areas with high rates of injection drug use or prevalence of STDs.[12]

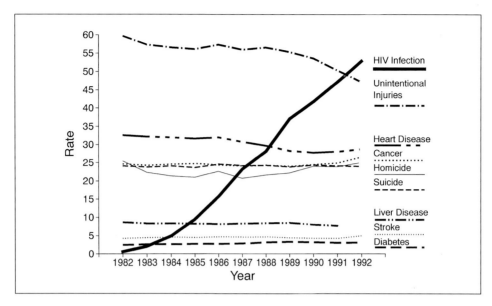

Fig 3-5a. Death rates (per 100,000 population) for leading causes of death among men aged 25 to 44 years, by year, United States, 1982–92. National vital statistics based on underlying cause of death, using final data for 1982–91 and provisional data for 1992. Data for liver disease in 1992 were unavailable.

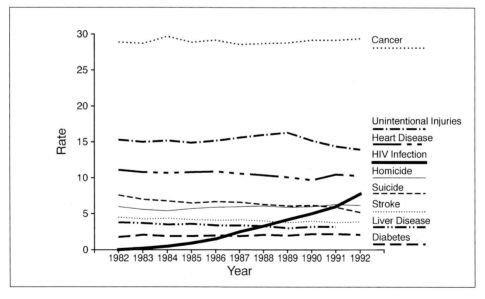

Fig 3-5b. Death rates (per 100,000 population) for leading causes of death among women aged 25 to 44 years, by year, United States, 1982–92. National vital statistics based on underlying cause of death, using final data for 1982–91 and provisional data for 1992. Data for liver disease in 1992 were unavailable.

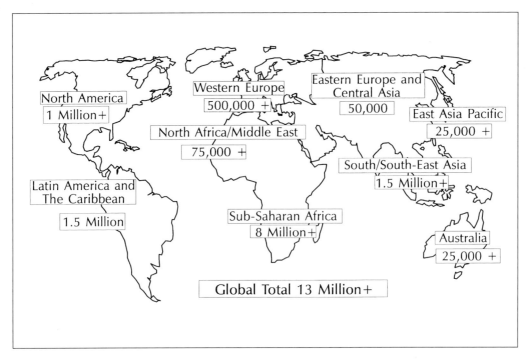

Fig 3-6. Estimated global distribution of cumulative adult HIV infections, mid-1993. (WHO Global Programme on AIDS, Geneva, July 1993.)

In South America, increasing heterosexual transmission has been noted among bisexual men and their female sex partners and among female prostitutes and their clients.[12,64] In Brazil, for example, the percentage of reported AIDS cases due to heterosexual transmission increased from 7.5% in 1987 to 23% in 1992.[12]

In sub-Saharan Africa, heterosexual contact has been the primary route of transmission since extensive spread of HIV began in this region in the late 1970s.[63] Numbers of men and women with HIV are approximately equal. Because more than 4 million women of childbearing age in this region are estimated to have HIV, perinatal transmission will continue to increase.[12]

Transmission through injection drug use or homosexual or bisexual contact is rare.[63] Transmission through receipt of contaminated blood, however, remains a significant problem in many areas of sub-Saharan Africa.[12]

By 1993, WHO estimated that 8 million persons were infected with HIV in sub-Saharan Africa.[11,12] Most infected persons reside in East and Central Africa, which account for only one-sixth of the total population of the sub-Saharan region. Recent serologic data indicate that in some areas, particularly in western and southern Africa, rates of HIV infection are increasing.[12] In 1992, in Nigeria, a country with almost one fifth of the sub-Saharan population, results of

HIV serosurveys indicated that up to 20% of some groups of female prostitutes[12,65] and up to 22% of persons attending STD clinics were infected with HIV.[12]

In Asia, the Middle East, North Africa, and eastern Europe, HIV was introduced later than in other regions. Among these areas, major modes of transmission vary and in many (eg, the Middle East, North Africa, eastern Europe, East Asia and the Pacific), HIV seroprevalence rates remain low. Recent explosive increases in HIV infections in South and South-East Asia, however, demonstrate the potential for rapid increase in the rate of HIV transmission.[66,67]

In Bangkok, HIV seroprevalence rates among persons who inject drugs rose from about 1% at the start of 1988[66] to more than 40% by 1992.[12] In 1991, the median HIV seroprevalence among persons who inject drugs in Thailand was 30%.[66] Among female prostitutes, rates increased from 3.5% in 1989 to 15% in 1991.[66] Routine testing of young men entering the Thai military found that HIV infection rates have increased rapidly among heterosexual men. HIV seroprevalence among these young men rose from 0.5% in 1989 to 3.6% in 1992.[67]

Rapid increases in HIV infection among populations at risk, such as persons who inject drugs, prostitutes or persons with sexually transmitted diseases, also have been found in Myanmar (Burma), India and neighboring provinces, Malaysia, and southwest China.[68–72] In Korea and Japan, populations at risk continue to have low rates of HIV infection.[73,74]

Prevention of HIV Infection in the Community

Recommendations for prevention are intended to reduce or eliminate transmission of HIV through the sexual, bloodborne, or perinatal routes. These recommendations target behaviors that are very difficult for individuals to change, or once changed, to maintain. Effective prevention strategies must be based on the epidemiology of HIV infection in the population and the science of human behavior.

Prevention of Sexual Transmission of HIV

The most effective way to prevent sexual transmission of HIV infection and other STDs is to avoid sexual intercourse with an infected partner. If a person chooses to have sexual intercourse with a partner whose infection status is unknown or who is infected with HIV or other STDs, the man should use a new latex condom with each act of intercourse.[75–77]

Multiple studies of heterosexual couples in which one partner has HIV and the other does not have confirmed that consistent and correct condom usage can substantially reduce transmission of HIV and other STDs.[78,79] For example, in one prospective study of 343 women without HIV, the risk of acquiring HIV infection was six times greater for women whose HIV-infected male partners either did not use or inconsistently used condoms than for women who reported that their partners always used condoms.[80]

Condom failure usually results from inconsistent or incorrect use rather than condom breakage. Several studies have shown that condom breakage is uncommon, particularly in developed countries where breakage rates of 2% or less have been found.[78] A recent laboratory study indicated that latex condoms are an effective mechanical barrier to fluid containing HIV-sized particles.[81]

When a male condom cannot be used, couples should consider using a female condom, which is an intravaginal pouch or sheath made of polyurethane or latex.[75–77] Although laboratory studies indicate that the female condom is an effective mechanical barrier to viruses, including HIV, no clinical studies defining the efficacy of female condoms in preventing HIV transmission have been completed. In one study, the female condom contraceptive failure rate ranged from 11% to 26%, depending on the consistency and correctness of usage.[77]

The effectiveness of spermicides in preventing HIV transmission is unknown. No data exist to indicate that condoms lubricated with spermicides are more effective than other lubricated condoms in protecting against the transmission of HIV infection and other STDs. Therefore, latex condoms with or without spermicides are recommended.[76,77]

Despite the widespread understanding that HIV infection is transmitted sexually and that condom use can reduce this risk, moderate rates of consistent condom use have been found among sexually active homosexual men and relatively low rates among heterosexual men and women.[75] Factors that contribute to low use of condoms are complex and not well understood.[75] Studies have suggested that concern about decreased sexual pleasure, lack of partner endorsement, and use of alcohol and drugs at the time of intercourse may be among the factors adversely influencing condom use.[82–84]

Partner notification and counseling are other strategies to prevent HIV transmission.[76,85,86] Partners of persons infected with HIV may already be infected or may be at high risk of being infected. Notification provides partners with the opportunity for early diagnosis and treatment of HIV infection and adoption of risk-reducing behaviors. Persons who have HIV should be encouraged to notify their partners and to refer them for counseling and testing.[76] If persons with HIV are unwilling to notify their partners or if it cannot be assured that their partners will seek counseling, physicians or trained health-department personnel should use confidential procedures to assure that partners are notified.[76] In most states, health-department personnel can assist in notifying partners of infected patients.[76] The success of testing and counseling efforts, including partner counseling, depends upon the quality of services provided and the continual availability of prevention services that are tailored to the individual's needs.

Prevention of HIV Transmission to Persons Who Inject Drugs

To prevent HIV transmission, it is necessary to help persons stop injecting drugs or using contaminated injection equipment. The primary prevention strategy for persons who inject drugs is to urge them to enter into or continue effective drug-treatment programs.[87] In many areas of the country, the capacity of drug treatment programs is far exceeded by the number of addicted drug users who need and would use these services. It is estimated, however, that about 80% of persons who inject drugs are not enrolled in drug treatment.[88] Within this context, additional strategies to reduce HIV transmission among injection drug users have been implemented. For persons who cannot or will not stop injecting drugs, prevention messages stress that injection equipment, such as needles or syringes, should not be shared with another person.[87,89] If injection equipment has been previously used or is shared by others, the equipment should be thoroughly cleaned with bleach and water before re-use.[87,89]

Other approaches to the prevention of HIV transmission to persons who inject drugs include removal of restrictions on the legal purchase of needles and syringes,[90] needle and syringe exchange programs,[91,92] interim methadone maintenance,[93] and community outreach to educate injection drug users about risk reduction. Decreases in some drug risk behaviors such as sharing injection equipment have been reported.[94,95] In some communities, HIV prevalence has stabilized following implementation of prevention efforts.[96] Recent reviews of needle exchange programs found that most programs did not increase drug injection use and may have decreased rates of HIV-related drug risk behaviors among clients.[91,92]

Prevention of Transmission through Blood and Other Tissues

Transfusion-associated AIDS was first reported in 1982, before the causative agent, HIV, had been identified.[97] In 1983, the U.S. Public Health Service recommended that persons at increased risk of AIDS refrain from donating blood.[98] In 1985, serologic tests for HIV antibody became available. With the initiation of screening of all blood and plasma donations, the risk of transfusion-associated HIV transmission was dramatically decreased.[40,99,100]

Currently, a three-step process minimizes the risk of HIV transmission through donated blood.[101] First, community-based media campaigns and educational programs discourage persons at risk of HIV infection from donating blood. Second, prospective donors are screened for HIV risk behaviors by blood bank personnel. Persons reporting high-risk behaviors for HIV infection are not permitted to donate. Finally, all blood donations are screened for HIV antibody. In the United States, lower rates of transfusion, increases in autologous blood donations, and screening of blood donations for hepatitis B core antibody and hepatitis C, among other measures, have further minimized transfusion-associated risks.[101,102]

For persons with hemophilia, the risk of HIV transmission through pooled plasma products has been virtually eliminated by the implementation of viral inactivation procedures such as heat and solvent/detergent treatments, donor deferral, and antibody screening. Organ and tissue donors also should be screened serologically and evaluated for risk behaviors associated with HIV infection.[103,104] Tissues, such as semen and bone that are obtained from living donors and can be stored, should be quarantined until subsequent testing confirms that the donor was not infected when the tissue was removed. Other approaches currently being studied to further prevent HIV transmission by organ and tissue transplantation include inactivation or removal of HIV by allograft processing, and donor testing for other laboratory markers of early HIV infection, such as p24 antigen.[101]

Prevention of HIV Transmission in Health-Care Settings

To prevent transmission of HIV in health-care settings, the CDC recommends that infection-control programs should incorporate principles of universal precautions.[105] Universal precautions include the appropriate use of handwashing, protective barriers (gloves, masks, and eyewear), and care in the use and disposal of needles and other sharp instruments in all health-care settings. In addition, instruments and other reusable equipment used in performing dental procedures should be appropriately disinfected and/or sterilized between each patient use.[105,106]

Skin and mucous membrane blood contacts can frequently be prevented with barrier precautions. Most percutaneous injuries, however, are not preventable by currently available barriers. As the nature, frequency, and circumstances of percutaneous injuries in health-care settings (including dental settings) are characterized, exposure prevention can be enhanced.[107] Prevention strategies will include engineering controls that do not require worker compliance, such as self-sheathing needles; changes in work practices and techniques; additional personal protective equipment during certain procedures; and modification of worker training.[107] (Chapters 14 and 15 address infection control and the management of occupational exposures, respectively.)

Prevention of HIV Transmission by Perinatal Infection

Prevention of perinatal transmission of HIV begins with the prevention of infection in women of childbearing age.[108] Preventive efforts focus on the provision of routine, voluntary counseling, and HIV antibody testing.[109,110] Voluntary counseling and testing services should be readily available and considered a standard of care for women of childbearing age in all health-care settings, particularly in areas of high HIV prevalence and for women with identified risks for HIV infection. Women infected with HIV should be advised to consider the risk of perinatal transmission of HIV in making reproductive choices.

An interim analysis of a randomized clinical trial, AIDS Clinical Trial Group (ACTG) protocol 076, found that a zidovudine regimen, including administration during pregnancy, labor, and to the newborn, was effective in substantially reducing the risk of perinatal transmission in a select group of HIV-infected women who met the trial entry criteria.[111] Women of childbearing age and all health-care workers providing care to pregnant women should be informed of the results of this clinical trial. HIV-infected pregnant women should be informed of the potential benefits but unknown long-term risks of zidovudine administration. A woman's decision to use zidovudine for prevention of perinatal transmission should be made with her physician.[111]

Although most perinatal transmission occurs during pregnancy and delivery, transmission during breast-feeding has been reported.[112,113] In the United States, where safe and nutritious alternative feeding methods are available, the CDC has recommended that mothers with HIV be advised against breast-feeding to avoid HIV transmission to a child who may not be infected.[114] In 1992, WHO and UNICEF developed a consensus statement on HIV transmission and breast-feeding, primarily for situations in developing countries where infant mortality was very high. This statement recommended that in settings where the primary causes of infant deaths are infectious diseases and malnutrition, breast-feeding should remain the standard advice to pregnant women, including those who are HIV-infected. . . . Their baby's risk of becoming infected through breast milk is likely to be lower than its risk of dying of other causes if deprived of breast-feeding. . . . In settings where infectious diseases are not the primary causes of death during infancy, pregnant women known to be infected with HIV should be advised not to breast feed but to use a safe feeding alternative for their babies.[115]

Counseling and HIV Antibody Testing

In the United States, counseling and HIV antibody testing are large and essential components of HIV prevention programs. Based on the results of antibody testing, persons with HIV can be referred for medical evaluation, treatment, and other social services. Counseling helps persons without HIV adopt and maintain safer behaviors, and assists those already infected to avoid infecting others. Dentists can have a role in these public health efforts, which include patient-risk assessment, voluntary antibody testing, and counseling (see Chapter 10, HIV Testing). An educational module to train dentists to routinely assess patient risks of HIV infection and to refer at-risk patients for counseling and antibody testing has been developed.[116]

References

1. CDC. *Pneumocystis* pneumonia—Los Angeles. MMWR 1981;30:250–252.

2. CDC. Kaposi's sarcoma and *Pneumocystis* pneumonia among homosexual men—New York City and California. MMWR 1981;30:305–308.

3. CDC. Update: acquired immunodeficiency syndrome—United States, 1992. MMWR 1993;42:547–551,557.

4. CDC. HIV prevalence estimates and AIDS case projections for the United States: report based upon a workshop. MMWR 1990;39:1–31.

5. Selik RM, Chu SY, Buehler JW. Human immunodeficiency virus (HIV) infection as a leading cause of death among young adults in U.S. cities and states. JAMA 1993;269:2991–2994.

6. CDC. Update on acquired immune deficiency syndrome (AIDS)—United States. MMWR 1982;31:507–508,513–514.

7. CDC. HIV/AIDS surveillance report, February 1993:1–23.

8. CDC. Update: mortality attributable to HIV infection among persons aged 25–44 years—United States, 1991 and 1992. MMWR 1993;42:869–872.

9. Brookmeyer R. Reconstruction and future trends of the AIDS epidemic in the United States. Science 1991;253:37–42.

10. Green TA, Karon JM, Nwanyanwu OC. Changes in AIDS incidence trends in the United States. J Acquired Immune Deficiency Syndrome 1992;5:547–555.

11. World Health Organization. The current global situation of the HIV/AIDS pandemic. Wkly Epidemiol Rec 1993;68:195–196.

12. World Health Organization. The HIV/AIDS Pandemic: 1993 Overview. Global Programme on AIDS. 1993.

13. Merson MH. The HIV pandemic: global spread and global response (Abstract PS-01-1). In: Abstracts of the IX International Conference on AIDS/IVth STD World Congress, v1; June 6–11, 1993; Berlin:9.

14. Buehler JW, Berkelman RL, Stehr-Green JK. The completeness of AIDS surveillance. J Acquired Immune Deficiency Syndrome 1992;5:257–264.

15. CDC. Revision of the case definition of acquired immunodeficiency syndrome for national reporting—United States. MMWR 1985;34:373–375.

16. CDC. Revision of the CDC surveillance case definition for acquired immunodeficiency syndrome. MMWR 1987;36:1–15.

17. CDC. 1993 Revised classification system for HIV infection and expanded surveillance case definition for AIDS among adolescents and adults. MMWR 1992;41: 1–19.

18. CDC. National HIV serosurveillance summary—results through 1992, vol. 3. Atlanta, GA: U.S. Department of Health and Human Services, Public Health Service, 1994.

19. CDC. Update: Public health surveillance for HIV infection—United States, 1989 and 1990. MMWR 1990;39:853,859–861.

20. CDC. Public health uses of HIV-infection reports—South Carolina, 1986–1991. MMWR 1992;41:245–249.

21. CDC. Update: acquired immunodeficiency syndrome—United States, 1989. MMWR 1990;39:81–86.

22. CDC. Use of race and ethnicity in public health surveillance. Summary of the CDC/ATSDR Workshop. MMWR 1993; 42:1–17.

23. CDC. Update: acquired immunodeficiency syndrome—United States, 1991. MMWR 1992;41:463–468.

24. Fleming PL, Ward JW, Morgan MW, et al. Mandatory HIV reporting: characteristics of adults reported with HIV compared to AIDS in the United States (Abstract WS-C17-2). In: Abstracts of the IXth International Conference on AIDS/IVth STD World Congress, v1; June 6–11, 1993; Berlin:98

25. Brundage JF, Burke DS, Gardner LI, et al. Tracking the spread of the HIV infection epidemic among young adults in the United States: results of the first four years of screening among civilian applicants for U.S. military service. J Acquired Immune Deficiency Syndrome 1990; 3:1168–1180.

26. Kennedy M, Petersen L, Doll L, et al. Five year trends in HIV seroprevalence and risk behaviors among U.S. blood donors: a multicenter study (Abstract P0-C21-3118). In: Abstracts of the IXth International Conference on AIDS/IVth STD World Congress, v2; June 6–11, 1993: Berlin:737

27. St. Louis ME, Conway GA, Hayman CR, et al. Human immunodeficiency virus infection in disadvantaged adolescents. JAMA 1991;266:2387–2391.

28. Conway GA, Epstein MR, Hayman CR, et al. Trends in HIV prevalence among disadvantaged youth. JAMA 1993; 269:2887–2889.

29. Gwinn M, Pappaioanou M, George JR, et al. Prevalence of HIV infection in childbearing women in the United States. JAMA 1991;265:1704–1708.

30. Davis S, Gwinn M, Wasser S, et al. HIV prevalence among U.S. childbearing women, 1989-1992 (Abstract 27). In: Program and Abstracts of the First National Conference on Human Retroviruses and Related Infections, December 12–16, 1993:Washington, D.C:60.

31. CDC. AIDS and human immunodeficiency virus infection in the United States: 1988 Update. MMWR 1989;38: 353–358,363.

32. Winkelstein W Jr, Wiley JA, Padian NS, et al. The San Francisco Men's Health Study: continued decline in HIV seroconversion rates among homosexual/bisexual men. Am J Public Health 1988; 78:1472–1474.

33. Kingsley LA, Bacellar H, Zhou S, et al. Temporal trends in HIV seroconversion: a report from the multicenter AIDS cohort study (MACS) (Abstract F.C.550). In: Final Program and Abstracts of the VIth International Conference on AIDS, v2. June 20–24, 1990; San Francisco, CA:218.

34. Peterson JL, Coates TJ, Catania JA, et al. High-risk sexual behavior and condom use among gay and bisexual African-American men. Am J Public Health 1992; 82:1490–1494.

35. Hays RB, Kegeles SM, Coates TJ. High HIV risk-taking among young gay men. AIDS 1990;4:901–907.

36. McCray E, Onorato IM, The Field Services Branch. Sentinel surveillance of human immunodeficiency virus infection in sexually transmitted disease clinics in the United States. Sex Transm Dis 1992; 19:235–241.

37. Selik RM, Castro KG, Pappaioanou M. Racial/ethnic differences in the risk of AIDS in the United States. Am J Public Health 1988;78:1539–1545.

38. Allen DM, Onorato IM, Green TA, et al. HIV infection in intravenous drug users entering drug treatment, United States, 1988 to 1989. Am J Public Health 1992; 82:541–546.

39. CDC. Update: acquired immunodeficiency syndrome—United States, 1981–1990. MMWR 1991;40:358–363,369.

40. Selik RM, Ward JW, Buehler JW. Trends in transfusion-associated acquired immune deficiency syndrome in the United States: 1982–1991. Transfusion 1993;33: 890–893.

41. Conley LJ, Holmberg SD. Transmission of AIDS from blood screened negative for antibody to the human immunodeficiency virus (Letter). N Engl J Med 1992; 326:1499–1500.

42. Petersen L, Satten G, Dodd R, et al. Time period from infectiousness as blood donor to development of detectable antibody and the risk of HIV transmission from transfusion of screened blood (Abstract MoC0091). In: Abstracts of VIII International Conference on AIDS/III STD World Congress v1;July 19–24, 1992; Amsterdam, the Netherlands.

43. Chiasson MA, Stoneburner RL, Hildebrandt DS, et al. Heterosexual transmission of HIV-1 associated with the use of smokable freebase cocaine (crack). AIDS 1991;5:1121–1126.

44. Chirgwin K, DeHovitz JA, Dillon S, et al. HIV infection, genital ulcer disease, and crack cocaine use among patients attending a clinic for sexually transmitted diseases. Am J Public Health 1992;81:1576–1579.

45. Chamberland ME, Conley LJ, Bush TJ, et al. Health care workers with AIDS. National surveillance update. JAMA 1991; 266:3459–3462.

46. Tokars JI, Bell DM, Culver DH, et al. Percutaneous injuries during surgical procedures. JAMA 1992;267:2899–2904.

47. Siew C, Chang S-B, Gruninger SE, et al. Self-reported percutaneous injuries in dentists: implications for HBV, HIV transmission risk. J Am Dent Assoc 1992;123 (7):37–44.

48. Marcus R, Culver DH, Bell DM, et al. Risk of human immunodeficiency virus infection among emergency department workers. Am J Med 1993;94:363–370.

49. Wong ES, Stotka JL, Chinchilli VM, et al. Are universal precautions effective in reducing the number of occupational exposures among health care workers? A prospective study of physicians on a medical service. JAMA 1991;265:1123–1128.

50. Tokars JI, Marcus R, Culver DH, et al. Surveillance of HIV infection and zidovudine use among health care workers after occupational exposure to HIV-infected blood. Ann Intern Med 1993;118:913–919.

51. Henderson DK, Fahey BJ, Willy M, et al. Risk for occupational transmission of human immunodeficiency virus type 1 (HIV-1) associated with clinical exposures. A prospective evaluation. Ann Intern Med 1990;113:740–746.

52. CDC. HIV/AIDS surveillance report, 1993;5:13.

53. Ippolito G, Puro V, De Carli G. The risk of occupational human immunodeficiency virus infection in health care workers. Italian multicenter study. Arch Intern Med 1993;153:1451–1458.

54. Chamberland ME, Bell DM. HIV transmission from health care worker to patient: what is the risk (Editorial). Ann Intern Med 1992;116:871–873.

55. Ciesielski C, Marianos D, Ou C-Y, et al. Transmission of human immunodeficiency virus in a dental practice. Ann Intern Med 1992;116:798–805.

56. Update: investigations of patients who have been treated by HIV-infected healthcare workers—United States. MMWR 1993;42:329–331,337.

57. Bell DM, Shapiro CN, Gooch BF. Preventing HIV transmission to patients during invasive procedures. J Public Health Dent 1993;53:170–173.

58. Chant K, Lowe D, Rubin G, et al. Patient-to-patient transmission of HIV in private surgical consulting rooms (Letter). Lancet 1993;342:1548–1549.

59. Patient exposures to HIV during nuclear medicine procedures. MMWR 1992;41: 575–578.

60. HIV infection in two brothers receiving intravenous therapy for hemophilia. MMWR 1992;41:228–231.

61. Hersh BS, Popovici F, Apetrei RC, et al. Acquired immunodeficiency syndrome in Romania. Lancet 1991;338:645–649.

62. Pokrovsky W, Eramova EU. Nosocomial outbreak of HIV infection in Elista, USSR (Abstract WA05). In: Abstracts of the V International Conference on AIDS;June 4–9, 1989;Montreal, Canada:63.

63. Chin J, Mann JM. The global patterns and prevalence of AIDS and HIV infection. AIDS 1988;2(Suppl l):247–252.

64. Cortes E, Detels R, Aboulafia D, et al. HIV-1, HIV-2, and HTLV-l infection in high risk groups in Brazil. N Engl J Med 1989;320:953–958.

65. Dada AJ, Oyewole F, Onofowokan R, et al. Lagos Nigeria-New Delhi India HIV-1 connection among high class prostitutes (Abstract PO-C07-2744). In: Abstracts of the IXth International Conference on AIDS/IVth STD World Congress v2; June 6–11, 1993;Berlin:674.

66. Weniger BG, Limpakarnjanarat K, Ungchusak K, et al. The epidemiology of HIV infection and AIDS in Thailand. AIDS 1991;5(Suppl 2):71–85.

67. Sirisopana N, Torugsa K, Carr J, et al. Prevalence of HIV-1 infection in young men entering the Royal Thai Army (Abstract PO-CO8-2778) In: Abstracts of the IXth International Conference on AIDS/IVth STD World Congress v2; June 6–11, 1993; Berlin:680.

68. Brajachand SN, Ibotomba SY, Naik TN, et al. Spread of HIV infection in Manipur, a border state of India (Abstract PO–C08-2763). In: Abstracts of the IXth International Conference on AIDS/IVth STD World Congress v2; June 6–11, 1993; Berlin:677.

69. Tripathy S, Banerjee K, Rodrigues J, et al. Increasing HIV infection in western India (Abstract PO-C08-2764). In: Abstracts of the IXth International Conference on AIDS/IVth STD World Congress v2; June 6–11, 1993:Berlin:678.

70. Singh YN, Malaviya AN, Tripathy SP, et al. HIV serosurveillance among prostitutes and patients from a sexually transmitted diseases clinic in Delhi, India. J Acquired Immune Deficiency Syndrome 1990;3: 287–289.

71. Singh S, Crofts N, Gertig D. HIV infection among IDU's in northeast Malaysia (Abstract PO-C08-2777). In: Abstracts of the IXth International Conference on AIDS/IVth STD World Congress v2; June 6–11, 1993:Berlin:680.

72. Zheng X, Tian C, Zhang J, et al. Rapid spread of HIV among drug users and their wives in southwest China (Abstract PO-C08-2766). In: Abstracts of the IXth International Conference on AIDS/IVth STD World Congress v2; June 6–11, 1993:Berlin:678.

73. Oh M-d, Choe K, Shin Y, et al. Current status of HIV/AIDS epidemic in South Korea (Abstract PO-C08-2769). In: Abstracts of the IXth International Conference on AIDS/IVth STD World Congress v2; June 6–11, 1993:Berlin:678.

74. Soda K, Fukutomi K, Hashimoto S, et al. Temporal trend and projection of HIV/AIDS epidemic in Japan (Abstract PO-C08-2779). In: Abstracts of the IXth International Conference on AIDS/IVth STD World Congress v2; June 6–11, 1993:Berlin:680.

75. Roper WL, Peterson HB, Curran JW. Commentary: condoms and HIV/STD prevention—clarifying the message. Am J Public Health 1993;83:501–503.

76. CDC. 1993 Sexually transmitted diseases treatment guidelines. MMWR 1993;42: 1–19.

77. CDC. Update: barrier protection against HIV infection and other sexually transmitted diseases. MMWR 1993;42:589–591, 597.

78. Cates W Jr, Stone KM. Family planning, sexually transmitted diseases and contraceptive choice: a literature update—part I. Family Planning Perspectives 1992;24: 75–84.

79. Weller SC. A meta-analysis of condom effectiveness in reducing sexually transmitted HIV. Soc Sci Med 1993;36:1635–1644.

80. Saracco A, Musicco M, Nicolosi A, et al. Man-to-woman sexual transmission of HIV: longitudinal study of 343 steady partners of infected men. J Acquired Immune Deficiency Syndrome 1993;6: 497–502.

81. Carey RF, Herman WA, Retta SM, et al. Effectiveness of latex condoms as a barrier to human immunodeficiency virus-sized particles under conditions of simulated use. Sex Transm Dis 1992;19:230–234.

82. CDC. Heterosexual behaviors and factors that influence condom use among patients attending a sexually transmitted disease clinic—San Francisco. MMWR 1990;39:685–689.

83. Peterson JL, Coates TJ, Catania JA, et al. High-risk sexual behavior and condom use among gay and bisexual African-American men. Am J Public Health 1992; 82:1490–1494.

84. Catania JA, Coates TJ, Kegeles S, et al. Condom use in multi-ethnic neighborhoods of San Francisco: the population-based AMEN (AIDS in multi-ethnic neighborhoods) Study. Am J Public Health 1991;81:284–287.

85. Roper WL. Current approaches to prevention of HIV infections. Public Health Rep 1991;106:111–115.

86. Hinman AR. Strategies to prevent HIV infection in the United States. Am J Public Health 1991;81:1557–1559.

87. CDC, CSAT, NIDA. HIV/AIDS Prevention Bulletin, April 19, 1993.

88. CDC. Update: reducing HIV transmission in intravenous-drug users not in drug treatment—United States. MMWR 1990; 39:97–101.

89. CDC. Use of bleach for disinfection of drug injection equipment. MMWR 1993; 42:418–419.

90. Groseclose SL, Weinstein B, Jones S, et al. Legal purchase and possession of clean needles and syringes in Connecticut: do they make a difference (Abstract PO-D27-4185)? In: Abstracts of the IX International Conference on AIDS/IVth STD World Congress v2; June 6–11, 1993: Berlin:915.

91. U.S. General Accounting Office. Needle exchange programs: research suggests promise as an AIDS prevention strategy. Washington, DC: USGAO, Human Resources Division; 1993. Report to the Chairman, Select Committee on Narcotics Abuse and Control, House of Representatives.

92. The public health impact of needle exchange programs in the United States and abroad. Summary, conclusions, and recommendations. School of Public Health, University of California, Berkeley; Institute for Health Policy Studies, University of California, San Francisco. Report prepared for the Centers for Disease Control and Prevention. October 1993.

93. Yancovitz SR, Des Jarlais DC, Peyser NP, et al. A randomized trial of an interim methadone maintenance clinic. Am J Public Health 1991;81:1185–1191.

94. Stephens RC, Feucht TE, Roman SW. Effects of an intervention program on AIDS-related drug and needle behavior among intravenous drug users. Am J Public Health 1991;81:568–571.

95. Watters JK, Estilo MJ, Clark GL, et al. Syringe and needle exchange as HIV/AIDS prevention for injection drug users. JAMA 1994;271:115–120.

96. Des Jarlais DC, Friedman SR, Sotheran JL, et al. Continuity and change within an HIV epidemic: injecting drug users in New York City, 1984 through 1992. JAMA 1994;271:121–127.

97. CDC. Possible transfusion-associated acquired immune deficiency syndrome (AIDS)—California. MMWR 1982;31:652–654.

98. CDC. Prevention of acquired immune deficiency syndrome (AIDS): report of inter-agency recommendations. MMWR 1983;32:101–103.

99. CDC. Provisional Public Health Service inter-agency recommendations for screening donated blood and plasma for antibody to the virus causing acquired immunodeficiency syndrome. MMWR 1985;34:1–5.

100. Ward JW, Holmberg SD, Allen JR, et al. Transmission of human immunodeficiency virus (HIV) by blood transfusions screened as negative for HIV antibody. N Engl J Med 1988;318:473–478.

101. Petersen LR, Simonds RJ, Koistinen J. HIV transmission through blood, tissues and organs. AIDS 1993;7(suppl l):99–107.

102. Surgenor DM, Wallace EL, Hao SHS, et al. Collection and transfusion of blood in the United States, 1982–1988. N Engl J Med 1990;322:1646–1651.

103. CDC. Semen banking, organ and tissue transplantation, and HIV antibody testing. MMWR 1988;37:57–58,63.

104. CDC. Transmission of HIV through bone transplantation: case report and public health recommendations. MMWR 1988;37:597–599.

105. Recommendations for prevention of HIV transmission in health care settings. MMWR 1987;36(Suppl No. 2S):1–18.

106. CDC. Recommended infection-control practices for dentistry, 1993. MMWR 1993;42(No. RR-8):4–8.

107. Bell DM. Human immunodeficiency virus transmission in health care settings: risk and risk reduction. Am J Med 1991;91(Suppl 3B):294–300.

108. Rogers MF. The epidemiology of pediatric HIV infections. In: Wormser GP, Stahl RE, Bottone EJ, eds. AIDS and Other Manifestations of HIV Infection. Park Ridge, NJ: Noyes Publications; 1987:36–47.

109. Public Health Service guidelines for counseling and antibody testing to prevent HIV infection and AIDS. MMWR 1987;36:509–515.

110. Working Group on HIV Testing of Pregnant Women and Newborns. HIV infection, pregnant women, and newborns. JAMA 1990;264:2416–2420.

111. CDC. Zidovudine for the prevention of HIV transmission from mother to infant. MMWR 1994;43:285–287.

112. World Health Organization. Consensus statement from the WHO/UNICEF consultation on HIV transmission and breast-feeding. Wkly Epidemiol Rec 1992;67: 177–179.

113. Oxtoby MJ. Human immunodeficiency virus and other viruses in human milk: placing the issues in broader perspective. Pediatr Infect Dis J 1988;7:825–835.

114. Recommendations for assisting in the prevention of perinatal transmission of human T-lymphotrophic type III/lymphadenopathy-associated virus. MMWR 1985; 34:721–726,731–732.

115. World Health Organization. Consensus statement from the WHO/UNICEF consultation on HIV transmission and breast-feeding. Wkly Epidemiol Rec 1992;67: 177–179.

116. Fine J, Bruerd B, Alexander G. A vital opportunity—dentistry's role in the prevention of HIV transmission through health history review. Presentation at the National Primary Care Networking Conference; January, 1993; Atlanta.

4

Transmission of HIV

Michael Glick

With emerging changes in the legal and ethical aspects of HIV and increased knowledge in the area of the disease's pathogenesis, the transmission of HIV still remains the primary concern for dental providers who treat infected patients.[1] The fear of contracting HIV is also a major concern in the community at large, and providers need to be well informed regarding known modes of transmission. They also should be familiar with fictitious and hypothetical modes of transmission that are being put forward mainly by the popular media. This chapter reviews the main theories about the transmission of HIV, and surveys the facts and fictions surrounding this issue.

There are three principal modes of HIV transmission: through sexual contact, through exposure to infected blood and blood products, and through perinatal contact from infected mothers to their children. Other possible routes of transmission of concern to dental health-care providers include saliva and cross-contamination with dental handpieces.

A variety of modes of exposures that have and have not been implicated in HIV transmission will be discussed (Table).

Successful transmission of HIV is influenced by several variables, such as the amount of infectious virus in a particular body fluid, the virulence of the virus, the ability of the infected fluid

Table. Documented and Undocumented Modes of HIV Transmission

- Documented modes of transmission
  - Sexual transmission
  - Exposure to blood and blood products
  - Vertical transmission from mother to fetus/child
- Undocumented modes of transmission
  - Aerosol
  - Dental rotary instrument
  - Tears
  - Urine
  - Sweat
  - Hepatitis B vaccine
  - Insect bites
  - Casual contact

to penetrate skin and mucosa, and the extent of contact with the infected fluid. Intimate sexual contact and contaminated blood were recognized early in the epidemic as sources for HIV transmission.[2] Subsequently, transmission from infected mothers to their children was documented.[3] More than a decade into the epidemic, the vast majority of HIV transmissions still occur by these three main routes.

Sexual Transmission

At the beginning of the epidemic, AIDS was described as a sexually transmitted disease. In the early 1980s, mainly homosexual/bisexual men were thought to be infected but over a decade later we know that the majority of infections worldwide occur via inti-mate heterosexual contacts.[4,5] Today, we recognize that transmission occurs both from men to women and from women to men.[6–8]

Several studies have attempted to evaluate the degree of risk involved with different sexual practices. Anal-receptive intercourse is associated with a high degree of risk for HIV transmission, because of trauma and subsequent abrasions of the rectal mucosa and as a result of direct HIV infection of the bowel mucosa with infected semen.[9] Semen, with 10 to 50 infectious particles per milliliter, has a higher concentration of infectious viruses than vaginal fluid, where free infectious viruses are rarely found[10–11]; however, HIV DNA in cervical and vaginal secretions has been documented.[12]

The presence of HIV-infected cells appears to be the main source for sexual transmission. Between 0.01% and 5% of cells in the seminal fluid may be infected,[13] but this percentage increases in patients with venereal diseases.[6–8] Venereal diseases not only increase the number of inflammatory cells infected with HIV, enhancing viral replication, but cause breaks in the mucosa, facilitating entry of the virus into the body. Studies in the United States have supported this finding, where the presence of venereal diseases such as herpes simplex virus and syphilis has been associated with an increased risk for HIV transmission among heterosexual couples.[14] Vaginal mucosal cells may be directly infected by HIV, increasing the risk for infections in women.[15] However, anal intercourse and bleeding as a result of intercourse are major determinants for heterosexual sexual transmission of HIV to women.[16]

The health of the infected sexual partner may be an even stronger predictor for infection rate during sexual transmission of HIV to women, since partners with more advanced stages of HIV disease can transmit HIV more readily.[16] It is not known if women are at a higher risk than men for infection during vaginal intercourse with an infected partner. However, genital tract secretion of HIV increases in infected women who use oral contraceptives, rendering these women more able to transmit the virus during heterosexual intercourse.[12] Epidemiologic studies seem to indicate no significant difference in women-to-men vs men-to-women transmission.[17]

Transmission of HIV between women has been suggested, but other than two possible cases,[18,19] little data exist to substantiate this mode of transmission. Moreover, a large study of 960,000 women blood donors failed to identify female-to-female transmission by sexual contact between women.[20]

Transmission of HIV during oral intercourse between men has also been reported.[21–24] Although these reports are anecdotal, unprotected oral-receptive intercourse cannot be considered safe until other risk factors facilitating transmission by this route have been elucidated.

Blood

It is clear that the concentration of virus in different body fluids plays an important role in transmission. Infected individuals carry HIV within infected cells and as a free virus (see Chapter 5). Free HIV has been isolated in quantities of 1 to 5,000 infectious particles per milliliter of plasma. Individuals with more advanced stages of disease and during the first couple of weeks after infection will show a high concentration of infectious viruses. However, asymptomatic patients have very low plasma concentrations, averaging approximately 100 infectious particles per milliliter of plasma.[25,26] Interestingly, there are an estimated 100,000 more noninfectious viruses compared to infectious viruses in the plasma.[27] Thus, to estimate the infectiousness of HIV fluids, it is important to consider the number of infectious viruses and not the total number of viruses. The classic example is that of saliva, where relatively large numbers of viral particles can be found but very few infectious viruses are present. Human immunodeficiency virus is found in even greater numbers within infected cells than as free viruses in the plasma.

It is possible that 1 in every 10 to 1,000 peripheral blood mononuclear cells (PBMC) harbor HIV in infected individuals.[28] This translates to 5,000 to 500,000 infected PBMC/mL in patients with a normal leukocyte count of 5×10^6 cells/mL. Furthermore, each infected cell can harbor and produce several thousand infectious viruses.[29] Again, asymptomatic individuals have much lower serum concentrations of HIV than symptomatic individuals and patients with more advanced stages of disease.

The high concentration of HIV in plasma makes this fluid one of the principal routes of transmission of HIV; however, in countries where precautions are taken to protect the blood supply from HIV, the blood supply has never been safer. Various methods have been implemented to make transfusion of blood and blood products safe. Hospitals encourage patients to donate blood before elective surgery to provide the patient with his or her own blood in case a transfusion is needed (autologous transfusion). All blood donors fill out a comprehensive health questionnaire that helps screen for individuals with potential risks of being carriers of infectious diseases. This is not a fail-safe method to detect diseases such as HIV, but it reduces the risk for other diseases, such as malaria, where rapid laboratory parameters may not be available.

The American Association of Blood Banks standards require testing of donated blood for hepatitis B surface antigen, anti-human T-cell leukemia/lymphoma virus I and II, HIV-1 antibodies, hepatitis C virus antibodies, hepatitis B core antigen antibodies, alanine aminotransferase, and syphilis.[30] In addition to regular laboratory tests to detect infectious agents, other safety measures such as viral inactivation factors are being used. Still, the risk for acquiring HIV through a blood transfusion is estimated to be 1 in 225,000 transfused units of blood,[31] ranging from 1 in 36,000 to 1 in 300,000.[32] Thus, the estimated risk of contracting HIV disease from a blood transfusion is 0.0025% to 0.0003% per unit transfused. Since testing for HIV was only instituted in the United States in May 1985, individuals who received multiple blood transfusions before this date are considered at high risk for having acquired HIV infection.

Blood Products

Blood products are used for patients with specific factor deficiencies such as factor VIII (hemophilia A), factor IX (hemophilia B), and von Willebrand factor (von Willebrand's disease). Unlike components of whole blood such as red blood cells, plasma, cryoprecipitate, or platelets, coagulation factors are extracted from plasma and cryoprecipitate from pools of thousands of donors. This obviously increases the risk of undetectable HIV. Before the implementation of specific safety measures, commercial clotting concentrates transmitted hepatitis viruses to 100% and HIV to 60% to 80% of patients with hemophilia.[33] For this reason, another safety measure was used, taking advantage of the heat labile characteristic of HIV. Factor concentrates were dry-heated (60°C for 30 hours), but HIV transmission still occurred.[34]

Dry-heated factor VIII concentrates are no longer available except in the United Kingdom, where a method of higher heat for a longer period—80°C for 72 hours—has been shown to be safe.[33] Other inactivation procedures are now being used, such as pasteurization, solvent/detergent sterilization, monoclonal antibody purification with subsequent sterilization, ion-exchange chromatography, and recombinant DNA technology. This last method produces a nonhuman source of the factor. Available testing for HIV and viral inactivation methods have virtually eliminated all risks for HIV transmission to patients with hemophilia A.

For patients with hemophilia B, methods to improve the safety for factor IX concentrate transfusion is not as developed as those with factor VIII. However, dry-heated factor IX complex is available after being treated at a temperature of 80°C. Other methods are also being used, making transfusion of factor IX concentrates safe from HIV contamination.[35]

Mother to Child

Transmission of HIV from mother to child is becoming more common with increasing numbers of women of childbearing age who have HIV (see Chapter 3). It is estimated that infected mothers transmit the virus on an average of 30% to their newborns, with numbers ranging from 7% to 71%.[36–38] Many factors have been suggested to explain the wide variation in transmission rate, but it is generally believed that a higher percentage of children born to mothers with more advanced disease will become infected. One study evaluating the risk for perinatal transmission of HIV indicated that four major factors are associated with an increased transmission rate.[38] The highest risk, 71%, was associated with the presence of maternal p24 antigenemia. (This laboratory parameter indicates active HIV replication; see Chapter 5.) The risk for perinatal transmission was estimated to be 50% in mothers with CD8+ cell counts of at least 1,800 cells/mm³, and 29% in women with CD4+ cell counts below 600 cells/mm³. In women with normal CD4+ and CD8+ cell counts but with placental inflammation, the risk for perinatal transmission was estimated to be 40%.

It is not clear how or when transmission of HIV from the mother to the child occurs. Apparently, viral transmission takes place in utero, during delivery, or after delivery.[39,40] HIV has been found in placentas and fetuses, and has been isolated from cord blood and amniotic fluid, supporting in utero transmission. However, in some instances HIV cannot be isolated from cord blood but is instead recovered in infected infants older than 1 month.[41,42] This suggests that HIV is transmitted at birth or shortly afterward. HIV transmission during delivery is also supported by data indicating that only one monozygotic twin may be infected[43] and that there is a higher risk of infection for the first born of twins.[44] This indicates that transmission during delivery is associated with contact between amniotic fluid, genital secretions, or blood from the mother and the newborn.

Transmission after delivery has also been suggested to occur through breast feeding.[45] Studies of women infected via blood transfusions after

and, second, the virus needs to be incubated with susceptible cells to determine if it has retained its ability to infect. These steps were not performed in this experiment. Instead, another virus was used that does not have the same survival characteristics of HIV. Although the study showed that HIV DNA was expelled from the dental equipment, this does not mean that viable viruses survived. Furthermore, from a highly concentrated suspension (10^9 viruses per milliliter), only 0.001% to 0.1% survived. In a patient with advanced HIV disease, 5,000 free viruses per milliliter and 5×10^5 infected cells may be present. In assuming that HIV survives inside a dental handpiece at the same rate as a bacteriophage suspension, we can similarly assume that the handpiece will contain 5 to 500 free viruses and 500 to 50,000 infected cells per milliliter. As the amount of blood inside a contaminated handpiece is probably only 1/100 to 1/1,000 of a milliliter, the amount of HIV would at the most be 0.5 to 5 free viruses and 50 to 500 infected cells. Since it is impossible to draw any conclusions about the survival rate of infectious HIV or the amount of viruses necessarily expelled from a handpiece into the oral cavity to cause infection, the previously mentioned study at best indicates only a very rare mode of HIV transmission.

Another study that used herpes simplex virus to assess possible transmission from a dental rotary instrument, found that when contaminated instruments were treated only with external chemical disinfectants, viable viruses were eliminated.[69]

Aerosol

Aerosolization of infectious human papilloma virus has been documented during removal of warts with the carbon dioxide laser and with electrocoagulation.[70] No published study has evaluated the potential for HIV transmission via this route. However, preliminary data from a pilot study conducted in a clinical dental setting did not indicate survival of HIV-1 in aerosol generated by high-speed handpieces, cavitrons, or Nd:Yag lasers (Glick M., unpublished data).

Tears

HIV has been isolated from tears[71] as well as from contact lenses worn by infected individuals.[72] Possibly because of the extremely low concentration of HIV in tears, less than one infected virus per milliliter, transmission of HIV has not been documented via this route. However, guidelines for ophthalmologic procedures have been developed.[73]

Urine

Although HIV has been recovered from the urine[74] of infected individuals, this fluid has never been implicated in the transmission of the virus.[75]

Sweat

Sweat has never been implicated in HIV transmission and probably does not contain infectious particles.[76]

Hepatitis B Vaccine

An initial hepatitis B vaccine (Heptavax-B) was developed in early 1980 from plasma donated by a large cohort of homosexual/bisexual men from San Francisco. This vaccine became available to the public in 1982, but because of concerns of the recipients that HIV transmission may occur via this route, recombinant vaccines (Engerix-B, Recombivax-HB) were developed. Concerns about an association between the initial vaccine and HIV transmission were not warranted since the process to develop this vaccine removes and inactivates HIV.[77] Long-term epidemiologic studies have reconfirmed the safety of this vaccine.[78]

Insect Bites

Transmission of HIV through biting or blood-sucking insects has not been proved. Theoretically, such transmission could occur if the virus can multiply within the insect or survives in the mouthpiece of the insect, enabling a mechanical spread of the virus. In African insects, DNA sequences homologous to HIV have been found,[79] but there is no evidence indicating that free virus or viral replication can survive inside arthropods.[80] Mechanical transmission of HIV was assessed in experiments where mosquitoes and bedbugs gorged on HIV-contaminated blood. Even with concentrations 100 times that found in individuals with HIV, transmission from the insects could not be accomplished.[81] Arthropod infection was suggested as a route of transmission in multiple cases of HIV infection in Palm Beach County and the town of Belle Glade, Florida.[82] Extensive epidemiologic investigations, however, failed to confirm this hypothesis.[83]

Casual Contact

The concern for casual spread of HIV has accompanied HIV disease and AIDS since the onset of this epidemic. However, studies from over 700 households and boarding schools in the United States and Europe could not document transmission of HIV by routes previously known and described.[65,84] Nonsexual contacts of HIV-infected individuals in 314 households in Africa also failed to document casual transmission of HIV.[85] Because of the lack of evidence indicating casual transmission of HIV, the Public Health Service has issued guidelines for offices, schools, food service establishments, and factories barring restrictions of infected individuals solely based on their HIV status.[86] According to these guidelines, infected individuals should have unrestricted use of telephones, office equipment, toilets, showers, eating facilities, and water fountains. Furthermore, infected individuals should be allowed to both serve and prepare food and beverages.

A frequent query concerns the survival of HIV outside the body. One study indicated that HIV may survive and retain its infectivity for approximately 30 hours even in dried specimens at room temperature.[87] This finding is in accordance with other studies.[88] However, HIV transmission from inert objects has not been demonstrated.

HIV Transmission in Health-Care Settings

All health-care providers have pondered the question of occupational HIV transmission. Numerous books, monographs, and articles have discussed infection and exposure control, and updated guidelines are continually published by professional organizations and the Centers for Disease Control and Prevention (CDC).[89] Each of these protocols emphasizes how proper precautions minimize the risk of transmission of infectious pathogens. Yet transmission still occurs. The perception of risk embodied in each health-care setting can only be determined by each individual worker, even though the perception may not be the same as the actual risk involved. The risk for HIV transmission in health-care settings is discussed in Chapter 15.

Many instances have been documented in which health-care providers were exposed to patients' HIV-contaminated blood. Very few of these cases result in HIV infection but apprehensions may remain for long periods after all tests show that transmission did not occur. Overall, 39 documented occupational exposures among health-care providers have resulted in HIV transmission. No dental worker is included in this group. An additional 81 possible occupational HIV transmissions have been reported to the CDC, including six dental providers.[90] It is not known how many of these individuals are dentists, dental assistants, or dental hygienists. A large study of 1,309 dental providers concluded that despite poor infection control, the risk for occupational transmission of HIV was very low among this professional group.[91]

Transmission of HIV in a dental setting is a two-way street. Theoretically, transmission from HIV-infected health-care providers to patients is possible. But has it ever been documented, and what is the proven mode of transmission? In July 1990, the CDC reported a possible transmission of HIV during a dental procedure to a patient from an HIV-positive dentist.[92] This report resulted in a massive public reaction culminating in new proposed CDC infection control guidelines limiting providers with HIV to perform only specific, noninvasive medical and dental procedures. Yet, the only case of possible transmission from a health-care worker to a patient was that of the Florida dental case. In May 1992, four separate articles were published establishing CDC's conclusions concerning the transmission of HIV from infected health-care providers to patients.[93–96] Two main conclusions were reached: dentist-to-patient transmission had occurred in the case of the Florida dentist but the mode of transmission could not be established; and no other instances of health-care worker-to-patient transmission have been documented. Since this time, the CDC has conducted a large retrospective study, including over 22,032 patients treated by 63 HIV-positive health-care providers, 34 of them dentists and dental students. In that study, the CDC was not able to document any HIV transmission from health-care providers to patients.[97]

In lieu of known data, the risk of HIV transmission in a dental setting is a highly unlikely event. However, the outcome of transmission is so severe that the perceived risk of transmission overshadows the documented factual risk.

In conclusion, existing knowledge of HIV transmission has remained the same, despite the fact that other areas of knowledge about the disease are constantly evolving. Transmission of HIV occurs by intimate sexual contact, exchange of contaminated blood and blood products, and perinatally between infected mothers and their newborn offspring. Although HIV can be isolated from other body fluids, such as saliva, tears, and urine, these fluids have not been implicated in HIV transmission. Additional body fluids like sweat have not been shown to harbor HIV and have not been associated with virus transmission. Other suggested modes of transmission, including casual contacts, insect bites, and dental prophylaxis angles and high-speed handpieces, have also not been confirmed. For HIV transmission to occur, a sufficient amount of infectious virus needs to be present. But it is not clear how many infectious particles are necessary to achieve infection. Infection is probably also dependent on an individual's ability to mount an appropriate immune response. If alternative modes of HIV transmission exist, they need to be confirmed with epidemiologic studies. The most illustrative example of this concerns dentistry. If dental equipment could truly transmit HIV, there would be several clusters of HIV-infected patients who had become infected by attending clinics that treat HIV-infected individuals. Since this has not been found, this mode of transmission is either extremely rare or does not exist, and, at best, remains a reflection of public fear about this disease.

References

1. Kunzel C, Sadowsky D. Comparing dentists' attitudes and knowledge concerning AIDS: differences and similarities by locale. J Am Dent Assoc 1991;122:55–61.

2. Jaffe HW, Bregman DJ, Selik RM. Acquired immune deficiency syndrome in the United States: the first 1,000 cases. J Infect Dis 1983;148:339–345.

3. Ammann AJ, Cowan MJ, Wara DW, et al. Acquired immunodeficiency in an infant: possible transmission by means of blood products. Lancet 1983;i:956–958.

4. Nkowane BM. Prevalence and incidence of HIV infection in Africa: a review of data published in 1990. AIDS 1991;5:7–16.

5. Stoneburner RL, Chiasson M, Weisfuse IB, Thomas PA. The epidemic of AIDS and HIV-1 infection among heterosexuals in New York City. AIDS 1990;4:99–106.

6. Plummer FA, Simonsen JN, Cameron DW, et al. Cofactors in male-female sexual transmission of human immunodeficiency virus type 1. J Infect Dis 1991;163:233–239.

7. Padian NS, Shiboski S, Jewell NP. Female-to-male transmission of human immunodeficiency virus. JAMA 1991;266:1664–1667.

8. Cameron DW, Simonsen JN, D'Costa LJ, et al. Female to male transmission of human immunodeficiency virus type 1: risk factors for seroconversion in men. Lancet 1989;2:403–407.

9. Heise C, Dandekar S, Kumar P, Duplantier R, Donovan RM, Halsted CH. Human immunodeficiency virus infection of enterocytes and mononuclear cells in human jejunal mucosa. Gastroenterology 1991;100:1521–1527.

10. Pudney J, Oneta M, Mayer K, Seage III G, Anderson D. Pre-ejaculation fluid as a potential vector for sexual transmission of HIV-1. Lancet 1992;93:651–656.

11. Wofsy CB, Cohen JB, Hauer LB, et al. Isolation of the AIDS-associated retrovirus from genital secretions from women with antibodies to the virus. Lancet 1986;i:527–529.

12. Clemetson DBA, Moss GB, Willerford DM, et al. Detection of HIV DNA in cervical and vaginal secretions. JAMA 1993;269:2860–2864.

13. Levy JA. The transmission of AIDS: the case of the infected cell. JAMA 1988;259:3037–3038.

14. Hook III EW, Cannon RO, Nahmias AJ, et al. Herpes simplex virus infection as a risk factor for human immunodeficiency virus infection in heterosexuals. J Infect Dis 1992;165:251–255.

15. Pomerantz RJ, de la Monte SM, Donegan SP, et al. Human immunodeficiency virus (HIV) infection of the uterine cervix. Ann Intern Med 1987;108:321–327.

16. Seidlin M, Vogler M, Lee E, Lee YS, Dubin N. Heterosexual transmission of HIV in a cohort of couples in New York City. AIDS 1993;7:1247–1254.

17. van der Graaf, Diepersloot R. Sexual transmission of HIV: routes, efficiency, cofactors and prevention. A survey of the literature. Infection 1989;17:210–215.

18. Marmor M, Weiss LR, Lyden M, et al. Possible female-to-female transmission of human immunodeficiency virus. Ann Intern Med 1986;105:969.

19. Monzon OT, Capellan JMB. Female-to-female transmission of HIV (letter). Lancet 1987;2:40-41.

20. Petersen LR, Doll L, White C, Chu S. The HIV Blood Donor Study Group. No evidence for female-to-female HIV transmission among 960,000 female blood donors. J Acquired Immune Deficiency Syndrome 1992;5:853–855.

21. Detels R, English P, Visscher BR, et al. Seroconversion, sexual activity and condom use among 2915 HIV seronegative men followed for up to 2 years. J Acquired Immune Deficiency Syndrome 1989;2:77–83.

22. Lifson AR, O'Malley PM, Hessol NA, Buchbinder SP, Cannon L, Rutherford GW. HIV seroconversion in two homosexual men after receptive oral intercourse with ejaculation: implications for counseling concerning safe sexual practices. Am J Public Health 1990;80:1509–1511.

23. DeGruttola V, Mayer KH. Human immunodeficiency virus and oral intercourse. Ann Intern Med 1987;107:428–429.

24. Rozenbaum W, Gharakhanian S, Cardon B, Duval E, Coulaud JP. HIV transmission by oral sex. Lancet 1988;1:1395.

25. Ho DD, Moudgil T, Alam M. Quantitation of human immunodeficiency virus type 1 in the blood of infected persons. N Engl J Med 1989;321:1621–1625.

26. Pan L-Z, Werner A, Levy JA. Detection of plasma viremia in human immunodeficiency virus-infected individuals at all clinical stages. J Clin Microbiol 1993;31:283–288.

27. Layne SP, Merges MJ, Dembo M, et al. Factors underlying spontaneous inactivation and susceptibility to neutralization of human immunodeficiency virus. Virology 1992;189:695–714.

28. Bagasra O, Hauptman SP, Lischner HW, Sachs M, Pomerantz RJ. Detection of human immunodeficiency virus type 1 provirus in mononuclear cells by in situ polymerase chain reaction. N Engl J Med 1992;326:1385–1391.

29. Levy JA. The transmission of HIV and factors influencing progression to AIDS. Am J Med 1993;95:86–100.

30. Widmann FK. Standards for Blood Banks and Transfusion Services, ed 14. Arlington, VA: American Association of Blood Banks; 1991.

31. Dodd RY. The risk of transfusion-transmitted infection. N Engl J Med 1992;327:419–421.

32. Menitove JE. Current risk of transfusion-associated human immunodeficiency virus infection. Arch Pathol Lab Med 1990;114:330–334.

33. Epstein JS, Fricke WA. Current safety of clotting factor concentrates. Arch Pathol Lab Med 1990;114:335–340.

34. CDC. Perspectives in disease prevention and health promotion: safety of therapeutic products used for hemophilia patients. MMWR 1988;37:441–450.

35. Julius C, Westphal RG. The safety of blood components and derivatives. Hematol Oncol Clin North Am 1992;6:1057–1077.

36. Oxtoby MJ. Perinatally acquired human immunodeficiency virus infection. Pediatr Infect Dis J 1990;9:609–619.

37. Rogers MF, Ou C-Y, Kilbourne B, Schochetman G. Advances and problems in the diagnosis of human immunodeficiency virus infection in infants. Pediatr Infect Dis J 1991;10:523–531.

38. St. Louis ME, Kamenga M, Brown C, et al. Risk for perinatal HIV-1 transmission according to maternal immunologic, virologic, and placental factors. JAMA 1993;269:2853–2859.

39. Rossi P. Maternal factors involved in mother-to-child transmission of HIV-1. Report of a Consensus Workshop, Siena, Italy, Jan 1992. J Acquired Immune Deficiency Syndrome 1992;5:1019–1029.

40. Douglas GC, King BF. Maternal-fetal transmission of human immunodeficiency virus: a review of possible routes and cellular mechanisms of infection. Clin Infect Dis 1992;15:678–691.

41. Krivine AG, Firtion G, Cao L, Francoual C, Henrion R, Lebon P. HIV replication during the first weeks of life. Lancet 1992;339:1187–1189.

42. Ehrnst A, Lindgren S, Dictor M, et al. HIV replication in pregnant women and their offspring: evidence for late transmission. Lancet 1991;338:203–207.

43. Menez-Bautista R, Fikrig SM, Pahwa S, Sarangadharan MG, Stoneburner RL. Monozygotic twins discordant for the acquired immunodeficiency syndrome. Am J Dis Child 1986;140:678–679.

44. Goedert JJ, Duliege A-M, Amos CI, Felton S, Biggar RJ. High risk of HIV-1 infection for first-born twins. Lancet 1991;338:1471–1475.

45. Oxtoby MJ. Human immunodeficiency virus and other viruses in human milk: placing the issue in broader perspective. Pediatr Infect Dis 1988;7:825–835.

46. Palasanthirn P, Ziegler JB, Stewart GJ, et al. Breast-feeding during primary maternal human immunodeficiency virus infection and risk of transmission from mother to child. J Infect Dis 1993;167:441–444.

47. Goldfarb J. Breastfeeding. AIDS and other infectious diseases. Clin Perinatol 1993;20:225–243.

48. Nicoll A, Killewo JZJ, Mgone C. HIV and infant feeding practices: epidemiological implications for sub-Saharan African countries. AIDS 1990;4:661–665.

49. CDC. Zidovudine for the prevention of HIV transmission from mother to infant. MMWR 1994;43:285–287.

50. Levy JA, Greenspan D. HIV in saliva. Lancet 1988;ii:1248.

51. Ho DD, Byington RE, Schooley RT, Flynn T, Rota TR, Hirsch MS. Infrequency of isolation of HTLV-III virus from saliva in AIDS. N Engl J Med 1985;313:1306.

52. Groopman JE, Salahuddin SZ, Sarngadharan MG, et al. HTLV-III in saliva of people with AIDS-related complex and healthy homosexual men at risk for AIDS. Science 1984;226:447–449.

53. Barr CE, Miller LK, Lopez MR, et al. Recovery of infectious HIV-1 from whole saliva. J Am Dent Assoc 1992;123:37–45.

54. Fox PC, Wolff A, Yeh C-K, Atkinson JC, Baum BJ. Saliva inhibits HIV-1 infectivity. J Am Dent Assoc 1988;116:635–637.

55. Archibald DW, Cole GA. In vitro inhibition of HIV-1 infectivity by human salivas. AIDS Res Hum Retroviruses 1990;6:1425–1432.

56. Yeh C-K, Handelman B, Fox PC, Baum BJ. Further studies of salivary inhibition of HIV-1 infectivity. J Acquired Immune Deficiency Syndrome 1992;5:898–903.

57. CDC. Recommendations for prevention of HIV transmission in health-care settings. MMWR 1987;36(suppl 2S):1-19.

58. Tsoukas CM, Hadjis T, Shuster J, Theberge L, Feorino P, O'Shaughness M. Lack of transmission of HIV through human bites and scratches. J Acquired Immune Deficiency Syndrome 1988;1:505-507.

59. Drummond JA. Seronegative 18 months after being bitten by a patient with AIDS. JAMA 1986;256:2342–2343.

60. Rogers MF, White CR, Sanders R. Can children transmit HTLV-III/LAV infection? Presented at the 26th Interscience Conference on Antimicrobial Agents and Chemotherapy, New Orleans, Oct 1, 1986.

61. Wahn V, Kramer HH, Voit T, Broster HT, Scrampical B, Scheid A. Horizontal transmission of HIV infection between two siblings. Lancet 1986;2:694.

62. Piazza M, Chirianni A, Picciotto L, Guadagnino V, Orlando R, Cataldo PT. Passionate kissing and microlesions of the oral mucosa: possible role in AIDS transmission. JAMA 1989;261:244–245.

63. Woolley RJ. The biologic possibility of HIV transmission during passionate kissing. JAMA 1989;262:2230.

64. Salahuddin SZ, Groopman JE, Markham PD, et al. HTLV-III in symptom-free seronegative persons. Lancet 1984;2:1418–1420.

65. Lifson AR. Do alternative modes for transmission of human immunodeficiency virus exist? JAMA 1988;259:1353–1356.

66. Yeung SCH, Kazazi F, Randle CGM, et al. Patients infected with human immunodeficiency virus type 1 have low levels of virus in saliva even in the presence of periodontal disease. J Infect Dis 1993;167:803–807.

67. Lewis DL, Boe RK. Cross-infection associated with current procedures for using high-speed dental handpieces. J Clin Microbiol 1992;30:401–406.

68. Lewis DL, Arens M, Appleton SS, et al. Cross-contamination potential with dental equipment. Lancet 1992;340:1252–1254.

69. Epstein JB, Rea G, Sibau L, Sherlock CH. Rotary dental instruments and the potential risk of transmission of infection: herpes simplex virus. J Am Dent Assoc 1993;124(12):55–59.

70. Sawchuk WS, Weber PJ, Lowy DR, Dzubov LM. Infectious papillomavirus in the vapor of warts treated with carbon dioxide laser or electrocoagulation: detection and protection. J Am Acad Dermatol 1989;21:41-49.

71. Fujikawa LS, Salahuddin SZ, Palestine AG, Nussenblatt RB, Gallo RC. Isolation of human T-lymphotropic virus type III from tears of a patient with the acquired immunodeficiency syndrome. Lancet 1985;2:529–530.

72. Tervo T, Lahdevirta J, Vaheri A, Valle SL, Suni J. Recovery of HTLV-III from contact lenses. Lancet 1986;1:379–380.

73. CDC. Recommendations for preventing possible transmission of human T-lymphotropic virus type III/lymphadenopathy-associated virus from tears. MMWR 1985;34:533–534.

74. Levy JA, Kaminsky LS, Morrow WJW, et al. Infection by the retrovirus associated with the acquired immunodeficiency syndrome. Ann Intern Med 1985;103:694–699.

75. Gerberding JL, Bryant-LeBlanc CE, Nelson K, et al. Risk of transmitting the human immunodeficiency virus, cytomegalovirus, and hepatitis B virus to health care workers exposed to patients with AIDS and AIDS-related conditions. J Infect Dis 1987;156:1–8.

76. Wormser GP, Bittker S, Forester G, et al. Absence of infectious human immunodeficiency virus type 1 in natural eccrine sweat. J Infect Dis 1992;165:155-158.

77. Francis DP, Feorino PM, McDougal S , et al. The safety of hepatitis B vaccine: inactivation of the AIDS virus during routine vaccine manufacture. JAMA 1986;256:869–872.

78. CDC. Hepatitis B vaccine: evidence confirming lack of AIDS transmission. MMWR 1984;33:685–687.

79. Chermann JC, Becker JL, Hazan U, et al. HIV related sequences in insects from central Africa. Presented at the Third International Conference on AIDS, Washington, DC, June 1, 1987.

80. Srinivasan A, York D, Bohan C. Lack of HIV replication in arthropod cells. Lancet 1987;2:1094–1095.

81. Jupp PG, Lyons SF. Experimental assessment of bedbugs (*Cimex lecturalius* and *Cimex hemipterus*) and mosquitoes (*Aedes aegypti formosus*) as vectors of human immunodeficiency virus. AIDS 1987;1:171–174.

82. Whiteside ME, Withum D, Tavris D, et al. Outbreak of no identifiable risk for acquired immunodeficiency syndrome (AIDS) in Belle Glade, Florida. Presented at the First International Conference on AIDS, Atlanta, April 17, 1985.

83. Castro KG, Lieb S, Jaffe HW, et al. Transmission of HIV in Belle Glade, Florida: lessons for other communities in the United States. Science 1988;239:193-197.

84. Gershon RRM, Vlahov D, Nelson KE. The risk of transmission of HIV-1 through nonpercutaneous, non-sexual modes: a review. AIDS 1990;4:645–650.

85. Mann JM, Quinn TC, Francis H, et al. Prevalence of HTLV-III/LAV in household contacts of patients with confirmed AIDS and controls in Kinshasa, Zaire. JAMA 1986;256:721–724.

86. CDC. Recommendations for preventing transmission of infection with human T-lymphotropic virus type III/lymphadenopathy-associated virus in the workplace. MMWR 1985;34:681–686, 691–695.

87. Tjotta E, Hungnes O, Grinde B. Survival of HIV-1 activity after disinfection, temperature and pH changes, or drying. J Med Virol 1991;35:223–227.

88. Resnick L, Veren K, Salahuddin SZ, Tondreau S, Markham PD. Stability and inactivation of HTLV-III/LAV under clinical and laboratory environments. JAMA 1986;255:1887–1891.

89. CDC. Recommended infection-control practices for dentistry, 1993. MMWR 1993;42:1–12.

90. CDC. HIV/AIDS surveillance report. 1993;5(3):13.

91. Klein RS, Phelan JA, Freeman K, et al. Low occupational risk of human immunodeficiency virus infection among dental professionals. N Engl J Med 1988;318:86–90.

92. CDC. Possible transmission of human immunodeficiency virus to a patient during an invasive dental procedure. MMWR 1990;39:489–493.

93. CDC. Update: investigations of patients who have been treated by HIV-infected health-care workers. MMWR 1992;41:344–346.

94. Tokars JI, Bell DM, Culver DH, et al. Percutaneous injuries during surgical procedures. JAMA 1992;267:2899–2904.

95. Ciesielski C, Marianos D, Ou C-Y. Transmission of human immunodeficiency virus in a dental practice. Ann Intern Med 1992;116:798–805.

96. Ou C-Y, Ciesielski C, Myers G, et al. Molecular epidemiology of HIV transmission in a dental practice. Science 1992;256:1165–1171.

97. Robert M, Bell DM. HIV transmission in the health-care setting. In Glatt AE (ed): Infect Dis Clin North Am 1994;8:319–329.

5

Pathogenesis of HIV

Michael Glick

Early in the epidemic, the search for a causative agent for AIDS focused on a variety of viruses known to cause immune deficiency. Today, well into the epidemic's second decade, we are still trying to accurately establish the pathogenesis of HIV disease.

The discovery of the pathways of HIV infection has been systematic and continuous. In 1983, French researchers recovered reverse transcriptase (RT), an enzyme responsible for transcribing RNA into DNA, in a lymph node from a man with signs and symptoms of what was then known as lymphadenopathy syndrome (LAS).[1] This syndrome was recognized as an early manifestation of AIDS. The identification of reverse transcriptase was the first indication that a virus, preserving its genetic information in the form of RNA, might be responsible for the immune deficiency described in affected individuals. The presence of reverse transcriptase, together with signs and symptoms of the disease, also suggested that the causative agent of AIDS belonged to a family of viruses called retroviruses. Further evidence for the causal status of this virus was provided by the same French research team that demonstrated how the virus could infect and kill CD4+ T-helper lymphocytes.[2]

This virus was initially given three different names. The French group led by Montagnier called it lymphadenopathy-associated virus (LAV); a group from the National Institutes of Health (NIH) in the United States, led by Gallo, called the virus human T-lymphotropic virus type III (HTLV-III)[3,4]; and a third group of researchers from San Francisco led by Levy called it AIDS-associated retrovirus (ARV).[5] In 1986, to reduce the confusion created by having different names for the same virus, the International Committee on Taxonomy of Viruses recommended human immunodeficiency virus (HIV).[6]

Further research has established that HIV belongs to the family of lentiviruses. As the name implies, infections caused by lentiviruses progress slowly with long incubation periods.[7] With HIV disease, this refers to a potential incubation period of more than 15 years, from initial infection to signs and symptoms of AIDS, with a median time of 10 years.[8–11]

After the initial recovery of viruses from lymph nodes, HIV was isolated from peripheral blood mononuclear cells (PBMC) both in patients with clinical manifestations of AIDS as well as in patients without any clinical signs or symptoms.[12,13] Not long after its discovery, a separate viral subtype was discovered in individuals from Western Africa.[14] To distinguish these two viruses, the initial HIV was named HIV type 1 (HIV-1), while the second virus was called HIV type 2 (HIV-2). The course of the disease appears to be much longer with HIV-2.

This chapter presents the characteristics of HIV-1, the mechanism for HIV infection of cells, and the host immune response to the infection.

Viral Structure and Cellular Infection

The viral structure of HIV (Fig 5-1) is simple, yet complex. The virus is specifically suited to infect specific cells and subsequently replicate within these cells. Human immunodeficiency virus has a lipid membrane, or envelope, surrounding a bullet-shaped core characteristic of retroviruses. The outside envelope of the virus is coated with 72 knob-like glycoproteins, gp120, connected to the viral membrane with another glycoprotein, gp41.[15] The numbers assigned to these proteins are based on their molecular weights in kilodaltons. The surface protein, gp120, contains sites that recognize and subsequently attach to a specific cellular receptor, CD4, on the surface of a target cell (Fig 5-2).[16]

The main target for HIV is T-helper lymphocytes, which express CD4 surface receptors. However, other cells, such as monocytes and macrophages, also express these surface receptors,[17] although to a lesser extent.[18] While lymphocytes may express 40,000 to 100,000 CD4 receptors per cell, macrophages have less than 200 receptors per cell. Recent in vitro studies have identified an increasing number of different CD4-positive cells throughout the body, including neural and endothelial cells of the brain, intestinal epithelial cells, bone marrow precursor cells, placental cells, and Langerhans' cells in the epidermis. This may explain the wide range of HIV-related symptoms exhibited in different body systems as well as the various clinical manifestations among HIV-positive individuals.[19]

Fig 5-1. HIV contains the viral genetic information in RNA strands (HIV RNA) located within the core of the virus (p24). The enzyme responsible for transcribing HIV RNA into proviral DNA (reverse transcriptase) is also located within the viral core. A surrounding lipid membrane and a matrix (p17) protects the internal structures of the virus. Seventy-two protruding knob-like proteins (gp120) are connected to the outside of the lipid membrane by a transmembrane protein (gp41).

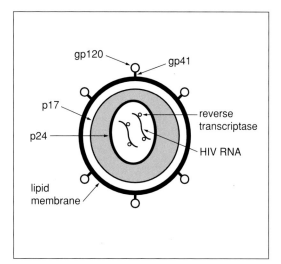

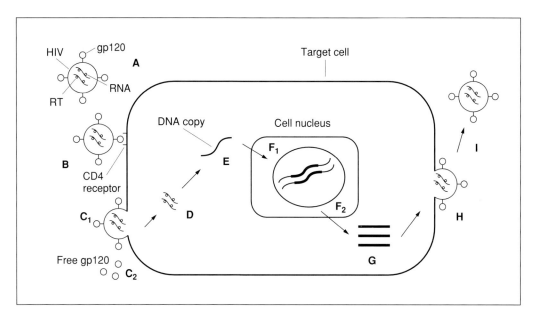

Fig 5-2. A, Free, extracellular HIV; **B**, Gp120 recognizes and attaches to a CD4 receptor of a target cell; **C$_1$**, The viral membrane fuses with the target cell membrane enabling HIV RNA to enter the cytoplasm of the target cell; **C$_2$**, During the process of virus-to-target membrane fusion, gp120 is released from the virus, creating free circulating gp120s; **D**, HIV RNA is transcribed with the help of reverse transcriptase; **E**, Linear and later double-stranded circular proviral DNA will be created; **F$_1$**, The proviral DNA migrates into the nucleus of the host cell and is integrated into the cell's chromosome; **F$_2$**, Stimulation of viral replication creates HIV-mRNA; **G**, Translation of the HIV-mRNA produces long proteins that need to be cleaved into viral structural proteins; **H**, Assembly and budding of the virus; and, **I**, Continuous assembly of the internal structures of the virus eventually result in a new formed virus.

The presence of infected cells and circulating free viruses plays an important role in explaining the routes and modes of HIV transmission (see Chapter 4). After viral attachment, gp120 is cleaved from gp41, which hooks onto the target cell membrane and facilitates fusion of the viral membrane and the target cell (see Fig 5-2, C_1).[20] Some of the cleaved gp120 moieties remain on the surface of the target cell, while others detach and circulate freely as independent proteins (see Fig 5-2, C_2).[21] The virus-to-target cell membrane fusion enables viral RNA to enter into the target cell's cytoplasm. As previously mentioned, retroviruses maintain their genetic material in the form of RNA within the core of the virus. This core consists of a protein designated as p24. In addition, the core also contains the enzyme reverse transcriptase, which is necessary to convert viral RNA into proviral DNA (see Fig 5-2, D).

Transcription of viral RNA into single-stranded and later double-stranded DNA takes place in the cytoplasm (see Fig 5-2, E). These DNA copies (complementary DNA, cDNA) of the viral RNA migrate into the nucleus and become integrated into the genome of the infected cell (see Fig 5-2, F_1). The integrated proviral DNA stays relatively latent until the host cell is stimulated (see Fig 5-2, F_2).[22] Such stimulation normally initiates production of cellular proteins but in infected cells, with integrated viral genomes, viral proteins are also produced (see Fig 5-2, G). These viral proteins are broken down by proteases into building-blocks for viral assembly.

The infected cell, or target cell, provides the necessary environment for viral reproduction as well as protection for the virus against the body's humoral (antibody) immune response. Newly formed viruses are subsequently released from the host cell (see Fig 5-2, H) and can infect other susceptible cells (see Fig 5-2, I). Much research is focused on the nature of HIV activation and latency. If it is possible to determine the mechanism for viral activation or how latency is achieved, it might also be possible to artificially reproduce long-term asymptomatic periods in infected individuals.

In vitro experiments suggest that other viruses, such as herpes simplex virus, Epstein-Barr virus, cytomegalovirus, human herpes virus 6, papovavirus, hepatitis B virus, and even other strains of HIV, may be partially responsible for activation of HIV replication.[23] This activation is probably achieved by induction of cytokines and by stimulation of a transactivating gene called Tat.

Some cells without CD4 surface receptors can apparently also be infected by HIV.[24] However, very low viral replication is noted within these cells, possibly due to inefficient viral entry.[25] Even cells within the dental pulp, probably fibroblasts which generally lack CD4 receptors, have been shown to be infected with HIV.[26] It has been proposed that a special fusion receptor may be responsible for HIV entry into CD4-negative cells.[27]

Macrophages

The role of macrophages in HIV infection deserves special mention. Although HIV infection of macrophages occurs via its CD4 receptor, other mechanisms for cell infection, such as viral entry by phagocytosis and antibody-mediated endocytosis, have also been described.[28] Replication of HIV in macrophages is different from that described in lymphocytes. During HIV replication in lymphocytes, virus continuously buds out of the cell (see Fig 5-3). In contrast, HIV replication inside macrophages results in a continuous accumulation of infectious and noninfectious viruses. This amassing of viruses continues until lysis of the cell occurs. Consequently, it has been proposed that macrophages serve as the reservoir for HIV in the body and facilitate the transport of the virus to different tissues, including the brain.[29] Release of infectious viruses from macrophages and subsequent dissemination of HIV in the body could be initiated by any agent that stimulates macrophage function, including a normal inflammatory response. The release of many viruses at the same time results in a rapid infusion of a large amount of highly virulent viruses. Such a massive viral attack overwhelms the host's already debilitated immune response, resulting in faster disease progression.

It is generally believed that the initial infection with HIV can be sup-

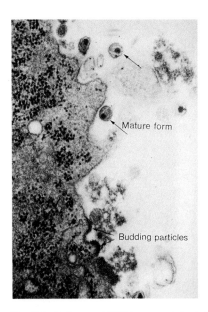

Mature form

Budding particles

Fig 5-3. Release of HIV from an infected lymphocyte. Courtesy of CDC.

pressed by the cellular and/or humoral immune response. However, less virulent viruses are not recognized by the immune response and are instead picked up by macrophages. As such, a state of relative latency is established. However, HIV replication continues within the lymph nodes and inside macrophages.[30] Because of the high rate of mutational changes of HIV, more virulent variants are continuously produced and eventually overwhelm the immune system. Thus, although clinical latency may be present for many years, a true viral latent state, where no HIV replication takes place, does not exist in HIV disease.[31,32]

CD4+ T-Helper Lymphocyte Depletion and Dysfunction

The hallmark of HIV infection is the progressive decline of CD4+ T-helper lymphocytes during the course of the disease. It is not clear what causes this cellular depletion and dysfunction, but several hypotheses have been presented.[33] The enigma surrounding CD4+ cell depletion becomes even more intriguing when considering that perhaps only one of every 1,000 PBMC harbor HIV in infected individuals.[34] Thus, although few cells are directly infected by HIV, uninfected CD4+ cells are also destroyed. Single-cell killing[35] of infected cells cannot account for all the destruction of CD4+ cells. It has been observed that syncytial formations occur in individuals with advanced stages of HIV disease.[36] The formation of syncytia, or giant cells, results from fusion of the cell membranes of infected cells with the cell membranes of uninfected cells. These giant cells become nonfunctional and are later destroyed. Another proposed mechanism for CD4+ cell dysfunction and depletion occurs when complexes of circulating gp120 antigens, released when the virus connected with the CD4 receptor of the target cell, and antibodies bind to the CD4 receptor of uninfected cells. This results in anergy, a state in which these cells cannot be activated. Such cells are recognized as infected and therefore destroyed by the host immune response. Other mechanisms of CD4+ cell destruction have been proposed, but it is clear that more

than one method is needed to achieve the observed depletion.[33]

Many studies have attempted to assess the rate of CD4+ cell depletion during the course of HIV disease. It is generally believed that the CD4 cell count declines rapidly during the first couple of weeks after infection but increases to almost normal levels after seroconversion. (Seroconversion is the production and subsequent appearance of antibodies in the blood.) A steady decrease of an estimated 67 to 84 CD4+ T lymphocytes per milliliter per year continues until approximately 18 months prior to AIDS, when a more rapid decrease in CD4+ cell number is observed.[37,38] Studies in which patients showed a rapid cell depletion prior to AIDS diagnosis suggest a change of HIV virulence during disease progression. The continuous changes of the HIV phenotype within infected individuals during disease progression, such as a high proportion of syncytial-inducing (SI) phenotypic HIV found during the later but not during the earlier stages of HIV disease,[39] enables the virus to elude the body's attempt to eliminate the pathogen.

Acute HIV Infection

The progressive depletion of CD4+ T lymphocytes enables the development of opportunistic infections characteristic of HIV disease and eventually AIDS. However, this chronic infection starts with an acute viral syndrome. The first cases of acute HIV infection, or seroconversion syndrome, were described in 1985 among 11 homosexual men.[40] This syndrome appears, on average, 3 to 4 weeks after initial HIV infection and is characterized as a mononucleosis-like illness.[41] Signs and symptoms include fever, pharyngitis, adenopathy, rash, myalgias, arthralgias, vomiting, diarrhea, headache, leukopenia, lymphopenia, thrombocytopenia, and increased levels of serum aminotransferase. Studies have also described the presence of esophageal and oral ulcerations.[42] Between 50% and 80% of infected adults will develop this acute illness, which lasts for 7 to 10 days. It is important to recognize these clinical manifestations of acute HIV infection since these signs and symptoms can occur after occupational exposure to HIV. As an increased number of prevention strategies become available, the early identification of HIV infection can prolong life.

Clinical vs Viral Latency

Following the acute HIV infection, there is a short period of intense viral replication, heavy viremia, seeding of the virus to various organs such as the brain and lymphoid tissues, and an accompanied host immune response[43–45] that parallels clinical signs and symptoms. Within weeks to months, very few viruses and almost no viral replication can be detected in the serum (Fig 5-4). This state persists for several years during the clinical latency period.[46] However, a humoral and cellular immune response can be detected.

There is a high burden of HIV in the lymphoid tissues, both as extracellular virus trapped in the follicular dendritic cell network of the germinal centers and as intracellular virus during all various stages of HIV disease.[46] The major lymphoid organ in the body is the gastrointestinal tract, where 50% to 60% of all lymphocytes are distributed as Peyer's patches, lamina propria lymphoid cells and aggregates, and intraepithelial lymphocytes.[47] Accordingly, the lymphoid tissues of the gastrointestinal tract as well as the peripheral lymph nodes serve as reservoirs for latent and replicating HIV.[48] This has been corroborated in other studies showing that HIV accumulates in lymphoid organs during the clinically asymptomatic period.[49]

The chronic stimulation of the immune system by HIV results in spontaneous hyperactivation of B lymphocytes, activation of monocytes, lymph node hyperplasia, autoimmune phenomenon, and other immune-related expressions.[50] It is also possible that the persistent activation of the immune system ultimately leads to the observed immune dysfunction and loss of its ability to appropriately react to antigens.[50]

A progressive increase in the number of HIV-infected PBMC is noted during the later stages of HIV disease, when profound immune suppression is present.[46] During periods of viral replication, an increased level of p24 antigens can be detected in the serum. The presence of p24 antigenemia is sometimes used as a surrogate marker for disease progression.

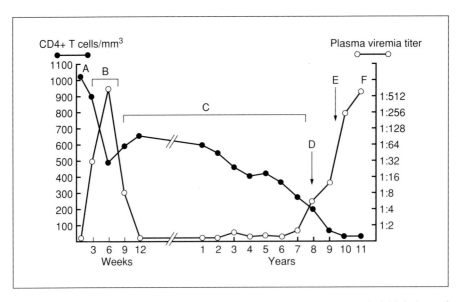

Fig 5-4. A, Initial infection with HIV. **B,** Acute HIV syndrome. During this period, high titers of HIV (5,000 infected particles/mL of blood) can be detected in the blood. There is also a drop and a subsequent increase of detectable CD4+ T lymphocytes in the peripheral blood during the first 3 months after the initial HIV infection. The CD4+ T lymphocyte level will usually stabilize at a lower level than before the acute HIV infection. **C,** Clinical latency period. An immune response to HIV reduces detectable viruses to less than one infected particle/mL of blood. Although no signs or symptoms associated with HIV disease occur, viral replication continues mostly within lymphoid tissues, and a continuous decline of peripheral CD4+ T lymphocytes (average of 67 to 84 cells per year) is noticed. **D,** Constitutional signs and symptoms start to occur when the CD4+ T lymphocyte count drops below 250 to 300 cells/mm[3]. **E,** When the CD4+ T lymphocyte count drops below 200 cells/mm[3], opportunistic infections start to occur and at this time plasma viremia starts to be noticed. Manifestations of infections with a high degree of mortality are more common when CD4+ cell T lymphocyte count drop below 100 cells/mm[3]. **F,** Patients with a CD4+ T lymphocyte count below 50 cells/mm[3] have an average of 12 months to survive. (From Pantoleo G, Graziosi C, Fauci AS. N Engl J Med 1993;328:329. Used with permission.)

HIV Virulence

The number of both infected cells and free viruses increases during the progression of HIV disease. Furthermore, the virus also undergoes changes during the course of the disease. Strains of HIV recovered from the same individual in the early stages of infection differ from viruses isolated from the same person during the clinical stages of the disease.[36,51] An increased virulence of HIV is especially observed in the later stages of infection. The virulence of HIV is characterized by the virus' ability to infect a larger range of cells, a faster rate of replication with high titers of virus production, an increased ability to form syncytia, more efficient killing of target cells, lack of latency, and sensitivity to enhancing antibodies and not neutralizing antibodies. All of these features increase the rate of disease progression.

Although a constant replication of HIV, increasingly virulent strains, and progressive immune deterioration are present in infected individuals, the body's immune response can suppress HIV expression to a certain extent.

Immune Response Against HIV

During most viral infections, the progression of infections is arrested and the pathogens eliminated by the cell-mediated immune response. This immune response is associated with the recognition and killing of virus-infected cells by natural killer (NK) cells. However in HIV infection, NK cells appear to have a reduced function, particularly in the later stages of the disease.[52,53] The mechanism of HIV killing by NK cells is accompanied by an antibody-dependent cellular cytotoxicity (ADCC). Thus, HIV coated by antibodies is recognized and destroyed by NK cells.

CD4+ T-helper lymphocytes have an important role in the elimination and regulation of HIV expression. It appears that human CD4+ T-helper lymphocytes can respond in more than one manner when antigen-presenting cells (APC), such as macrophages, present them with antigens such as HIV. The different responses are measured by a shift in the type and level of cytokines (chemicals produced by cells of the immune system to regulate immune response) produced by stimulated CD4+ cells. These responses have been named T-helper cell type 1 or TH1 and T-helper cell type 2 or TH2 responses. The presence and activation of these two responses of T lymphocytes are apparently associated with the course of HIV disease.[54,55]

A TH1 response is found in healthy asymptomatic individuals and in individuals at high risk for HIV but without evidence of infection.[53] This response is associated with the release of cytokines such as interleukin-2 (IL-2), gamma-interferon, and IL-12, which seems to promote the growth of cytotoxic CD8+ T lymphocytes. Since the TH1 response enhances CD8+ cell activity, which has been associated with reduced HIV replication,[56] reduced TH1 activity may result in decreased immune surveillance of viral replication. An increased TH2 response, on the other hand, is noted in patients with AIDS. This type of response is associated with the release of IL-4, IL-5, IL-6, and IL-10, which results in B-cell activation and hypergammaglobulinemia as well as suppression of TH1 and subsequent reduction in CD8+ cell activity.

CD8+ T-cytotoxic/suppressor lymphocytes are often associated with killing of virus-infected cells. This type of cellular destruction requires cell-to-cell contact. These cells destroy HIV-infected cells, but the role of the antiviral activity of CD8+ cells in HIV disease is not completely understood. Although some studies indicate an increased survival rate in individuals with high levels of peripheral CD8+ cells,[57] disease progression occurs even in the presence of these cells. As mentioned, CD8+ cells may also directly suppress HIV replication.

Humoral immune response is associated with B lymphocyte activation and subsequent antibody production. The response of B lymphocytes to HIV is reduced by a lack of T lymphocyte regulation. This leads to polyclonal proliferation and increased production of antibodies. These antibodies seldom neutralize HIV infection but instead appear to act against platelets, T lymphocytes, and peripheral nerves.[58] It has been proposed that the initial immune response against HIV infection can produce neutralizing antibodies against gp120 and gp41.[59,60] At this point, a specific viral strain is usually present, but with progression of disease more viral strains are being produced and will elude antibody neutralization. Thus, even patients with AIDS may have high titers of neutralizing antibodies[61] but apparently not against all infected strains. Furthermore, the response to neutralizing antibodies appears to be most beneficial directly after the initial infection with HIV. This has also been demonstrated in chimpanzees receiving low-dose HIV inoculum or passive immunization (with HIV-specific antibodies) 1 day prior to infection.[62,63] The protection against HIV was strain-specific and could not be noticed if the same passive immunization was given after a longer delay after infection. This lack of protection can be explained by the increased number of strains present after longer periods of infection. Fur-

thermore, it has been suggested that activated B lymphocytes secrete cytokines, such as tumor necrosis factor (TNF) alpha and IL-6, which upregulate virus expression possibly leading to increased virus spread.[64] Thus, in contrast to other viral diseases, such as hepatitis B infection where the presence of antibodies indicates immunity, the presence of antibodies in HIV disease indicates active infection.

In conclusion, a model of HIV pathogenesis can be proposed based on our present knowledge of the immunologic response to HIV and the inherit ability of HIV to elude the immune response. The virus enters the body either within infected T lymphocytes or macrophages but also as free viruses. Initial infection of HIV results in viremia, high levels of HIV in the bloodstream, and subsequent trapping of the virus within the lymphoid tissues. Within lymph nodes, HIV is caught by follicular dendritic cells in the germinal layer and presented to CD4+ T-helper lymphocytes and macrophages. This causes a redistribution of CD4+ T-helper lymphocytes from the peripheral blood into the lymphoid tissue, which results in a noticeable decrease of peripheral CD4+ cells. At this stage, an increased level of CD8+ T-cytotoxic lymphocytes can also be noted in the peripheral blood, similar to that noted in other viral infections. Neutralizing antibodies against HIV, together with a cell-mediated immune response, initially controls the HIV infection. Clinically, signs and symptoms of the acute HIV infection, or seroconversion syndrome, emerge approximately 3 weeks after infection and last for 1 to 2 weeks. While the CD8+ cell count remains slightly elevated during the course of the disease, the peripheral CD4+ cell count usually increases to normal or near-normal levels 3 to 4 months after the initial infection.

Progressive CD4+ cell count depletion and dysfunction are the hallmark of HIV disease and result in an overall immune deterioration over time. Interestingly, long-term HIV-infected survivors show a persistent CD4+ cell count that is approximately 400 cells/mm³ below normal and an increased CD8+ cell count that is approximately 250 cells/mm³ above normal levels.[65] The clinical latent stage of the disease is estimated to be approximately 10 years but it may range from 2 to 4 months to at least over 15 years.[8,11,66,67] Since HIV replication occurs throughout the clinical latent period, a true viral latency does not exist. With an ongoing reduction in immune regulation, the virus takes on more virulent characteristics and eventually destroys large numbers of CD4+ cells. All mechanisms involved in CD4+ cell dysfunction and depletion have not been elucidated, but this characteristic of HIV disease correlates with disease progression and results in the eventual development of opportunistic infections and neoplasms.

References

1. Barre-Sinoussi F, Chermann J-C, Rey F, et al. Isolation of a T-lymphotropic retrovirus from a patient at risk for acquired immune deficiency syndrome (AIDS). Science 1983;220:868–871.

2. Montagnier L, Chermann J-C, Barre-Sinoussi F, et al. A new human T-lymphotropic retrovirus: characterization and possible role in lymphadenopathy and acquired immune deficiency syndrome. In Gallo RC, Essex ME, Gross L (eds): Human T-cell leukemia/lymphoma virus. Cold Spring Harbor, NY: Cold Spring Harbor Laboratory; 1984:363–379.

3. Popovic M, Sarngadharan MG, Read E, Gallo RC. Detection, isolation and continuous production of cytopathic retroviruses (HTLV-III) from patients with AIDS and pre-AIDS. Science 1984;224:497–500.

4. Gallo RC, Salahuddin SZ, Popovic M, et al. Frequent detection and isolation of cytopathic retroviruses (HTLV-III) from patients with AIDS and at risk for AIDS. Science 1984;224:500–503.

5. Levy JA, Hoffman AD, Kramer SM, Landis JA, Shimabukuro JM, Oshiro LS. Isolation of lymphocytopathic retroviruses from San Francisco patients with AIDS. Science 1984;225:840–842.

6. Coffin JM, Haase A, Ley JA, et al. Human immunodeficiency viruses (Letter). Science 1986;232:697.

7. Haase AT. Pathogenesis of lentivirus infection. Nature 1986;322:130–136.

8. Lifson AR, Buchbinder SP, Sheppard HW, et al. Long-term human immunodeficiency virus infection in asymptomatic homosexual and bisexual men with normal CD4+ lymphocyte counts: immunologic and virologic characteristics. J Infec Dis 1991;163:959–965.

9. Rutherford GW, Lifson AR, Hessol NA. Course of HIV-1 infection in a cohort of homosexual and bisexual men: an 11 year follow up study. Br Med J 1990;301:1183–1188.

10. Longini Jr IM, Clark WS, Gardner LI, et al. The dynamics of CD4+ T-lymphocyte decline in HIV-infected individuals: a Markov modeling approach. J Acquired Immune Deficiency Syndrome 1991;4:1141–1147.

11. Levy JA. HIV pathogenesis and long-term survival. AIDS 1993;7:1401–1410.

12. Levy JA, Shimabukuro J, McHugh T, Casavant C, Stites D, Oshiro L. AIDS-associated retroviruses (ARV) can productively infect other cells besides human T helper cells. Virology 1985;147:441–448.

13. Salahuddin SZ, Markham PD, Popovic M, et al. Isolation of infectious human T-cell leukemia/lymphotropic virus type III (HTLV-III) from patients with acquired immunodeficiency syndrome (AIDS) or AIDS-related complex (ARC) and from healthy carriers: a study of risk groups and tissue sources. Proc Natl Acad Sci USA 1985;82:5530–5534.

14. Clavel F, Guetard D, Brun-Vezinet F, et al. Isolation of a new human retrovirus from West African patients with AIDS. Science 1986;233:343–346.

15. Ozel M, Pauli G, Gelderblom HR. The organization of the envelope projections on the surface of HIV. Arch Virol 1988; 100:255–266.

16. Dalgleish AG, Beverley PC, Clapham PR, Crawford DH, Greaves MF, Weiss RA. The CD4 (T4) antigen is an essential component of the receptor for the AIDS retrovirus. Nature 1984;312:763–767.

17. Clapham PR, Weber JN, Whitby D, et al. Soluble CD4 blocks the infectivity of diverse strains of HIV and SIV for T cells and monocytes but not for brain and muscle cells. Nature 1989;337:368–370.

18. Meltzer MS, Skillman DR, Hoover DL, et al. Macrophages and the human immunodeficiency virus. Immunol Today 1990;11: 217–223.

19. Rabson AB. HIV virology: implications for the pathogenesis of HIV infection. J Am Acad Dermatol 1990;22:1196–1202.

20. Kowalski M, Potz J, Basiripour L, et al. Functional regions of HIV type 1. Science 1987;237:1351–1355.

21. Schneider J, Kaaden O, Copeland TD, Oroszlan S, Hunsmann G. Shedding and interspecies type sero-reactivity of the envelope glycopeptide gp120 and the human immunodeficiency virus. J Gen Virol 1986;67:2533–2538.

22. Cann AJ, Karn J. Molecular biology of HIV: insights into the virus life-cycle. AIDS 1989;3(Suppl 1):19–34.

23. Rosenberg ZF, Fauci AS. Induction and expression of HIV in latently or chronically infected cells. AIDS Res Hum Retroviruses 1989;5:1–4.

24. Levy JA. Pathogenesis of human immunodeficiency virus infection. Microbiol Rev 1993;57:183–289.

25. Mellert W, Kleinschmidt A, Schmidt J, et al. Infection of human fibroblasts and osteoblast-like cells with HIV-1. AIDS 1990; 4:5327–5335.

26. Glick M, Trope M, Bagasra O, Pliskin ME. Dental pulp HIV infection in serum positive patients. Oral Surg Oral Med Oral Pathol 1991;71:733–736.

27. Tateno MF, Gonzalez-Scarano F, Levy JA. The human immunodeficiency virus can infect CD4-negative human fibroblastoid cells. Proc Natl Acad Sci USA 1989;86: 4287–4290.

28. Homsy J, Meyer M, Tateno M, Clarkson S, Levy JA. The Fc and not the CD4 receptor mediates antibody enhancement of HIV infection in human cells. Science 1989; 244:1357–1360.

29. Gendelman HE, Orenstein JM, Martin MA, et al. Efficient isolation and propagation of human immunodeficiency virus on recombinant colony-stimulating factor 1-treated monocyte. J Exp Med 1988;167: 1428–1441.

30. Embretson J, Zupanic M, Ribas JL, et al. Massive covert infection of helper T lymphocytes and macrophages by HIV during the incubation period of AIDS. Nature 1993;362:359–362.

31. Pantaleo G, Graziozi C, Demarest JF, et al. HIV infection is active and progressive in lymphoid tissue during the clinically latent stage of disease. Nature 1993;362:355–358.

32. Miedema F, Tersmette M, van Lier RAW. AIDS pathogenesis: a dynamic interaction between HIV and the immune system. Immunol Today 1990;11:293–297.

33. Pantaleo G, Graziosi C, Fauci AS. The immunopathogenesis of human immunodeficiency virus infection. N Engl J Med 1993;328:327–335.

34. Bagasra O, Hauptman SP, Lischner HW, Sachs M, Pomerantz RJ. Detection of human immunodeficiency virus type 1 provirus in mononuclear cells by in situ polymerase chain reaction. N Engl J Med 1992;326:1385–1391.

35. Garry RF. Potential mechanisms for the cytopathic properties of HIV. AIDS 1989;3:683–694.

36. Tersmette M, Gruters RA, de Wolf F, et al. Evidence for a role of virulent human immunodeficiency virus (HIV) variants in the pathogenesis of acquired immunodeficiency syndrome: studies of sequential HIV isolates. J Virol 1989;63:2118–2125.

37. Lang W, Perkins H, Anderson RE, Royce R, Jewell N, Winkelstein Jr W. Patterns of T lymphocyte changes with human immunodeficiency virus infection: from seroconversion to the development of AIDS. J Acquired Immune Deficiency Syndrome 1989;2:63–69.

38. Schellekens PA, Tersmette M, Roos ML, et al. Biphasic rate of CD4 + cell count decline during progression to AIDS correlates with HIV-1 phenotype. AIDS 1992;6:665–669.

39. Phillips AN, Elford J, Sabin C, Janossy G, Lee CA. Pattern of CD4+ T-cell loss in HIV infection. J Acquired Immune Deficiency Syndrome 1992;5:950–951.

40. Cooper DA, Gold J, Maclean P, et al. Acute AIDS retrovirus infection. Definition of a clinical illness associated with seroconversion. Lancet 1985;i:537–540.

41. Clark SJ, Shaw GM. The acute retroviral syndrome and the pathogenesis of HIV-1 infection. Sem Immunol 1993;5:149–155.

42. Tindall B, Cooper DA. Primary HIV infection: host response and intervention strategies. AIDS 1991;5:1–14.

43. Daar ES, Moudgil T, Meyer RD, Ho DD. Transient high levels of viremia in patients with primary human immunodeficiency virus type 1 infection. N Engl J Med 1991; 324:961–964.

44. Clark SJ, Saag MS, Decker WD, et al. High titers of cytopathic virus in plasma of patients with symptomatic primary HIV-1 infection. N Engl J Med 1991;324:954–960.

45. Graziozi C, Pantaleo G, Butini L, et al. Kinetics of HIV DNA and RNA synthesis during primary HIV-1 infection. Proc Natl Acad Sci USA 1993;90:6405–6409.

46. Fauci AS, Schnittman SM, Poli G, Koenig S, Pantaleo G. Immunopathogenic mechanisms in human immunodeficiency virus (HIV) infection. Ann Intern Med 1991; 114:678–693.

47. Kagnoff MF. In Sleisenger MH, Fordtran JS (eds): Gastrointestinal Disease: Pathophysiology, Diagnosis, Management. Philadelphia: WB Saunders; 1981:114.

48. Racz P, Moncada LA, Schmidt H, et al. Lymphatic follicles of rectal mucosa harbor HIV-1 (abstract). Lab Invest 1993; 68:106.

49. Lafeuillade A, Tamalet C, Pellegrino P, et al. High viral burden in lymph nodes during early stages of HIV-1 infection. AIDS 1993;11:1527–1541.

50. Fauci AS. Multifactorial nature of human immunodeficiency virus disease: implications for therapy. Science 1993;262:1011–1018.

51. Cheng-Mayer C, Seto D, Tateno M, Levy JA. Biologic features of HIV that correlate with virulence in the host. Science 1988; 240:80–82.

52. Fontana L, Sirianni MC, de Sanctis G, Carbonari M, Ensoli B, Aiuti F. Deficiency of natural killer activity, but not of natural killer binding, in patients with lymphadenopathy syndrome positive for antibodies to HTLV-III. Immunobiology 1986;171: 425–435.

53. Cai Q, Huang X-L, Rappocciolo G, Rinaldo CR Jr. Natural killer cell responses in homosexual men with early HIV infection. J Acquired Immune Deficiency Syndrome 1990;3:669–676.

54. Shearer GM, Clerici M. Early T-helper cell defects in HIV infection. AIDS 1991;5:245–253.

55. Sher A, Gazzinelli RT, Oswalg IP, et al. Role of T-cell derived cytokines in the downregulation of immune responses in parasitic and retroviral infection. Immunol Rev 1992;127:183–204.

56. Walker CM, Levy JA. A diffuse lymphokine produced by CD8+ t lymphocytes suppresses HIV replication. Immunology 1989;66:628–630.

57. Autran B, Plata F, Debre P. MHC-restricted cytotoxicity against HIV. J Acquired Immune Deficiency Syndrome 1991;4:361–367.

58. Morrow WJW, Isenberg DA, Sobol RE, Stricker RB, Kieber-Emmons T. AIDS virus infection and autoimmunity: a perspective of the clinical, immunological, and molecular origins of the autoallergenic pathologies associated with HIV disease. Clin Immunol Immunopathol 1991;58:163–180.

59. Haigwood NL, Shuster JR, Moore GK, et al. Importance of hypervariable regions of HIV-1 gp120 in the generation of virus-neutralizing antibodies. AIDS Res Hum Retroviruses 1990;6:855–869.

60. Broliden P-A, von Gegerfelt A, Clapham P, et al. Identification of human neutralization-inducing regions of the human immunodeficiency virus type 1 envelope glycoproteins. Proc Natl Acad Sci USA 1992;89:461–465.

61. Robert-Guroff M, Brown M, Gallo RC. HTLV-III neutralizing antibodies in patients with AIDS and AIDS-related complex. Nature 1985;316:72–74.

62. Prince AM, Reesink H, Pascual D, et al. Prevention of HIV infection by passive immunization with HIV immunoglobulin. AIDS Res Hum Retroviruses 1991:7:971–973.

63. Emini EA, Schleif WA, Nunberg JH, et al. Prevention of HIV-1 infection in chimpanzees by gp120 V3 domain-specific monoclonal antibody. Nature 1992;355:728–730.

64. Amadori A, Chieco-Bianchi L. B-cell activation and HIV-1 infection: deeds and misdeeds. Immunol Today 1990;11:374–379.

65. Sheppard HW, Lang W, Ascher MS, Vittinghoff E, Winkelstein W. The characterization of non-progressor: long-term HIV-1 infection with stable CD4+ T-cell levels. AIDS 1993;7:1159–1166.

66. Isaksson B, Albert J, Chiodi F, Furucrona A, Krook A, Putkonen P. AIDS two months after primary human immunodeficiency virus infection. J Infect Dis 1988;158:866–868.

67. McLean KA, Holmes DA, Evans BA, et al. Rapid clinical and laboratory progression of HIV infection. AIDS 1990;4:369–371.

6

Clinical Manifestations of HIV Disease

Michael Glick

The clinical manifestations associated with HIV disease remain the most visible indicator of a patient's disease progression. Patients infected with HIV eventually develop opportunistic infections, some of which can be successfully treated, but others will lead to severe debilitation and eventual death. The introduction of prophylactic antiretroviral and other therapies has delayed certain infections associated with high mortality and has resulted in prolonged survival. However, this early intervention is changing the pattern of opportunistic infections among people with HIV. Specifically, since the introduction of prophylaxis against *Pneumocystis carinii* pneumonia in patients with CD4+ cell counts below 200 cells/mm^3, patients are surviving longer and the collective incidence of other opportunistic infections such as *Mycobacterium avium* complex disease, wasting syndrome, cytomegalovirus disease, and esophageal candidiasis has quadrupled.[1]

This chapter describes the more common infections associated with HIV disease to facilitate the dental practitioner's grasp of the clinical spectrum of HIV. The infections are presented in alphabetical order.

Aspergillosis

Infection with *Aspergillus,* a common mold, is a rare fungal infection in patients with AIDS. It usually manifests during the late stages of the disease and presents as bronchial obstruction and pulmonary invasion.[2,3] Infected individuals have cough, chest pain, fever, night sweats, sinus pain, facial swelling, and are often neutropenic. Oral manifestations have also been reported.[4] Patients with aspergillosis have a very poor prognosis, with a median survival of 3 months. Treatment consists of the administration of intravenous amphotericin B.

B19 Parvovirus

This virus has recently been identified as the causative agent for erythema infectiosum (EI or fifth disease).[5,6] In adults with AIDS, this virus infection may cause anemia,[7] while in children with AIDS, EI causes pancytopenia.[8] Experimental treatment with intravenous immunoglobulin has been successful.[7]

Candidiasis

Candida species is the most common fungal infection in HIV disease. Almost all infected individuals develop oral candidiasis during the progression of disease (see Chapter 8). Although oral candidiasis frequently manifests in patients with CD4+ cell counts above 200 cells/mm³, candidiasis of the esophagus, trachea, bronchi, and lung occurs when CD4+ cell counts drop below 100 cells/mm³.[9] Esophageal candidiasis is included as a

diagnosis for AIDS,[10] and it typically presents with dysphagia and odynophagia, although 10% to 15% of patients may be asymptomatic.[11] Vaginal candidiasis may be present in a large number of HIV-infected women, sometimes with oropharyngeal candidiasis.[12] Nail dystrophies caused by candidal infections are also found in a large percentage of HIV-positive individuals.[13]

Disseminated candidiasis is uncommon in patients with HIV and usually occurs only in patients with severe neutropenia caused by antineoplastic or myelosuppressive-associated antiviral therapy,[14] or in patients with indwelling catheters. Treatment for candidiasis, not necessarily intraoral disease, includes oral administration of ketoconazole, fluconazole, and intravenous administration of amphotericin B. Intravenous therapy is usually only instituted in patients with CD4+ cell counts below 100 cells/mm³.

Coccidioidomycosis

Coccidioidomycosis is a fungal infection caused by *Coccidioides immitis*. It is more common in endemic areas such as North, Central, and South America. This infection mostly affects the lungs but also disseminates to the kidneys, spleen, lymph nodes, brain, and thyroid gland. The symptoms are usually nonspecific, including malaise, weight loss, fatigue, and cough.[15,16] Patients with diffuse pulmonary involvement have a very poor prognosis. One study reported a median survival of only 1 month.[15] Standard treatment consists of the administration of intravenous amphotericin B.

Cryptococcosis

Among individuals with HIV, infection with *Cryptococcus neoformans,* a fungus, mainly involves the brain and lungs. This fungal infection is the major cause of meningitis in patients with AIDS; however, disseminated disease is common. Between 6% to 12% of HIV-infected patients will develop cryptococcal infection, and cryptococcosis is the defining illness for AIDS in 1.5% of all reported AIDS cases.[17,18] This fungal infection usually manifests only in individuals with CD4+ cell counts below 100 cells/mm3.[19,20]

Cryptococcal meningitis presents with fatigue, fever, headache, nausea, seizures, and neurologic changes, while pulmonary cryptococcal infections may be asymptomatic. Oral manifestations of cryptococcosis have been reported.[21] Standard treatment consists of intravenous amphotericin B or fluconazole. Fluconazole is also approved for prophylactic use.[22]

Cryptosporidiosis

Cryptosporidium parvum, the causative agent of cryptosporidiosis, is the most common enteric pathogen in patients with AIDS and is responsible for up to 10% of all cases of severe diarrhea in patients with AIDS in the United States.[23] The same pathogen is responsible for "slim" disease, described among African patients with AIDS.[24] Before 1982, only 11 cases of cryptosporidiosis were reported in the world literature,[25] but a few years later an estimated 16% of all the patients with AIDS in the United States and 50% of patients with AIDS in Haiti and Africa were found to be infected with *Cryptosporidium.*[26–28] Retrospective studies of HIV-infected patients indicate that cryptosporidiosis occurs in patients with both high and low CD4+ cell counts.[29] *Cryptosporidium* has been detected in sputum,[30] and nosocomial transmissions have been documented.[31,32]

Treatment modalities available for patients with cryptosporidiosis are limited. Symptomatic treatment with anti-diarrheal agents, such as loperamide (Imodium) or diphenoxylate (Lomotil), is not effective in immunosuppressed patients. Experimental therapy with various medications, including hyperimmune bovine colostrum, azithromycin, diclazuril, and paromomycin (Humatin), have shown limited success.[33–35]

Cytomegalovirus

Infection with cytomegalovirus (CMV) is the most common multiorgan viral opportunistic infection in HIV disease. Serologic evidence of previous exposure to CMV can be found in 60% to 80% of the general population but approaches 100% in homosexual men.[36–38] One autopsy series showed that 73% of 75 HIV-infected patients had histopathologic evidence of CMV disease.[39] As with other herpes viruses, CMV causes a primary disease and then remains latent for many years. Reactivation usually occurs only when the host's cell-mediated immune response is impaired.[40] Subsequently, clinical manifestations of HIV-associated CMV disease are only present in individuals with severe immunosuppression,[41] particularly among those with CD4+ cell counts below 50 cells/mm^3.[42] Furthermore, in a study among hemophiliacs, CMV infection was strongly associated with a more rapid progression of HIV disease.[43]

Although CMV infection has been implicated in esophagitis, gastritis, hepatitis, pneumonia, central nervous system infection, and infection of the adrenal glands, the most common clinical manifestation in HIV disease is CMV retinitis.[43,44] CMV retinitis is usually painless with a progressive unilateral loss of vision. This type of retinal infection has fairly distinct characteristics and can be detected during opthalmoscopic examination. Untreated cases result in blindness. Severe cases involve the optic nerve, potentially resulting in blindness within days. The gastrointestinal (GI) tract is the second most common area of CMV infection and, as with CMV retinitis, clinical manifestations are usually present only in individuals with severe immunosuppression. The entire GI tract can exhibit CMV-associated pathologic states, including the oral cavity.

In the oral cavity, the most common manifestation of CMV disease is mucosal ulcerations.[45] Adrenal insufficiency associated with CMV infection has also been reported.[46] This is significant since dental therapy may necessitate replacement therapy with corticosteroids before initiating treatment. Standard therapy for CMV infections consists of intravenous administration of ganciclovir or foscarnet.[47] Lifelong maintenance therapy is generally required. Cytomegalovirus is spread through blood transfusions, sexual contacts, and respiratory secretion. Although CMV is spread via saliva, no increased incidence has been documented among health-care professionals.[48]

Herpes Simplex Virus

Early reports of HIV disease described oral and perianal herpes simplex virus (HSV) infections.[49] These infections are associated with increased morbidity both directly and indirectly as they break down the mucosal barrier, facilitating the entry for HIV and opportunistic infections into the body. Herpes simplex virus has also been implicated in the activation of HIV replication. Most commonly, clinical signs of HSV infection occur in the oral cavity and in the genital area. However, HSV-associated esophagitis is a common manifestation in advanced HIV disease.[50] Oral and labial lesions are discussed in Chapter 8.

A relatively overlooked manifestation of HSV in HIV disease is herpetic whitlow. This cutaneous herpes infection of the fingers can become progressive and persist during the disease's more advanced stages.[51] Treatment for HSV infections consists of the administration of acyclovir. According to the severity and site of infection, either intravenous, oral, or topical formulations are used. Although this drug is very well tolerated and causes few side effects, HSV resistance has been described in HIV-infected individuals.[52] In such cases, foscarnet is the alternate drug of choice.[53]

Histoplasmosis

Infection with *Histoplasma capsulatum,* the causative pathogen of histoplasmosis, is endemic in certain geographic areas, such as those surrounding the Mississippi River in the United States, portions of Central and South America, Europe, Africa, and Asia.[54] Individuals with HIV who reside in these endemic areas more commonly present with disseminated histoplasmosis as compared to other infected individuals.[55] Still, the overall incidence of histoplasmosis among individuals with HIV in endemic areas is approximately 5%.[56] Many individuals with HIV and disseminated histoplasmosis develop this infection prior to other AIDS-defining illnesses,[57] but CD4+ cell counts below 100 cells/mm^3 are present in over 90% of all cases. One study cited a series of patients with a median CD4+ cell count of 30 cells/mm^3.[58]

Manifestations of disseminated his-

toplasmosis are nonspecific and include fever, weight loss, respiratory complaints, splenomegaly, hepatomegaly, cutaneous lesions, and neurologic abnormalities. Oral manifestations have also been reported.[59] Amphotericin B and itraconazole are approved medications for disseminated histoplasmosis, but fluconazole is also used for treatment as well as prophylaxis.[22]

Kaposi's Sarcoma

Kaposi's sarcoma (KS) is a tumor of endothelial and/or spindle cell origin, first described as a malignancy by Hungarian dermatologist Moritz Kaposi in 1872.[60] The classic type of KS is described as a rare multicentric, pigmented angiosarcoma. Before the AIDS epidemic, this lesion was most commonly found on the lower extremities of older men of Jewish and/or Mediterranean ancestry, with an incidence rate in the United States of approximately 1:50,000 before 1980.[61]

The development of KS has also been associated with iatrogenic immunosuppression, particularly in patients undergoing organ transplantations, where it accounts for approximately 4% of all malignancies.[62,63] Since the first report of KS in homosexual/bisexual men in 1981, an AIDS-associated or epidemic type of KS has been recognized as the most common malignancy in HIV disease.[64] This condition is also included as an AIDS diagnosis.[10] Interestingly, the proportion of KS in patients with AIDS in San Francisco has declined from 58% at the beginning of the epidemic to 23% in 1989.[65] This may be a reflection of the decline in new HIV infections among homosexual/bisexual men in this area. Kaposi's sarcoma has been reported among individuals in all transmission categories, but in the United States, it is most commonly found among HIV-infected homosexual/bisexual men. Approximately 96% of all AIDS-associated KS has been reported in homosexual/bisexual men.[66] Nine percent of these patients were also injection drug users; heterosexual men and women comprise the remaining 4%. The incidence of epidemic KS among heterosexual injection drug users is estimated to be 3%, while 4% of transfusion recipients, 3% of women, 2% of children, and 1% of hemophiliacs with AIDS present with this lesion.[66,67]

The etiology of Kaposi's sarcoma has not been established, but speculations about the significance of cofactors, including oncogenic substances, non-HIV viral infections, and the possibility that KS is not a true neoplasm but a cellular proliferation in response to angiogenic substances, have all been proposed. It is not known why the incidence of KS is much higher among homosexual/bisexual men than in other risk groups for HIV disease.[68] Many theories have been put forward to explain this phenomenon. The use of nitrite inhalants, a practice more common among homosexual/bisexual men than among other risk groups for HIV disease, has been associated both clinically and by epidemiologic studies with the development of KS.[69] Such use both facilitates and enhances the efficiency of transmission of possible viral cofactors. The high incidence of CMV infection in the homosexual/bisexual community and the finding of CMV in tissue culture cell lines from KS lesions suggests that this herpes virus may be a cofactor in the development of this lesion.[70] Studies have also found strong associations between HIV risk factors, such as multiple partners and receptive anal intercourse, and the development of KS. This in turn suggests an etiology associated with a sexually transmitted pathogen.[69]

AIDS-associated KS is most commonly diagnosed as a cutaneous manifestation with a propensity for the extremities and the face (see Chapter 7). Initially, only a few localized lesions may be present. They usually present as painless, macular, bluish lesions resembling hematomas. As with hematomas they do not blanch upon pressure. However, unlike hematomas, they do not undergo color changes. The localized lesions become nodular and frequently progress to involve lymph nodes, solid visceral organs, and most commonly, the gastrointestinal tract. Oral KS lesions are common and may sometimes be the initial sign of this neoplasm (see Chapter 8). Patients with cutaneous manifestations of KS may present with CD4+ cell counts of 200 to 300 cells/mm³, but intraoral signs of this lesion are associated with a CD4+ cell count below 100 cells/mm³.[71]

An autopsy report indicated that KS was seldom found in a single organ.

Instead, multiple organ involvement was evident in over 90% of all cases.[72] Interestingly, only 26% of all cases in this study had cutaneous involvement. Patients with KS are much more likely to die of opportunistic infections than of KS. However, many of the fatal cases due to KS have pulmonary involvement. Patients with KS but without opportunistic infections survive for long periods. The median survival time among a group of mainly homosexual/bisexual men in San Francisco with KS but without any other opportunistic infection within 3 months of the KS diagnosis was reported to be 17.0 months.[73] The 5-year survival rate among these 1,015 individuals was 8.7 plus/minus 1.3%, with the longest survival of 7.3 years. Many patients with biopsy-verified cutaneous KS are still alive without any HIV-related complications, even 10 years after initial diagnosis (Glick M, unpublished data).

Treatment for KS is usually palliative and intended to reduce the size and number of lesions. A cure for KS does not exist, although spontaneous regression of lesions has been noted. Systemic single drug therapy is used for lesions without evidence of visceral involvement, while multiple drug therapy is instituted for more advanced disease. One successful regimen, with an overall response rate of 88%, is low-dose adriamycin, bleomycin, and vincristine (ABV).[74] Intramuscular injections with interferon-alpha (INF-a) have been approved by the Food and Drug Administration (FDA) for the treatment of KS. Success rates of 60% to 67% have been reported.[75] Early intervention with low doses of INF-a have also shown to be beneficial by reducing proliferation of the lesion over a long time.[76] Successful localized treatment with radiation therapy and intralesional injections with vinblastine[77] or with sodium tetradecyl sulfate[78] has also been reported.

Lymphoma

AIDS-related lymphomas, most commonly non-Hodgkin's lymphomas, are relatively late manifestations of HIV disease. Although an increasing number of cases is being reported, this may be due to the longer survival of patients with HIV infection.[79] The majority of lymphomas have been reported among homosexual/bisexual men, but cases occur in all transmission categories.[80–82]

Lymphomas in patients with AIDS are generally high-grade forms of B-cell lymphomas, such as B-immunoblastic or small noncleaved lymphomas, which include Burkitt's and non-Burkitt's variants.[83] A diagnosis is usually made from a biopsy specimen of bone marrow or lymph nodes. Extranodal disease occurs in up to 90% of all cases, commonly involving the central nervous system (32%), the gastrointestinal tract (26%), the bone marrow (25%), and the liver (12%).[84] Other sites can also be involved, including the oral cavity, but they are less common.[85] Approximately 75% of patients with AIDS-related lymphomas present with fever, drenching night sweats, and weight loss. These symptoms are referred to as systemic B symptoms. Site-specific complications can also occur depending on the size and involvement of the lymphoma. Patients already diagnosed with AIDS, with bone marrow involvement of the lymphoma, and low CD4+ cell counts, particularly below 100 cells/mm³, have a poor prognosis.[86] Treatment for AIDS-related non-Hodgkin's lymphoma consists of multiple drug chemotherapy, such as a modified mBACOD regimen[87] in conjunction with corticosteroids, radiation therapy, zidovudine, and prophylactic medication for *P. carinii* pneumonia (PCP). To prevent central nervous system (CNS) involvement, intrathecal (delivered directly into the CNS) prophylactic chemotherapy is administered.

Mycobacterium avium-intracellulare Complex

Disseminated infection due to *Mycobacterium avium-intracellulare* complex (MAC) is the most common systemic bacterial infection among patients with AIDS in the United States, occurring in up to 43% of all cases.[88] An estimated 5% of all patients diagnosed with AIDS have MAC bacteremia and this prevalence increases approximately 20% annually. Furthermore, patients receiving prophylaxis for *P. carinii* pneumonia are surviving longer and the incidence of MAC in this group has doubled.[1] The occurrence of this infection does not differ by gender or transmission category but is strongly associated with severe immunosuppression. In one study of 159 patients, all patients had CD4+ cell counts below 100 cells/mm³.[89]

The clinical signs and symptoms of MAC infection include fever, night sweats, diarrhea, weight loss and wasting, abdominal pain, nausea and vomiting, lymphadenopathy, and hepatosplenomegaly. Disseminated MAC infection may be the most frequent cause of fever of unknown origin in HIV-infected individuals (31.9%) (followed by tuberculosis [26.2%] and PCP [9.5%]).[90] Although pulmonary involvement of MAC infection, as seen on chest radiographs, is common in individuals with HIV, pulmonary symptoms are rare. Anemia, with hemoglobin levels below 8.5 g/dL, is very common and occurs in up to 85% of all patients with disseminated MAC infections.[91] More than 90% of patients with AIDS and symptomatic MAC infection also have evidence of disseminated disease, and autopsy reports indicate that disseminated MAC infection affects virtually all organs in the body. Although the mortality rate of MAC is difficult to estimate, multiple studies have indicated a poorer prognosis for patients with AIDS and MAC than patients with AIDS without MAC.[91] A definitive diagnosis of MAC infection is usually obtained by isolating the pathogen from blood culture specimens. The organism can be found in the sputum, but this is not always an indication of disseminated disease. Furthermore, detection of acid-fast bacilli on sputum smears is more likely associated with coinfection with *Mycobacterium tuberculosis*.

Treatment for MAC consists of

antibacterial therapy. The most commonly used medications are oral clarithromycin, azithromycin, rifamycin derivatives, ethambutol, clofazamine, ciprofloxacin, or sparfloxacin; parenteral amikacin and gentamicin are also used. Lifelong therapy is recommended. Lifetime prophylactic medication with daily doses of oral rifabutin has been recommended for patients with CD4+ cell counts below 100 cells/mm^3 and has been approved by the FDA for this purpose.[92] In contrast to tuberculosis, MAC is not believed to be transmittable from person to person but rather from environmental sources.

Neurologic Disorders, HIV Encephalopathy (AIDS dementia complex), and Progressive Multifocal Leukoencephalopathy

Neurologic complications associated with HIV disease are common and can clinically affect over 60% of infected individuals.[93] Postmortem examination reveals an even greater incidence of up to 90% of individuals with HIV and disorders of the nervous system.[94] Human immunodeficiency virus can directly infect the CNS and cause HIV encephalopathy. This HIV-associated motor-cognitive disorder is also called AIDS dementia complex (ADC). However, clinical manifestations of HIV encephalopathy usually occur only in patients with severe immunosuppression. Less than 1% of asymptomatic patients and 4% of patients with AIDS demonstrate signs of ADC; however,

up to 7% of patients show signs of ADC within 12 months and 14% within 2 years of an AIDS diagnosis.[95]

Common patient complaints surrounding ADC include fatigue, malaise, headaches, increasing forgetfulness, and slowness in thinking. Clinical motor dysfunctions typically reveal a fine tremor of the upper extremities, bradykinesia, postural instability, cogwheel rigidity, hypomimetic facies, and abnormal ocular movements.[96,97]

The diagnosis of HIV encephalopathy is based on exclusion of other possible causes. Serum levels of vitamin B$_{12}$ and folate, as well as a nontreponemal antibody test and thyroid function tests, rule out toxic-metabolic causes and neurosyphilis. Focal brain disease such as toxoplasmosis encephalitis, primary CNS lymphoma and progressive multifocal leukoencephalopathy (PML) should also be excluded. Lumbar punctures should be performed to rule out neurosyphilis and cryptococcal meningitis. Treatment for HIV encephalopathy consists of the administration of zidovudine to slow HIV replication.

Neurologic disorders may result not only directly from HIV infection but more commonly from opportunistic infections and neoplasms. One third of all patients with AIDS have opportunistic infections of the CNS due to toxoplasmosis, cryptococcal meningitis, cytomegalovirus encephalitis, and PML. The most common opportunistic neoplasm affecting the CNS is primary CNS lymphoma.

Progressive multifocal leukoencephalopathy is a less common opportunistic infection caused by a papova virus (JC virus). It is a demyelinating disease, causing personality changes, memory deficits, and cognitive impairment, and it is a progressive disease that causes increased focal deficits and severe cerebral dysfunction. No therapy is available to treat PML, and patients have a very poor prognosis.

Pneumocystis Carinii Pneumonia

P. carinii pneumonia (PCP) is caused by a protozoan agent and is the most common opportunistic infection in patients with AIDS not receiving PCP prophylactic medications. It is estimated that up to 80% of this patient group develops PCP during the course of the disease. Since PCP occurs almost exclusively in patients with a CD4+ cell count below 200 cells/mm[3],[20,98] prophylactic medications are instituted at this stage.[99] Yet, 28% of patients receiving prophylactic medications may still develop PCP during the course of HIV disease.[1] The disease generally manifests with fever, dry cough, chest pain, and shortness of breath, especially on exertion. As these manifestations are not specific, other pulmonary pathologic conditions need to be excluded. A definitive diagnosis is obtained by demonstrating the parasitic pathogen in bronchoalveolar lavage specimens.[100]

Treatment for PCP usually consists of the administration of antibiotic therapy with trimethoprim/sulfamethoxazole (oral or intravenously), trimethoprim/sulfamethoxazole togeth-er with dapsone (oral), primaquine together with clindamycin (oral), or pentamidine isethionate (intravenously). Patients treated with trimethoprim/sulfamethoxazole frequently develop severe side effects (see Chapter 9). In such instances, atovaquone can be instituted. Additional treatment with corticosteroids has also been used, however; trimethoprim/sulfamethoxazole, together with other medications such as dapsone, reduces the overall toxicity associated with therapy. Administration of intravenous pentamidine is also associated with severe side effects that often necessitate cessation of the drug.

Prophylactic therapy for PCP consists of lower and less frequent doses of trimethoprim/sulfamethoxazole, sometimes thrice weekly, or aerosolized pentamidine once monthly. As mentioned previously, prophylaxis for PCP is administered to patients with CD4+ cell counts below 200 cells/mm[3] or with a history of PCP. However, PCP is also a major threat to infants and children with HIV. Since CD4+ cell counts in children have different normal limits when compared to those of adult patients, prophylaxis for infants between 0 to 11 months should be instituted at CD4+ cell counts below 1,500 cells/mm[3]; at 12 to 23 months of age, below 750 cells/mm[3]; and in children between 24 months and 5 years of age, below 500 cells/mm[3].

Although the transmission of *P. carinii* between immunocompromised patients has been suggested in hospital settings,[101,102] transmission to health-care providers has not been reported.

Peripheral Neuropathy

Symptomatic peripheral neuropathies occur in close to 50% of all patients with AIDS, but they can occur during all stages of HIV disease. Autopsy results indicate histopathologic peripheral nerve disease in up to 95% of patients.[103] A wide variety of causes has been reported for peripheral neuropathy in HIV-infected individuals. These include inflammatory demyelinated polyneuropathy, CMV infection of peripheral nerves, and, most commonly, sensory neuropathy.

Peripheral neuropathy is found in virtually all patients during the most advanced stages of the disease. It is uncommon to find peripheral neuropathy in patients with CD4+ cell counts above 250 cells/mm^3. The clinical signs and symptoms usually start in the feet and slowly involve the knees and the rest of the legs. The arms and hands are less commonly involved. Although this type of neuropathy is mainly sensory, the pain may be so severe that it interferes with walking.

Syphilis

Complications associated with syphilis in HIV-infected patients are usually limited to neurosyphilis. The diagnosis of neurosyphilis is complicated by frequent cerebrospinal fluid abnormalities found in HIV-associated conditions. Furthermore, false-negative serologic test results for syphilis in patients with HIV have been reported.[104,105] Oral manifestations associated with syphilis in patients with HIV are rare but have been reported (see Chapter 8).[106] Standard treatment of syphilis consists of 2.4 million units of benzathine penicillin.[107]

Toxoplasmosis

Toxoplasmosis is caused by an intracellular protozoan, *Toxoplasma gondii.* Clinical disease is usually the result of reactivation of a previous infection acquired from ingestion of inadequately cooked meat or from contact with cat feces. Serologic surveys have indicated a prevalence of up to 68% of adults in the United States[108] and over 90% in adults in some European countries, such as Germany and France.[109] In the United States, toxoplasmosis develops in 3% to 10% of patients with AIDS but the incidence in Europe and Africa may be as high as 25% to 50% of all patients with AIDS.[110]

The diagnosis of toxoplasmosis is based on a combination of factors: positive serologic results for anti-toxoplasma antibodies; a CD4+ cell count below 200 cells/mm^3; psychiatric dysfunctions; characteristic computed tomography and magnetic resonance imaging findings indicative of toxoplasmosis; or signs and symptoms of CNS toxoplasmosis. The most common neurologic abnormalities are those in ambulation (73%), gait (51%), arm strength (65%), motor strength (63%), and language and speech (55%); headaches are also common(61%).[111] A definitive diagnosis necessitates a brain biopsy. Treatment for acute episodes of toxoplasmosis consists of pyrimethamine with sulfadiazine, or pyrimethamine with clindamycin. Leucovorin is often added to ameliorate the therapy-associated bone marrow suppression. Prophylactic therapy includes the same medications as those for the acute illness but in lower doses and with an occasional dose of dapsone. This disease usually occurs in patients with HIV and CD4+ cell counts below 100 cells/mm^3.[112]

Tuberculosis

The World Health Organization estimates that 1.7 billion individuals worldwide are infected with *M. tuberculosis*, the pathogen that causes tuberculosis (TB).[113] Eight million of these individuals develop active disease and three million die annually. Between 1953 and 1984, an annual decrease of 5% was noted for reported TB cases in the United States. In 1984, 22,255 cases were reported, down from more than 84,000 cases in 1953. However, this decline leveled off between 1984 and 1985 and has since steadily increased. From 1985 to 1990, the overall number of reported TB cases in the United States increased by 18%.[114] During the same time, a 44% increase was noted among individuals 25 to 44 years old and a 27% increase among children less than 15 years old.[115] Furthermore, an estimated 51,700 accumulated cases in excess of the projected number, if the annual decline had continued at the same

rate, were reported by the end of 1993.[116] In 1991, the number of reported TB cases in the United States was 26,283,[117] and in 1992 there was an additional increase of 390 cases (1.5%), totaling 26,673 cases.[118]

There is a direct relationship between the emergence of TB and the HIV epidemic. The states and cities with the highest incidence of TB are also the same states and cities with the highest numbers of reported AIDS cases. Furthermore, demographically, the highest increase in TB occurs in the same groups with a high prevalence of AIDS (African-Americans and nonwhite Hispanics in the age group of 24 to 44 years of age). It is believed that 3.8% of patients with AIDS in the United States are infected with *M. tuberculosis*[119] and a median 3.4% of patients with tuberculosis who attend tuberculosis clinics are coinfected with HIV.[120] This coinfection rate varies greatly geographically. The coinfection rate was 46% in New York City; 34% in Newark, New Jersey; 27% in Boston; 24% in Miami; and 13% in Baltimore. These rates are in accordance with other studies that indicate a 31% prevalence in Miami and a 28% prevalence among nonAsian patients in San Francisco.[121,122] The coinfection rate in New York City actually increased by 81% between 1984 and 1991, from 19.9 cases per 100,000 persons to 36 cases per 100,000 persons. In central Harlem, an increase of 232%, from 50.9 to 169 cases per 100,000 persons, was recorded between 1979 to 1989. Thus, a clear link between HIV infection and TB has been suggested. Furthermore, in

1990, 54.2% of deaths from tuberculosis in patients 20 to 49 years of age were in individuals with AIDS.[123] This is true in not only the United States but also in other geographic areas with a high incidence of HIV infection. It has been reported that between 20% and 67% of patients with TB in Africa are coinfected with HIV.[124]

Renewed attention on tuberculosis and HIV disease has been linked with recent outbreaks of multiple-drug-resistant tuberculosis (MDR-TB) among individuals with HIV.[125] Both MDR-TB and nonMDR-TB are more common in patients with HIV than among other immunocompetent and immunocompromised individuals. There are three characteristic modes for development of TB and MDR-TB: primary infection, reactivation of a previous infection, or exogenous reinfection with a different TB strain.

Tuberculosis is spread via the airborne route by 1- to 5-μm droplets that contain M. tuberculosis. These droplets are generated during coughing, talking, or sneezing from individuals with pulmonary and laryngeal infections. Normal air currents keep the droplets airborne, and these droplets can be spread throughout a room and even a building. Infection occurs when a susceptible individual inhales an infectious droplet. This enables the pathogen to enter the mouth, nasal passages, upper respiratory tract, and bronchi, eventually reaching the alveoli of the lungs. At this site, alveolar macrophages take up the pathogen and spread it to other sites in the body. The initial infection and spread of the pathogen is limited by the immune response within 2 to 10 weeks. However, dormant M. tuberculosis may be present for years, creating a latent infection. Individuals with latent TB infections have positive PPD skin tests (see following) but are not considered infectious.

Approximately 10% of non–HIV-infected individuals with latent TB develop disease during their lifetime. Individuals with concurrent latent TB and HIV infections have a much higher incidence of reactivation of TB. It is estimated that an individual with HIV has an 8% to 10% risk of developing active TB every year.[126] The infectious droplet is contagious until removed from the air or inactivated. Contaminated surfaces are not considered contagious. The most contagious clinical syndrome of TB is pulmonary and laryngeal disease.[127] Only 10% of infected individuals develop clinical signs and symptoms of TB, with half showing disease within the first 2 years of infection. Expression of clinical disease associated with TB is directly linked to the body's ability to respond to this infection. The cell-mediated immune response, mediated by the T lymphocytes, is primarily responsible to fight off new TB infections and keep these infections from being reactivated. Since patients with HIV have an impaired T-lymphocyte response, it is not surprising to find that these individuals are at increased risk for developing clinical disease. Although previous infections with TB usually assure protection against reinfections, this may not be the case in HIV-infected patients. Thus, individuals who have acquired TB infections before acquiring HIV, or are exposed to TB after acquiring HIV infection, have a higher propensity to develop clinical disease. It is not clear if the high incidence of TB in this patient population is the result of reactivation or new infections with TB[128]; however, it has been suggested that TB progresses more rapidly in individuals with HIV.[128,129]

The tuberculin skin test for TB with a purified protein derivative (PPD) utilizes the body's immune response against a simulated localized infection. A reaction at the injection site, usually the skin of an arm, determines if an individual is infected or has previously been exposed to *M. tuberculosis*. However, due to patients' impaired immune system during advanced stages of HIV disease, HIV-infected individuals may not have the ability to mount an appropriate response to the test. In individuals with a CD4+ cell count below 200 cells/mm[3] over 70% may not be able to respond to PPD due to anergy.[130] Thus, TB tests in individuals with HIV and a deteriorated immune response either have a blunted response to the test or no reaction at all. A reactive response in immunocompetent individuals is defined as an induration of 10 mm. In patients with HIV, it has been suggested that a 5-mm or even a 2-mm reaction is enough to define infection (See Table 12-2).[131]

Clinical manifestations of TB occur early in HIV disease. Among patients who develop TB before an AIDS diagnosis and before severe immune deterioration, the course and presentation of TB are similar to those among other individuals. Pulmonary infection is the most common site for TB. The clinical syndrome is characterized by cough, hemoptysis, fever, night sweats, weight loss, and malaise. During the more advanced stages of HIV disease, TB may disseminate, affecting extrapulmonary organs. Positive results on sputum smears and cultures indicate pulmonary TB, while biopsies of affected organs need to be performed to diagnose disseminated disease. Standard technique for culture of *M. tuberculosis* may take 8 to 12 weeks. However, newer radiometric culture techniques and polymerase chain reaction assays can shorten the time for pathogen identification to 7 to 10 days or even within hours.[132,133]

The recommended drug treatment for TB in HIV-infected patients consists of the administration of isoniazid, rifampin, ethambutol, and pyrazinamide for 2 months and then continuation of therapy with only isoniazid and rifampin for an additional 7 months.[119] The total time for therapy is usually 9 months beyond the time of a negative sputum culture. Compliance with therapy is very important, since the development of MDR-TB appears to be more common in noncompliant patients. One study indicated that noncompliance contributed to the development of resistance to rifampin in at least 43% of a cohort of 171 patients with MDR-TB.[134] In the United States, nearly 10% of TB patients have shown resistance to isoniazid and/or rifampin.[135]

Outbreaks of MDR-TB have been described in hospital facilities and correction institutions, mainly involving individuals with HIV; but also persons without HIV.[136,137] The fatality rate from MDR-TB is very high and has been reported to range from 72% to 89% within 4 to 16 weeks. One report showed a median survival time among patients with AIDS and MDR-TB to be only 1.5 months.[138] Among individuals with HIV but without AIDS, the median survival time was 14.8 months. One of the more distressing aspects of MDR-TB for health-care providers is the risk for nosocomial transmission. Today, TB is the only systemic opportunistic infection in HIV disease that can cause disease in healthy individuals. Furthermore, transmission of MDR-TB has been reported to occur between infected patients and health-care providers without HIV.[139,140] Treatment of MDR-TB includes combinations of known TB drugs such as isoniazid, rifampin, pyrazinamide, and ethambutol or streptomycin.[114] However, these drugs are usually poorly tolerated, very toxic, and need to be administered for 18 to 36 months.

Varicella-Zoster Virus

Primary infection with varicella-zoster virus (VZV) manifests as chickenpox (varicella), while reactivation clinically manifests as herpes zoster (shingles). Since herpes zoster is more common among individuals over the age of 50 years and among immunocompromised individuals, clinical manifestations of herpes zoster in younger individuals should alert the health-care

provider to possible HIV infection.[141,142] Herpes zoster infections manifest in HIV-infected patients as a unilateral cutaneous infection. However, in more advanced stages of immune deterioration, multiple dermatomes, prolonged infections, and increased severity can be present[143]; involvement of the central nervous system has been documented.[144] Treatment for herpes zoster infections is usually successful with oral acyclovir, but in more severely immunocompromised patients intravenous administration of acyclovir may be necessary. Resistance to acyclovir therapy has been documented and in such instances treatment with foscarnet therapy has been successful.[145]

Wasting Syndrome

Malnutrition is a very common finding in patients with HIV and contributes to the mortality of HIV disease.[146] Anorexia and decreased food intake among individuals with HIV are related to a wide variety of factors, such as depression and organic brain disease,[147] neurologic dysfunctions,[148] adrenal insufficiency, high fevers, infections, malabsorption,[149] dysphagia, and dysgeusia. The diagnosis of HIV wasting syndrome has been defined as involuntary weight loss of more than 10% of baseline body weight, together with either chronic diarrhea (at least two loose stools per day for greater than or equal to 30 days) or chronic weakness and documented fever (for greater than or equal to 30 days, intermittent or constant) related to HIV infection and not other conditions that can cause similar findings. Wasting syndrome is an AIDS-defining illness in over 10% of individuals receiving prophylactic medication for *P. carinii* pneumonia.[1]

The dental health-care provider plays an important role in assessing and treating some of the signs and symptoms of wasting syndrome, such as dysphagia and dysgeusia (see Chapter 8 and Chapter 12). Diarrhea and involuntary weight loss occur in up to 80% of HIV-infected individuals. They can occur at any stage of HIV disease but are usually indicators of disease progression. Diarrhea can be caused by several medications, such as acyclovir, amphotericin B and nystatin, and a wide variety of infectious agents.[150] Vitamin B_{12} malabsorption is not uncommon in patients with HIV infection[151] and can have manifestations in the oral cavity. Treatment of wasting syndrome in HIV-infected patients is based on management of associated symptoms and conditions as well as identification and treatment of causative pathogens. Nutritional supplements are common and recommended for patients who cannot preserve their lean body mass and absorb adequate amounts of nutrition.

1993 Revised Classification System for HIV Infection and Expanded Surveillance Case Definition for AIDS Among Adolescents and Adults

The 1993 revised CDC classification system for HIV-infected adolescents and adults,[10] which went into effect January 1, 1993, replaces the system published by the CDC in 1986.[152] In contrast to the 1986 classification system, which relied on clinical conditions only, the 1993 classification system includes three additional clinical conditions as well as immunologic criteria that are measured with CD4+ T lymphocyte counts (Tables 6-1 and 6-2). The expanded AIDS surveillance case definition, which was last revised in 1987,[153] includes individuals with severe immune suppression, as measured by a CD4+ T-lymphocyte cell count below 200 cells/mm³ or a CD4 percentage below 14. It is believed that this new definition of AIDS will better reflect the number of individuals infected with HIV who are at the highest risk for HIV-related morbidity. The expanded AIDS surveillance case definition will have a substanial impact on reported cases. It is important to realize that the criteria for an AIDS diagnosis prior to January 1, 1993, do not include individuals without clinical signs and symptoms of AIDS or with severe immune suppression; consequently, with the new AIDS definition many more individuals will be reported as having AIDS.

The range of clinical manifestations

Table 6-1. Revised CDC Classification for HIV Infection*

- CD4+ T-lymphocyte categories
  The lowest accurate CD4+ T-lymphocyte count should be used for classification purposes, even though more recent and possibly different counts may be available
- Clinical categories
  Clinical category A
    Asymptomatic HIV infection
    Persistent generalized lymphadenopathy
    Acute HIV infection with accompanying illness or history of acute HIV infection: conditions listed in categories B or C must not have occurred.
  Clinical category B
    Symptomatic conditions in adolescents or adults with HIV that are not included in clinical category C and meet at least one of the following criteria: a) the conditions are attributed to HIV infection or are indicative of a defect in cell-mediated immunity; b) the conditions are considered by physicians to have a clinical course or to require management that is complicated by HIV infection. Examples include, but are not limited to, the following conditions:
        Bacillary angiomatosis†
        Candidiasis, oropharyngeal (thrush)
        Candidiasis, vulvovaginal; persistent, frequent, or poorly responsive to therapy
        Cervical dysplasia (moderate or severe)/cervical carcinoma in situ
        Constitutional symptoms, such as fever (38.5°C) or diarrhea lasting greater than 1 mo
        Herpes zoster (shingles), involving at least two distinct episodes or more than one dermatome
        Idiopathic thrombocytopenia purpura
        Listeriosis
        Oral hairy leukoplakia

Pelvic inflammatory disease, particularly if complicated by tubo-ovarian abscess
Peripheral neuropathy
Clinical category C
  Candidiasis of bronchi, trachea, or lung
  Candidiasis, esophageal
  Cervical cancer, invasive
  Coccidioidomycosis, disseminated or extrapulmonary
  Cryptococcosis, extrapulmonary†
  Cryptosporidiosis, chronic intestinal (greater than 1 mo duration)
  Cytomegalovirus disease (other than liver, spleen, or nodes)†
  Cytomegalovirus retinitis (with loss of vision)
  Encephalopathy, HIV-related
  Herpes simplex†: chronic ulcer(s) (greater than 1 mo duration); or bronchitis, pneumonitis, or esophagitis
  Histoplasmosis, disseminated or extrapulmonary†
  Isosporiasis, chronic intestinal (greater than 1 mo duration)
  Kaposi's sarcoma†
  Lymphoma, Burkitt's (or equivalent term)†
  Lymphoma, immunoblastic (or equivalent term)
  Lymphoma, primary, of brain
  M. avium complex or M. kansaii, disseminated or extrapulmonary†
  M. tuberculosis, any site (pulmonary or extrapulmonary)†
  Mycobacterium, other species or unidentified species, disseminated or extrapulmonary
  P. carinii pneumonia
  Pneumonia, recurrent
  Progressive multifocal leukoencephalopathy
  Salmonella septicemia, recurrent
  Toxoplasmosis
  Wasting syndrome due to HIV

*Adapted from CDC: MMWR 1992;41:1–19. Used with permission.
†Can present as oral manifestations.

Table 6-2. Category of HIV Infection According to CD4+ T-Lymphocyte Count*

CD4+ T-cells/mm³ Categories or CD4+ Percentage	Clinical Categories		
	(A) Asymptomatic, Acute HIV or PGL	(B) Symptomatic, Not (A) or (C) Conditions	(C) AIDS-Indicator Conditions
(1) ≥ 500 or ≥ 29%	A1	B1	C1[†]
(2) 200–499 or 14%–28%	A2	B2	C2[†]
(3) < 200 or < 14%	A3[†]	B3[†]	C3[†]

*From CDC: MMWR 1992;41:1–19. Used with permission.
[†]Expanded AIDS surveillance case definition.

of HIV disease is broad and ever-changing. The dental practitioner's ability to recognize these presentations associated with HIV disease is an instrumental part in providing appropriate dental care for infected individuals.

References

1. Hoover DR, Saah AJ, Bacellar H, et al. Clinical manifestations of AIDS in the era of pneumocystis prophylaxis. N Engl J Med 1993;329:1922–1926.

2. Denning DW, Follansbee SE, Scolaro M, Norris S, Edelstein H, Stevens DA. Pulmonary aspergillosis in the acquired immunodeficiency syndrome. N Engl J Med 1991;324:654–662.

3. Minamoto GY, Barlam TF, Vanderels NJ. Invasive aspergillosis in patients with AIDS. Clin Infect Dis 1992;14:66–74.

4. Rubin MM, Jui V, Sadoff RS. Oral aspergillosis in a patient with acquired immunodeficiency syndrome. J Oral Maxillofac Surg 1990;48:997–999.

5. Anderson MJ, Jones SE, Fisher-Hoch SP, et al. Human parvovirus: the cause of erythema infectiosum (fifth disease)? Lancet 1983;1:1378.

6. Plummer FA, Hammond GW, Forward K, et al. An erythema infectiosum-like illness caused by human parvovirus infection. N Engl J Med 1985;313:74–79.

7. Frickhofen N, Abkowitz JL, Safford M, et al. Persistent B19 parvovirus infection in patients infected with human immunodeficiency virus type-1 (HIV-1): a treatable cause of anemia in AIDS. Ann Intern Med 1990;113:926–933.

8. Nigro G, Luzi G, Fridell E, et al. Parvovirus infection in children with AIDS: high prevalence of B19-specific immunoglobulin M and G antibodies. AIDS 1992;6:679–684.

9. Imam N, Carpenter CCJ, Mayer KH, Fisher A, Stein M, Danforth SB. Hierarchical pattern of mucosal candida infections in HIV-seropositive women. Am J Med 1990;89:142–146.

10. CDC. 1993 Revised classification system for HIV infection and expanded surveillance case definition for AIDS among adolescents and adults. MMWR 1992; 41:1–19.

11. Clotet B, Grifol M, Parra O, et al. Asymptomatic esophageal candidiasis in the acquired immunodeficiency syndrome related complex. Ann Intern Med 1986; 105:145.

12. Rhoads JL, Wright DC, Redfield RR, Burke DS. Chronic vaginal candidiasis in women with human immunodeficiency virus infection. JAMA 1987;257:3105–3107.

13. Macher AM, DeVinatea ML, Tuur SM, Angritt P. AIDS and the mycoses. Infect Dis Clin North Am 1988;2:827–839.

14. Rolston KVI, Radentz S, Rodriguez S. Bacterial and fungal infections in patients with the acquired immunodeficiency syndrome. Cancer Detect Prevent 1990;14:377–381.

15. Fish DG, Ampel NM, Galgiani JN, et al. Coccidioidomycosis during human immunodeficiency virus infection: a review of 77 patients. Medicine 1990;69:384–391.

16. Galgiani JN, Ampel NM. Coccidioidomycosis in human immunodeficiency virus-infected patients. J Infect Dis 1990;162:1165–1169.

17. Chuck SL, Sande MA. Infections with *Cryptococcus neoformans* in acquired immunodeficiency syndrome. N Engl J Med 1989;321:794–799.

18. Clark RA, Greer D, Atkinson W, Valainis GT, Hyslop N. Spectrum of *Cryptococcus neoformans* infection in 68 patients infected with human immunodeficiency virus. Rev Infect Dis 1990;12:768–777.

19. Lecomte I, Meyohas MC, De Sa M. Relation between decreasing serial CD4 lymphocytes count and the outcome of cryptococcosis in AIDS patients: a basis for new diagnosis strategy (abstract). In Proceedings of the VI International Conference on AIDS, San Francisco, CA 1990, p 235.

20. Masur H, Ognibene FP, Yarchoan R, et al. CD4 counts as predictors of opportunistic pneumonias in human immunodeficiency virus (HIV) infection. Ann Intern Med 1989;111:223–231.

21. Glick M, Cohen SG, Cheney RT, Crooks GW, Greenberg MS. Oral manifestations of disseminated *cryptococcus neoformans* in a patient with acquired immunodeficiency syndrome. Oral Surg Oral Med Oral Pathol 1987;64:454–459.

22. Nightingale SD, Cal SX, Peterson DM, et al. Primary prophylaxis with fluconazole against systemic fungal infections in HIV-positive patients. AIDS 1992;6:191–194.

23. Soave R. Cryptosporidiosis and isosporiasis in patients with AIDS. Infect Dis Clin North Am 1989;2:485–493.

24. Sewankambo N, Mugerwa RD, Goodgame RD, et al. Enteropathic AIDS in Uganda: an endoscopic, histologic and microbiologic study. AIDS 1987;1:9–13.

25. Fayer R, Ungar BLP. *Cryptosporidium* spp. and cryptosporidiosis. Microbiol Rev 1986;50:458–483.

26. Laughon BE, Druckman DA, Vernon A, et al. Prevalence of enteric pathogens in homosexual men with and without acquired immunodeficiency syndrome. Gastroenterology 1988;94:984–993.

27. Smith PD, Lane HC, Gill VJ, et al. Intestinal infections in patients with the acquired immunodeficiency syndrome (AIDS). Ann Intern Med 1988;108:328–333.

28. Quinn TC, Mann JM, Curran JW, Piot P. AIDS in Africa: an epidemiologic paradigm. Science 1986;234:955–963.

29. Flanigan T, Whalen C, Turner J, et al. *Cryptosporidium* infection and CD4 counts. Ann Intern Med 1992;116:840–842.

30. Miller RA, Wasserhait JN, Kirihara J, Coyle MB. Detection of *Cryptosporidium* oocysts in sputum during screening for mycobacterium. J Clin Microbiol 1984;20:1192–1193.

31. Koch KL, Phillips DJ, Aber RC, Current WL. Cryptosporidiosis in hospital personnel: evidence for person-to-person transmission. Ann Intern Med 1985;102:593–596.

32. Martino P, Gentile G, Caprioli A, et al. Hospital acquired cryptosporidiosis in a bone marrow transplantation unit. J Infect Dis 1988;158:647–648.

33. Nord J, Ma P, DiJohn D, Tzipori S, Tacket CO. Treatment with bovine hyperimmune colostrum in cryptosporidial diarrhea in AIDS patients. AIDS 1990;4:581–584.

34. Connolly GM, Youle M, Gazzard BG. Diclazuril in the treatment of severe cryptosporidial diarrhea in AIDS patients. AIDS 1990;4:700–701.

35. Marshall RJ, Flanigan TP. Paromycin inhibits *Cryptosporidium* infection of a human enterocyte cell line. J Infect Dis 1992;165:772–774.

36. Drew WL. Cytomegalovirus infection in patients with AIDS. J Infect Dis 1988;158:449–456.

37. Mintz L, Drew WL, Miner RC, Braff EH. Cytomegalovirus infection in homosexual men: an epidemiologic study. Ann Intern Med 1983;99:326–329.

38. Quinnan GV Jr, Masur H, Rook AH, et al. Herpes virus infections in the acquired immunodeficiency syndrome. JAMA 1984;252:72–77.

39. McKenzie R, Travis WD, Dolan SA, et al. The causes of death in patients with human immunodeficiency virus infection: a clinical and pathologic study with emphasis on pulmonary diseases. Medicine 1991;70:326–343.

40. Zaia JA. Epidemiology and pathogenesis of cytomegalovirus disease. Semin Hematol 1990;27(suppl. 1):5–10.

41. Crowe SM, Carlin JB, Stewart KI, Lucas CR, Hoy JF. Predictive value of CD4 lymphocyte numbers for the development of opportunistic infections and malignancies in HIV-infected persons. J Acquired Immune Deficiency Syndrome 1991;4:770–776.

42. Pertel P, Hirschtick R, Phair J, Chmiel J, Poggensee L, Murphy R. Risk of developing cytomegalovirus retinitis in persons infected with the human immunodeficiency virus. J Acquired Immune Deficiency Syndrome 1992;5:1069–1074.

43. Webster A, Lee CA, Cook DG, et al. Cytomegalovirus infection and progression towards AIDS in haemophiliacs with human immunodeficiency virus infection. Lancet 1989;2:63–66.

44. Gross J, Bozette S, Matthews W, et al. Longitudinal study of cytomegalovirus retinitis in acquired immunodeficiency syndrome. Ophthalmology 1990;97:681–686.

45. Jones AC, Freedman PD, Phelan JA, Baughman RA, Kerpel SM. Cytomegalovirus infections of the oral cavity. A report of six cases and review of the literature. Oral Surg Oral Med Oral Pathol 1993;75:76–85.

46. Tapper MI, Rotterdam HZ, Lerner CW, Al'Khafaji K, Seitzman PA. Adrenal necrosis in the acquired immunodeficiency syndrome. Ann Intern Med 1984;100:239–241.

47. SOCA Study Group. Mortality in patients with the acquired immunodeficiency syndrome treated with either foscarnet or ganciclovir for cytomegalovirus retinitis. N Engl J Med 1992;326:213–220.

48. Flowers RH, Torner JC, Farr BM. Primary cytomegalovirus infection in pediatric nurses: a metaanalysis. Infect Control Hosp Epidemiol 1988;9:491–496.

49. Siegal FP, Lopez C, Hammer GS, et al. Severe acquired immunodeficiency in male homosexuals manifested by chronic perianal ulcerative herpes simplex lesions. N Engl J Med 1981;305:1439–1444.

50. Levine MS, Woldenberg R, Herlinger H, Laufer I. Opportunistic esophagitis in AIDS: radiographic diagnosis. Radiology 1987;165:815–820.

51. Baden LA, Bigby M, Kwan T. Persistent necrotic digits in a patient with acquired immunodeficiency syndrome: herpes simplex virus infection. Arch Dermatol 1991;127:113.

52. Birch CJ, Tachedjian G, Doherty RR, Hayes K, Gust ID, Lucas CR. Altered sensitivity to antiviral drugs of herpes simplex virus isolates from a patient with the acquired immunodeficiency syndrome. J Infect Dis 1990;162:731–734.

53. Safrin S, Crumpacker C, Chatis P, et al. A controlled trial comparing foscarnet with vidarabine for acyclovir-resistant mucocutaneous herpes simplex in the acquired immunodeficiency syndrome. N Engl J Med 1991;325:551–555.

54. Goodwin RA, Des Pres RM. Histoplasmosis. Am Rev Respir Dis 1978;117:929–956.

55. Huang CT, McGarry T, Cooper S, Saunders R, Andavolu R. Disseminated histoplasmosis in the acquired immunodeficiency syndrome: report of five cases from a nonendemic area. Ann Intern Med 1987;147:1181–1184.

56. Johnson PC, Khardori N, Najjar AF, Butt F, Mansell PWA, Sarosi GA. Progressive disseminated histoplasmosis in patients with acquired immunodeficiency syndrome. Am J Med 1988;85:152–158.

57. Wheat LJ, Connolly-Stringfield PA, Baker RL, et al. Disseminated histoplasmosis in the acquired immunodeficiency syndrome: clinical findings, diagnosis and treatment, and review of the literature. Medicine 1990;69:361–374.

58. Nightingale SD, Parks JM, Pounders SM, Burns DK, Reynolds J, Hernandez JA. Disseminated histoplasmosis in patients with AIDS. South Med J 1990;83:624–630.

59. Heinic GS, Greenspan D, MacPhail LA, et al. Oral *Histoplasma capsulatum* infection in association with HIV infection: a case report. J Oral Pathol Med 1992;21:85–89.

60. Kaposi M. Idiopathisches multiples pigmentsarkom der haut. Arch Dermatol Syph 1872;4:265–273.

61. CDC. Epidemiologic aspects of the current outbreak of Kaposi's sarcoma and opportunistic infections. N Engl J Med 1982;306:248–252.

62. Penn I. Kaposi's sarcoma in organ transplant recipients. Report of 20 cases. Transplantation 1979;27:8–11.

63. Penn I. Kaposi's sarcoma in immunosuppressed patients. J Clin Lab Immunol 1983;11:47–52.

64. Groopman JE. Biology and therapy of epidemic Kaposi's sarcoma. Cancer 1987;58:633–637.

65. Rutherford GW, Payne SF, Lemp GF. The epidemiology of AIDS-related Kaposi's sarcoma in San Francisco. J Acquired Immune Deficiency Syndrome 1990;3:4–7.

66. Haverkos HW, Friedman-Kien AE, Drotman DP, Morgan WM. The changing incidence of Kaposi's sarcoma among patients with AIDS. J Am Acad Dermatol 1990;22:1250–1253.

67. Lifson AR, Darrow WW, Hessol NA, et al. Kaposi's sarcoma in a cohort of homosexual and bisexual men: epidemiology and analysis for cofactors. Am J Epidemiol 1990;131:221–231.

68. Beral V, Peterman TA, Berkelman RL, Jaffe HW. Kaposi's sarcoma in patients with AIDS: a sexual transmitted infection? Lancet 1990;335:123–128.

69. Archibald CP, Schechter MT, Craib KJP, et al. Risk factors for Kaposi's sarcoma in the Vancouver Lymphadenopathy—AIDS Study. Acquired Immune Deficiency Syndrome 1990;3(suppl. 1):18–23.

70. Drew WL, Mills J, Hauer LB, Miner RC, Rutherford GW. Declining prevalence of Kaposi's sarcoma in homosexual AIDS patients paralleled by fall in cytomegalovirus transmission. Lancet 1988;1:66.

71. Glick M, Muzyka BC, Lurie D, Salkin LM. Oral manifestations associated with HIV disease as markers for immune suppression and AIDS. Oral Surg Oral Med Oral Pathol 1994;77:344–349.

72. Moskowitz LB, Hensley GT, Gould EW, Weiss SDS. Frequency and anatomic distribution of lymphadenopathic Kaposi's sarcoma in the acquired immunodeficiency syndrome: an autopsy series. Human Pathol 1985;16:447–456.

73. Payne SF, Lemp GF, Rutherford GW. Survival following diagnosis of Kaposi's sarcoma for AIDS patients in San Francisco. J Acquired Immune Deficiency Syndrome 1990;3:(suppl. 1)4–7.

74. Gill PS, Rarick M, McCutchan LA, et al. Systemic treatment of AIDS-related Kaposi's sarcoma: results of a randomized trial. Am J Med 1991;90:427–433.

75. Fischl M, Lucas S, Gorowski E, et al. Inerferon alpha-N1 Welferon (WFN) in Kaposi's sarcoma: single agent or combination with vinblastine (VBL) (abstract). J Interferon Res 1986;6(suppl. 1):4.

76. Schaart FM, Bratzke B, Ruszczak Z, Stadler R, Ehlers G, Orfanos CE. Long-term therapy of HIV-associated Kaposi's sarcoma with recombinant interferon a-2a. Br J Dermatol 1991;124:62–68.

77. Northfelt DW, Kahn JO, Volberding PA. Treatment of AIDS-related Kaposi's sarcoma. Hematol Oncol Clin North Am 1991;5:297–310.

78. Muzyka BC, Glick M. Sclerotherapy for the treatment of nodular intraoral Kaposi's sarcoma in patients with AIDS. N Engl J Med 1993;328:210–211.

79. Pluda JM, Yarchoan R, Jaffe ES, et al. Development of non-Hodgkin's lymphoma in a cohort of patients with severe human immunodeficiency virus (HIV) infection on long term antiretroviral therapy. Ann Intern Med 1990;113:276–282.

80. Levine AM, Gill PS, Meyer PR, et al. Retrovirus and malignant lymphoma in homosexual men. JAMA 1985;254:1921–1925.

81. Monfardini S, Vaccher E, Tirelli U. AIDS associated non-Hodgkin's lymphoma in Italy: intravenous drug users versus homosexual men. Ann Oncol 1990;1:208–211.

82. Ragni M, Kingsley L, Duzyk A, Obrams I. HIV associated malignancy in hemophiliacs: preliminary report from hemophilia malignancy study (HMS). Blood 1988;74:38.

83. Kaplan LD, Abrams DI, Feigal E, et al. AIDS-associated non-Hodgkin's lymphoma in San Francisco. JAMA 1989;261:719–724.

84. Levine AM. Lymphoma and other miscellaneous cancers. In DeVita VT (ed): AIDS: Etiology, Diagnosis, Treatment and Prevention. Philadelphia: JB Lippincott; 1992:225–236.

85. Ziegler JL, Beckstead JA, Volberding PA, et al. Non-Hodgkin's lymphoma in 90 homosexual men: relation to generalized lymphadenopathy and the acquired immunodeficiency syndrome. N Engl J Med 1984;311:565–570.

86. Levine AM, Sullivan-Halley J, Pike MC, et al. Human immunodeficiency virus-related lymphoma: prognostic factors predictive of survival. Cancer 1991;68:2466–2472.

87. Levine AM, Wernz JC, Kaplan L, et al. Low dose chemotherapy with CNS prophylaxis and zidovudine maintenance in AIDS-related lymphoma: a multi-institutional trial. JAMA 1991;266:84–88.

88. Nightingale SD, Byrd LT, Southern PM, Jockusch JD, Cal SX, Wynne BA. Incidence of Mycobacterium avium-intracellulare complex bacteremia in human immunodeficiency virus-positive patients. J Infect Dis 1992;165:1082–1085.

89. Havlik JA Jr, Horsburgh CR Jr, Metchock B, Williams PP, Fann SA, Thompson SE III. Disseminated Mycobacterium avium complex infection: clinical identification and epidemiologic trends. J Infect Dis 1992;165:577–580.

90. Pierone G, Lin J, Masci J, et al. Fever of unknown origin in AIDS (Abstract Th.B.540) Sixth International Conference on AIDS, San Francisco, 1990:254.

91. Benson CA, Ellner JJ. Mycobacterium avium complex infection and AIDS: advances in theory and practice. J Infect Dis 1993;17:7–20.

92. CDC. Recommendations for counseling persons infected with human T-lymphotropic virus, type I and II. Recommendations on prophylaxis and therapy for disseminated Mycobacterium avium complex for adult and adolescents infected with human immunodeficiency virus. MMWR 1993;42:14–20.

93. Berger JR, Moskowitz L, Fischl M, Kelley RE. Neurologic disease as the presenting manifestation of acquired immunodeficiency syndrome. South Med J 1987;80:683–686.

94. Navia BA, Cho ES, Petito CK, Price RW. The AIDS dementia complex. II. Neuropathology. Ann Neurol 1986;19:525–535.

95. McArthur JC. Neurological manifestations of AIDS. Medicine 1987;19:517–524.

96. Navia BA, Jordan BD, Price RW. The AIDS dementia complex. I. Clinical features. Ann Neurol 1986;19:517–524.

97. Price RW, Brew B, Sidtis J, et al. The brain in AIDS: central nervous system HIV-1 infection and AIDS dementia complex. Science 1988;239:586–592.

98. Phair J, Munoz A, Detels R, Kaslow R, Rinaldo C, Saah A. The risk of *Pneumocystis carinii* pneumonia among men infected with human immunodeficiency virus type 1. N Engl J Med 1990;322:161–165.

99. CDC. Guidelines for prophylaxis against *Pneumocystis carinii* pneumonia for persons infected with human immunodeficiency virus. MMWR 1989;38(suppl. 5): 1–9.

100. Golden JA, Hollander H, Stulbarg MS, Gamsu G. Bronchoalveolar lavage as the exclusive diagnostic modality for *Pneumocystis carinii* pneumonia: a prospective study among patients with acquired immunodeficiency syndrome. Chest 1986; 90:18–22.

101. Bensousan T, Garo B, Islam S, Bourbigot B, Cledes J, Garre M. Possible transmission of *Pneumocystis carinii* between kidney transplant recipients (letter; comment). Lancet 1990;336:1066–1067.

102. Francioli P, Prod'hom G, Poloni C. Progress and problems in hospital infections: exemplified by pneumonia. Schweiz Med Wochensch 1991;121:1423–1428.

103. De la Monte SM, Gabuzda DH, Ho DD, et al. Peripheral neuropathy in the acquired immunodeficiency syndrome. Ann Neurol 1988;28:485–492.

104. Musher DM, Hamill RJ, Baughn RE. Effect of human immunodeficiency virus (HIV) infection on the course of syphilis and on response to treatment. Ann Intern Med 1990;113:872–881.

105. Johnson PDR, Graves SR, Stewart L, Warren R, Dwyer B, Lucas CR. Specific syphilis serological tests may become negative in HIV infection. AIDS 1991;5:419–423.

106. Ficarra G, Zaragoza AM, Stendardi L, Parri F, Cockerell CJ. Early oral presentation of lues maligna in a patient with HIV infection. Oral Surg Oral Med Oral Pathol 1993;75:728–732.

107. CDC. Recommendations for diagnosing and treating syphilis in HIV-infected patients. MMWR 1988;37:600–602.

108. Remington JS, Desmonts G. Toxoplasmosis. In Remington JS, Klein JO (eds): Infectious Diseases of the Fetus and Newborn Infant. Philadelphia: WB Saunders; 1983.

109. Holliman RE. Serological study of the prevalence of toxoplasmosis in asymptomatic patients infected with human immunodeficiency virus. Epidemiol Infect 1990;105:415–418.

110. Luft BJ, Remington JS. Toxoplasmic encephalitis in AIDS. Clin Infect Dis 1992:15:211–222.

111. Luft BJ, Hafner R, Korzun AH, et al. Toxoplasmic encephalitis in patients with acquired immunodeficiency syndrome. N Engl J Med 1993;329:995–1000.

112. Luft BJ, Brooks RG, Conley FK, McCabe RE, Remington JS. Toxoplasmosis encephalitis in patients with acquired imunodeficiency syndrome. JAMA 1984; 252:913–917.

113. Kochi A. The global tuberculosis situation and the new control strategy of the World Health Organization (editorial). Tubercle 1991;72:1–6.

114. CDC. Tuberculosis morbidity—United States, 1980–1992. MMWR 1993;42:699–704.

115. CDC. Prevention and control of tuberculosis in the the United States communities with at-risk minority populations and prevention and control of tuberculosis among homeless persons. Recommendations of the Advisory Council for the Elimination of Tuberculosis. MMWR 1992;41(No. RR-5):1–23.

116. CDC. Expanded Tuberculosis surveillance and tuberculosis morbidity—United States 1993. MMWR 1994;43:361–365.

117. CDC. Tuberculosis morbidity—United States, 1991. MMWR 1992;41:240.

118. CDC. Tuberculosis morbidity—United States, 1992. MMWR 1993;42:363.

119. CDC. Tuberculosis and human immunodeficiency virus infection: recommendation of the advisory committee for elimination of tuberculosis. MMWR 1989;38: 236–250.

120. Onorato IM, McCray E, the Field Service Branch. Prevalence of human immunodeficiency virus infection among patients attending tuberculosis clinics in the United States. J Infect Dis 1992;165:87–92.

121. Theur CP, Hopewell PC, Elias D, Schecter GF, Rutherford GW, Chaisson RE. Human immunodeficiency virus infection in tuberculosis patients. J Infect Dis 1990;162:8–12.

122. Pitchenik AE, Burr J, Suarez M, Fertel D, Gonzalez G, Moas C. Human T-cell lymphotropic virus-III (HTLV-III) seropositivity and related disease among 71 consecutive patients in whom tuberculosis was diagnosed. Am Rev Respir Dis 1987;135:875–879.

123. Braun MM, Cote TR, Rabkin CS. Trends in death with tuberculosis during the AIDS era. JAMA 1993;269:2865–2868.

124. DeCock KM, Soro B, Coulibaly AM, Lucas SB. Tuberculosis and HIV infection in Sub-Saharan Africa. JAMA 1992;268:1581–1587.

125. Frieden TR, Sterling T, Pablos-Mendez A, Kilburn JO, Cauthen GM, Dooley SW. The emergence of drug-resistant tuberculosis in New York City. N Engl J Med 1993;328:521–526.

126. Selwyn PA, Hartel D, Lewis VA, et al. A prospective study of the risk of tuberculosis among intravenous drug users with human immunodeficiency virus infection. N Engl J Med 1989;320:150–204.

127. American Thoracic Society. Control of tuberculosis in the United States. Am Rev Respir Dis 1992;146:1623–1633.

128. Daley CL, Small PM, Schecter GF, et al. An outbreak of tuberculosis with accelerated progression among persons infected with human immunodeficiency virus: an analysis using restriction-fragment-length polymorphisms. N Engl J Med 1992;326:231–235.

129. Di Perri G, Cruciani M, Danzi MC, et al. Nosocomial epidemic of active tuberculosis among HIV-infected patients. Lancet 1989;2:1502–1504.

130. Markovitz N, Hansen NI, Wilcosky TC, et al. Tuberculin and anergy testing in HIV-seropositive and HIV-seronegative persons. Ann Intern Med 1993;119:185–193.

131. Graham NMH, Nelson KE, Solomon L, et al. Prevalence of tuberculin positivity and skin test anergy in HIV-1-seropositive and -seronegative intravenous drug users. JAMA 1992;267:369–373.

132. Snider DE Jr, Good RC, Kilburn JO, et al. Rapid drug susceptibility testing of Mycobacterium tuberculosis. Am Rev Respir Dis 1981;123:402–406.

133. Eisenach KD, Sifford MD, Cave MD, Bates JH, Crawford JT. Detection of Mycobacterium tuberculosis in sputum samples using a polymerase chain reaction. Am Rev Respir Dis 1991;144:1160–1163.

134. Goble M, Iseman MD, Madsen LA, Waite D, Ackerson L, Horsburgh CR Jr. Treatment of 171 patients with pulmonary tuberculosis resistant to isoniazid and rifampin. N Engl J Med 1993;328:527–532.

135. Bloch AB, Canthen GM, Onorato IM, et al. Nationwide survey of drug-resistant tuberculosis in the United States. JAMA 1994;271:665–671.

136. CDC. Nosocomial transmission of multidrug resistant tuberculosis among HIV-infected patients. MMWR 1991;40:585–591.

137. Edlin BR, Tokars JI, Grieco MH, et al. An outbreak of multiple-drug resistant tuberculosis among hospitalized patients with acquired immunodeficiency syndrome. N Engl J Med 1992;326:514–521.

138. Fischl MA, Daikos GL, Uttamchandani RB, et al. Clinical presentation and outcome of patients with HIV infection and tuberculosis caused by multiple-drug-resistant bacilli. Ann Intern Med 1992;117:184–190.

139. Pearson ML, Jereb JA, Frieden TR, et al. Nosocomial transmission of multidrug-resistant Mycobacterium tuberculosis: a risk to patients and health care workers. Ann Intern Med 1992;117:191–196.

140. Iseman MD. Treatment of multidrug-resistant tuberculosis. N Engl J Med 1993;329:784–791.

141. Friedman-Kien AE, Lafleur FL, Gendler E, et al. Herpes zoster: a possible early sign for development of acquired immunodeficiency syndrome in high-risk individuals. J Am Acad Dermatol 1986;14:1023–1028.

142. Colebunders R, Mann JM, Francis H, et al. Herpes zoster in African patients: a clinical predictor of human immunodeficiency viral infection. J Infect Dis 1988; 157:314–318.

143. Hoppenjans WB, Bibler MR, Orme RL, Solinger AM. Prolonged cutaneous herpes zoster in acquired immunodeficiency syndrome. Arch Dermatol 1990;126: 1048–1050.

144. Gilden DH, Murray RS, Wellish M, Kleinschmidt-DeMasters BK, Vafai A. Chronic progressive varicella-zoster virus encephalitis in an AIDS patient. Neurology 1988; 38:1150–1153.

145. Safrin S, Berger TG, Gilson I, et al. Foscarnet therapy in five patients with AIDS and acyclovir-resistant varicella-zoster virus infections. Ann Intern Med 1991; 115:19–21.

146. Kotler DP, Tierney AR, Wang J, Pierson RN Jr. Magnitude of body-cell-mass depletion and the timing of death from wasting in AIDS. Am J Clin Nutr 1989;50:444–447.

147. Greene JB. Clinical approach to weight loss in the patient with HIV infection. Gastroenterol Clin North Am 1988;17: 573–586.

148. Resler SS. Nutrition care of AIDS patients. J Am Diet Assoc 1988;88:828–832.

149. Kotler DP. Intestinal and hepatic manifestations of AIDS. Adv Intern Med 1989;34: 43–71.

150. Ghiron L, Dwyer J, Stollman LB. Nutrition support of the HIV-positive, ARC and AIDS patient. Clin Nutr 1989;8:103–113.

151. Harriman GR, Smith PD, Horne MK, et al. Vitamin B_{12} malabsorption in patients with acquired immunodeficiency syndrome. Arch Intern Med 1989;149:2039–2041.

152. CDC. Classification system for human T-lymphotropic virus type III/lymphadenopathy-associated virus infections. MMWR 1986;35:334–339.

153. CDC. Revision of the CDC surveillance definition for acquired immunodeficiency syndrome. MMWR 1987;36:1–15.

Table. Cutaneous Disorders Associated with HIV Infection That May Present to Dental Health-Care Professionals

• Oral and labial herpes simplex	• Facial and scalp psoriasis; geographic tongue
• Facial zoster	• Reiter's syndrome
• Facial molluscum contagiosum	• Photodermatitis involving the face
• Oral and facial HPV infection	• Porphyria cutanea tarda
• Facial folliculitis	• Drug eruptions involving the face and oral mucosa
• Syphilis (mucous patches, split papules, papular and annular syphilides of facial skin, alopecia)	• Eosinophilic pustular folliculitis of the head and neck area
• Bacillary angiomatosis of the face, head, neck and, rarely, the oral mucosa	• Diffuse hyperpigmentation from wasting and CMV adrenal infection
• Atypical mycobacterial infection	• Trichomegaly of the eyelashes
• Tinea facei	• Alopecia
• Molluscum contagiosum–like papules of disseminated cryptococcosis	• Basal cell carcinoma of the head and neck
• Disseminated histoplasmosis, including oral ulcerations	• Malignant melanoma of the head and neck, especially lentigo maligna
• Facial scabies	• Facial and mucosal Kaposi's sarcoma
• Seborrheic dermatitis	• Metastatic lymphoma of the head and neck

Infectious Skin Diseases

Viral infections

Acute Exanthem of HIV Disease

The earliest cutaneous manifestation of HIV disease is the acute HIV exanthem.[1,2] This develops in up to 80% of patients who eventually acquire HIV infection[3] (see Chapter 5). In most patients it goes unnoticed, although when it is detected, the skin is involved in approximately 75% of cases.[4] Patients characteristically develop a febrile illness associated with pharyngitis, malaise, and lymphadenopathy 3 to 6 weeks after exposure to HIV. Following the onset of fever and pharyngitis, a slightly pruritic, erythematous eruption of macules and papules involving the trunk, extremities and head and neck area develops. Other manifestations include urticaria (hives), enanthemata (rash), perleche (fissures and desquamation at the corners of the mouth) and oral ulcers.[4] The process usually lasts for up to 1 week and resolves without incident. Some patients, however, develop a severe, rapidly progressive form associated with profound immunodeficiency, persistent p24 antigenemia, melena, pneumonitis, meningitis, and early demise.[4,5] This eruption is usually similar to other viral exanthemata (skin eruptions), such as rubella, and to morbilliform drug eruptions. The mean CD4+ cell count at the time of presentation is 495 cells/mm³.

Cytomegalovirus Infection

Cytomegalovirus (CMV) has been reported to cause disease in up to 95% of patients with advanced AIDS.[6,7] Cutaneous manifestations of CMV infection include petechiae (small, purplish, hematorrhagic spots that blanche on pressure) and purpura (hemorrhage into skin or mucosa that does not blanch on pressure), vesicles, bullae, a morbilliform skin eruption, hyperpigmented cutaneous plaques,[8,9] cutaneous papules and nodules,[10] and persistent perianal ulcers that resemble the perianal ulcerations seen with anogenital herpes simplex.[11] Ulcers from CMV usually do not respond to topical treatments such as sitz baths and compresses and are usually associated with intractable proctitis or colitis caused by enteric CMV infection. Most perianal ulcerations that contain CMV-infected cells are not caused by CMV. However, if CMV is the only pathogen identified, it may be a sign of systemic CMV infection.[12] This is similar to the scenario found in the oral cavity.

Light microscopic or electron microscopic examinations of biopsy specimens, or virus isolation, is required to confirm the diagnosis. The finding of true CMV-induced perianal ulcers confers a grave prognosis. Again, this is similar to situations in which CMV-associated lesions are present in the oral cavity. Treatment for perianal ulcers with ganciclovir has been effective in some cases.[13]

In patients with HIV infection and AIDS, ulcerations may be caused by more than one infectious agent. It is not uncommon to find cells containing inclusions of CMV along with characteristic multinucleated giant cells of herpes simplex.[14] Other cases have been reported in which skin lesions were found to contain acid-fast bacilli and herpesvirus.[15] Tissue samples from patients with AIDS should be searched carefully for multiple infectious agents since therapy for each disease differs.

Herpes Zoster and Herpes Simplex

Herpes zoster infection is the result of the reactivation of a latent varicella-zoster virus infection in the dorsal root ganglion of patients with previous varicella infection. It is usually manifest by painful clusters of vesicles on an erythematous patch of skin in a localized neurodermatomal distribution (Fig 7-1). In patients with HIV, initially localized zoster infection may become generalized with vesicles appearing at sites distant from the original dermatome involved. Lung and central nervous system involvement may develop with serious complications. Zoster in patients with HIV infection tends to leave residual deforming scars associated with persistent postherpetic pain.

The occurrence of herpes zoster infection in a patient with HIV infection should alert the physician to the possibility of the impending development of AIDS since 70% will progress to the complete syndrome within 2 years following its development.[16]

Patients with HIV infection often develop recurrent herpes simplex virus (HSV) infections. These infections are often more extensive, last longer, and are less responsive to

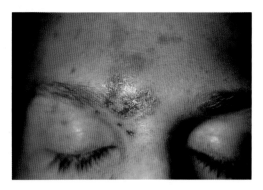

Fig 7-1. Herpes zoster in a young individual should cause concern about the possibility of underlying HIV infection.

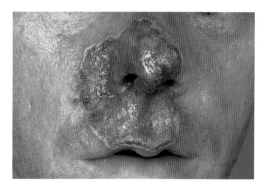

Fig 7-2. Severe necrotizing ulcerations of herpes simplex virus infection in a patient with advanced AIDS. Many such cases are resistant to acyclovir and require treatment with intravenous foscarnet.

antiviral therapy with acyclovir than HSV infections that occur in healthy hosts (Fig 7-2). Usually HSV infection is localized, but when dissemination occurs in immunocompromised patients, the entire skin surface may be covered with erythematous papules and vesicles. Anogenital herpetic infections may be prolonged and painful and may develop into extensive necrotizing perianal ulcerations that often become superinfected with bacterial organisms as a result of secondary contamination.[17] These severe forms of herpetic infection require treatment with intravenous acyclovir. In cases of acyclovir-resistant herpetic infections, intravenous treatment with foscarnet is often successful.[18,19]

Molluscum Contagiosum

Molluscum contagiosum is an infection of the skin characterized by pearly, yellowish, waxy papular lesions with central umbilications caused by a poxvirus and spread by close contact. In patients with HIV infection, the cutaneous lesions of molluscum contagiosum are usually widely disseminated and more numerous than those in immunocompetent hosts.[20] Individual lesions in adults can be several times larger than those seen in children and may occasionally be confused with basal cell carcinomas or nevi (Fig 7-3). Because of the clinical similarity to some examples of cutaneous cryptococcosis, it is important to consider this serious opportunistic fungal infection in the differential diagnosis and perform skin biopsies when indicated. Molluscum papules are easily eradicated by simple curettage or cryosurgery with the topical application of liquid nitrogen. Lesions in patients with AIDS tend to recur and spread with greater frequency so that treatment must often be continued indefinitely. Molluscum contagiosum infection is often more severe as CD4+ cell numbers fall below 250 cells/mm[3].[20] Furthermore, cells infected with the molluscum contagiosum virus may be demonstrated in

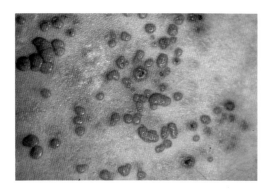

Fig 7-3. Molluscum contagiosum may give rise to multiple lesions as depicted here. Treatment usually consists of locally destructive measures such as liquid nitrogen cryosurgery.

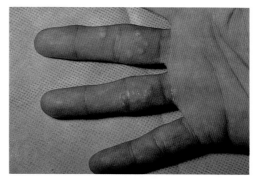

Fig 7-4. Multiple verrucae vulgares in an asymptomatic patient with HIV. Persistent HPV infection should cause concern about the possibility of occult HIV disease.

clinically unaffected skin adjacent to skin lesions, a sign that the virus affects the skin diffusely.[21]

Human Papilloma Virus Infections

Human papilloma virus (HPV) infections of the skin are common in patients with HIV infection. They are similar to those seen in healthy hosts but tend to occur in greater numbers and are often quite resistant to standard therapies. A possible reason for this phenomenon is that HIV tat protein secreted from HIV-infected cells exhibits a growth factor–like effect on HPV-infected cells, leading to enhanced survival, increased cell division, and abundant transcription of HPV DNA.[22,23] Some of the manifestations of HPV infection include extensive verrucae planae and filiform warts on the face; exuberant cauliflower-like plaques of condyloma accuminata of the anogenital region; hyperkeratotic verrucae vulgares on the fingers; multiple plantar warts; and HPV-induced malignancies, including bowenoid papulosis, epidermodysplasia verruciformis, and intraepithelial neoplasia of the anal and cervical mucosa[24,25] (Fig 7-4). This final complication may be found in up to 50% of patients with AIDS by exfoliative cytologic studies.[26] Extensive condylomata acuminata may pose an especially serious problem since it may involve mucosal surfaces as well as the external genitalia. Bowenoid papulosis is a form of squamous carcinoma in situ that may progress to fully developed squamous cell carcinoma. Surgery is usually required to treat this disorder.

In addition to the induction of epithelial malignancies, HPV has recently been associated with Kaposi's sarcoma. In a significant percentage of AIDS-related KS lesions, HPV-16–associated DNA sequences have been identified with the polymerase chain reaction.[27,28]

Treatment of HPV infection usually consists of local measures such as liquid nitrogen cryotherapy, intralesional interferon, or electrodessication and curettage. Podophyllum resin is effective for condylomata in some cases, but surgical therapy may be required.

Other Viral Infections

Several other viral infections may develop in patients with HIV infection with attendant complications. Parvovirus B19, the cause of erythema infectiosum (fifth disease) may lead to persistent and occasionally fatal aplastic anemia.[29] An adenovirus has been reported to cause palisaded granulomatous inflammatory dermatitis in one patient with AIDS.[30] Coxsackie and enteroviruses may also lead to extensive morbilliform or vesicular eruptions.

Localized Pyogenic Bacterial Infections

Common pyogenic bacterial organisms as well as more virulent bacteria may cause serious problems in individuals with HIV. Although the T lymphocytes are abnormal, abnormalities in B cells and in neutrophils have become increasingly recognized.[31] Some of the manifestations of these bacterial infections include: folliculitis usually caused by *Staphylococcus aureus* and *Streptococcus pyogenes;* cellulitis, pyomyositis, deep soft tissue abscesses, and toxic strep syndrome caused by Group A *Streptococcus;* and folliculitis, otitis externa, and ecthyma gangrenosum caused by *Pseudomonas aeruginosa.*[32-37] Like other infectious diseases in patients with HIV disease, these infections may be refractory to routine treatment with oral antibiotics so that hospitalization for treatment with intravenous antibiotics may be required.

When attempting to isolate the causative organism of a pyogenic bacterial infection in a patient with HIV, the physician should alert the microbiology laboratory that the patient is immunocompromised so that a search for unusual opportunistic infectious organisms will be undertaken. This may require special handling and culturing methods. Clinically, one may not be able to distinguish a pyogenic infection caused by *S. aureus* from one caused by a mycobacterium. Delays in accurate diagnosis can be detrimental.

Impetigo is another skin infection seen in patients with HIV disease. Impetigo is caused by coagulase-positive staphylococci and by beta-hemolytic streptococci. In patients with HIV, it may involve axillary, inguinal, and other intertriginous locations. It usually begins as painful red areas that often develop into vesicles and bullae that rupture, oozing serous or purulent fluid. The characteristic honey-colored crust eventually forms. Although the infection generally responds readily to treatment with antibiotics, in patients with AIDS therapeutic responses may be delayed.

Botryomycosis is a soft tissue infection usually caused by *S. aureus* and represents growth of colonies of bacteria in the tissue.[38] Clinically, this is manifest as a verrucous crusted papule or plaque. Treatment consists of antibiotics, local excision, or heat therapy.

A disorder similar to Job's syndrome has been described in patients with HIV disease,[39] manifest by recurrent staphylococcal abscesses with markedly increased serum immunoglobulin E levels and diminished polymorphonuclear leukocyte chemotaxis. A related disorder characterized by chronic diffuse dermatitis, elevated serum IgE levels, and eosinophilia with recurrent *S. aureus* and *Candida albicans* infections has also been observed.[40]

Corynebacterium diphtheriae may cause a cutaneous infection associated with septicemia in patients with HIV.[41] Cutaneous lesions are bullous and eventually become covered with a grayish pseudomembrane similar to that seen in pharyngeal diphtheria.

Syphilis

Syphilis is encountered commonly in patients with HIV infection, and it has been estimated that of all cases of reported syphilis, 25% occur in these patients.[42] The disease may respond poorly to treatment. Bizarre manifestations such as rapid progression from the primary chancre to gummatous tertiary lues,[43] lues maligna (syphilis with vasculitis), sclerodermatous lesions, and rupial lesion have all been described.[44] Serologic tests for syphilis may be negative despite the presence of spirochetes in tissues.[45,46] Seronegativity may be due both to prozone phenomena as well as true absence of antibody.

Increased severity of central nervous system lues has also been noted in patients with HIV infection.[42] Lancinating pain and meningovascular syphilis have developed following presumed adequate treatment of secondary syphilis. In one unusual case, a patient developed a relapse of syphilis after the administration of tetanus vaccine, implying that the alteration of the immune status may be sufficient to trigger latent yet viable treponemes.[43] Thus, in patients with HIV infection, the immune system may be unable to totally eradicate syphilis, even following recommended regimens of penicillin.

Mycobacterial infections

Patients with systemic mycobacterial infections may develop cutaneous lesions in 10% of cases.[47,48] Usually patients have CD4+ cell counts well below 200 cells/mm[3] when this complication develops. Skin lesions may assume different appearances such as small papules and pustules, an atopic-dermatitis–like eruption, localized cutaneous abscesses, ulcerations and sporotrichoid nodules.[49–53] Because of the nondescript nature of the lesions, tissue specimens for culture and special stains must be obtained to confirm the diagnosis. Any of the mycobacteria may lead to cutaneous lesions.[49–53]

Bacillary (Epithelioid) Angiomatosis

Bacillary (epithelioid) angiomatosis is a bacterial infection characterized by vascular proliferation seen most commonly in patients with HIV disease.[54–56] Clinically, lesions usually begin as pinpoint papules that gradually enlarge to form rounded, red-to-purple papules or nodules. Lesions may ulcerate and become encrusted. Most lesions are located in the superficial integument, although some lesions are located more deeply and may involve deep soft tissues and bone.

Disseminated lesions may involve the viscera as vascular lesions or as bacillary peliosis hepatis in the liver. Virtually every organ system may be affected. Histologically, lesions consist of lobules of capillaries and large, cuboidal, endothelial cells. In the interstitium, there are abundant aggregates of purplish granular material that represent colonies of *Rochalimaea henselae,* a rickettsia-like bacterium. There is also often an infiltrate of neutrophils that may be dense. Bacillary (epithelioid) angiomatosis can be distinguished from Kaposi's sarcoma histologically since there are no bizarre, jagged blood vessels and the inflammatory cell infiltrate in the lesions consists of lymphocytes, histiocytes, and neutrophils rather than plasma cells. Histologically, lesions have an appearance similar to that seen in pyogenic granuloma and verruga peruana lesions of bartonellosis.[56] When tissue sections of lesions are stained with the Warthin-Starry stain, clumps of darkly staining bacteria can usually be seen. Treatment with erythromycin at a dosage of 500 mg orally four times per day for 2 to 4 weeks, or doxycycline 100 mg orally twice a day for the same duration, is highly effective in eradicating the lesions. In some cases, these medications may need to be continued indefinitely, because when they are discontinued, lesions may recur.

The causative agent of bacillary angiomatosis has been identified as *R. henselae.*[57,58] Recent work has suggested that some cases may be caused by closely related organisms *R. quintana,* the causative agent of trench fever, and *R. elizabethae.*[59] While at one point, the disease was thought to be caused by *Afipia felis,* an unrelated organism, this has been shown not to be the case.[60] Other recent work has suggested that most cases of classical lymphadenopathic cat scratch disease is also caused by *R. henselae.*

Superficial Fungal Infections

While it is well known that candidiasis may affect patients with HIV, other fungi may also cause severe cutaneous or systemic infections. Widespread dermatophytosis caused by *Trichophyton rubrum* involving the palms, soles, nails, and intertriginous areas has been observed in individuals with or at high risk for AIDS.[61] Systemic griseofulvin and ketoconazole and topical antifungal medications have been found to be ineffective in completely eradicating such infections. Proximal white subungual onychomycosis also is a marker for immunodeficiency and is commonly encountered in patients with AIDS. This is manifest as a diffuse whiteness of the nail plates of multiple toes that extends from proximal to distal rather than the reverse, commonly seen in immunocompetent patients with tinea unguium.

Systemic Fungal Infections

Opportunistic systemic fungi commonly infect patients with HIV. Unless these infections are recognized and treated promptly, they may prove fatal. These infections are most likely to arise when patients are profoundly immunocompromised with CD4+ cell counts at or below 200 cells/mm³. Prophylactic antifungal therapy is routinely administered to immunocompromised patients to prevent these infections from developing.

Cryptococcus Neoformans

Cryptococcosis most often causes a meningitis, although the skin may be involved as single or multiple reddish 5-mm to greater than 1-cm papules, nodules, and/or indurated plaques.[62] Other manifestations that have been described include nodular herpes-like lesions and a rhinophyma-like tumoral growth on the nose.[63] One of the most common signs of cutaneous cryptococcosis is the presence of widespread, skin-colored, dome-shaped, and sometimes slightly umbilicated papules that bear a striking resemblance to the papules of molluscum contagiosum.[64] It is often necessary to biopsy and culture papular lesions thought to be molluscum contagiosum to exclude the more serious diagnosis of cryptococcosis. Patients with cryptococcosis may be asymptomatic. Treatment consists of itraconazole fluconazole or amphotericin B.

Histoplasma Capsulatum

Cutaneous histoplasmosis develops in approximately 10% of all cases of disseminated histoplasmosis.[65] This is slightly lower than the incidence of cutaneous cryptococcosis which is seen in 15% of cases of systemic cryp-

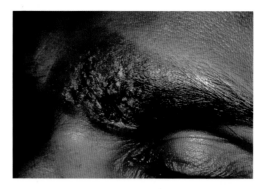

Fig 7-5. Histoplasmosis, a fairly common opportunistic infection in patients with HIV, involves the skin in up to 10% of patients with disseminated disease. Lesions may be nondescript and may mimic other disorders.

tococcosis, although in endemic areas it may be as high as 27%.[66] Skin lesions may appear as scattered acneiform papules, a widespread eruption of reddish macules and papules or one to a few indurated, pinkish red crusted plaques[67,68] (Fig 7-5). A specific diagnosis can be established only by culture and histopathologic examination.

Patients with cutaneous histoplasmosis may not be acutely ill or have any evidence of systemic or central nervous system involvement. Patients with AIDS and cutaneous histoplasmosis are often not aware of prior pulmonary disease.

Other manifestations of cutaneous histoplasmosis that have been observed include condyloma-like perianal nodules, caseating nodules on the forehead, and intranasal masses. Cutaneous histoplasmosis may coexist with other cutaneous disorders such as Kaposi's sarcoma, psoriasis, and psoriasiform dermatitis.[69,70] In a series of cases of disseminated histoplasmosis involving the skin, the diagnosis of histoplasmosis was first confirmed with skin biopsy in 25% of patients.[71] Thus, clinicians should maintain a high index of suspicion and should perform biopsies and viral, bacterial, and/or fungal cultures of any atypical skin lesion so that a potentially fatal infectious disease is not overlooked.

Other Systemic Mycoses

Penicillium marneffei, a fungus endemic in the Far East, may cause systemic disease in patients with HIV infection[72] with skin manifestations in up to 76% of cases. Signs of *P. marneffei* infection in the skin include umbilicated papules bearing similarity to molluscum contagiosum, ecthyma-like lesions, folliculitis, subcutaneous nodules, and morbilliform eruptions. The diagnosis is usually established with skin biopsy and culture.

Sporotrichosis may cause disseminated disease in patients with HIV infection. The classic lymphocutaneous form with lesions arranged in ascending fashion along lymphatics of the lower arm may be observed, although widespread verrucous papules and pustules has been noted.[73] Microorganisms in tissue may be numerous.

Other fungi that have been reported to cause disseminated infections in patients with HIV include *Scedosporium inflatum, Pseudoallescheria boydii, Microsporum canis,* and *Aspergillus* spp.[74–77]

Parasitic Infections and Ectoparasitic Infestations

Scabies

Scabies is common in patients with HIV infection. Norwegian (crusted) scabies manifest as hyperkeratotic plaques of the palms, soles, trunk, or extremities; as pruritic papules accompanied by slight scale on the trunk or extremities; or as a widespread papulosquamous eruption that may resemble atopic dermatitis.[78] In rare cases, scalp and facial scaling that may mimic seborrheic dermatitis may be noted. Severe forms have been associated with bacteremia and fatal septicemia, especially in severely compromised hosts.[79] Because scabies may have protean clinical features, it must be considered in the differential diagnosis of a wide variety of inflammatory dermatoses. Treatment consists of scabicidal medications such as 5% permethrin (Elimite) cream, gamma hexabenzene (Kwell) lotion, and lindane preparations, but because of the large number of organisms and the immunocompromised state of the patient, the condition may be difficult to eradicate. Often severe pruritus develops following destruction of the mites.

Demodicidosis

Marked proliferation of *Demodex folliculorum* may result in a persistent follicular eruption that may be confused with scabies.[80] The most common manifestation of this disorder is a widespread eruption of pruritic follicular reddish papules that may involve the face, trunk, and extremities. Antipruritic lotions and antihistamines are often ineffective at relieving the pruritus. The correct diagnosis is usually not made until mites are demonstrated on microscopic examination of scrapings or skin biopsies.

Treatment with 5% permethrin cream, benzoyl benzoate, or metrondazole is usually effective, although recurrences may develop.[81]

P. Carinii and Other Protozoans

Cutaneous pneumocystosis may develop in immunocompromised patients with HIV. The use of aerosolized pentamidine mist prophylaxis for pulmonary pneumocystosis has led to the development of systemic forms of this infection. Skin manifestations most commonly consist of friable reddish papules in the region of the external ear,[82] although lesions with features similar to molluscum contagiosum and Kaposi's sarcoma have been seen.[83,84] As with other opportunistic infections in individuals with HIV, biopsies and cultures of skin lesions are often required for diagnosis.

One case of cutaneous toxoplasmosis has been reported that was manifest by an eruption of papules involving the trunk and extremities.[85]

Acanthamoeba infections caused by *Acanthamoeba castellani* may develop in patients with HIV. Skin manifestations are painful, firm, red papules and nodules of the trunk and extremities that ulcerate.[86] Since lesions do not have a characteristic appearance, skin biopsies are generally required for diagnosis. Even after biopsy, the diagnosis may remain elusive since the number of organisms may be small and difficult to see.

Mucocutaneous leishmaniasis has been observed in patients with AIDS from Central America.[87] Hyperinfective strongyloidiasis may become disseminated and involve the skin, giving rise to a widespread livedo reticularis-like eruption. Careful observation of affected areas demonstrates the rapidly migrating nature to the eruption that has been designated larva currens. Severe forms of this infestation may be fatal.[88]

Noninfectious Skin Conditions

A number of secondary noninfectious cutaneous disorders have been described in patients with HIV disease. The presence of many of these conditions should alert the clinician to consider HIV infection in the differential diagnosis.

Seborrheic Dermatitis and Psoriasis

Seborrheic dermatitis is one of the most commonly observed skin conditions associated with HIV infection and AIDS; it has been reported in up to 85% of all patients with HIV.[89] The eruption is most commonly manifest as slightly indurated pink-to-red scaly plaques involving the face and scalp[90] (Fig 7-6). Other areas may be involved such as the intertriginous areas, the upper anterior chest, back, groin, and extremities. The eruption may be refractory to the usual treatment modalities used for seborrheic dermatitis, such as topical corticosteroids, especially when patients are profoundly immunocompromised. It may be the presenting complaint in an otherwise asymptomatic individual with HIV who may later develop AIDS.

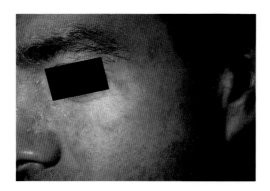

Fig 7-6. Seborrheic dermatitis, often of a severe and diffuse nature, occurs commonly in patients with HIV. It may serve as an early warning signal of HIV disease.

Patients with HIV infection may develop psoriasis that is often quite severe,[91] associated with pustule formation and arthritis in up to 35% of cases. Patients with a history of psoriasis may experience severe exacerbations of their disease although the condition may occur de novo with HIV infection. Most patients with HIV develop severe psoriasis with the onset of AIDS, especially when they have diminished CD4+ cell counts.

Psoriasis may exhibit different clinical courses ranging from partial remission in response to zidovudine to erythroderma. Some cases are unresponsive to all forms of treatment.

The coexistence of Reiter's syndrome and AIDS is well documented.[92] It may have its onset either concomitant with, preceding, or following the diagnosis of HIV disease. The development of this condition in patients without HIV is thought to be precipitated by infections with enteric bacteria, although whether these organisms play a role in patients with HIV has not been determined. Immunosuppressive therapy, especially methotrexate, commonly administered for Reiter's syndrome, may lead to profound immunodepression so that if it is used, it must be administered with caution (Odom R, personal communication, 1992). Alternate therapies include etretinate, dapsone, and exposure to low-level ultraviolet B irradiation.

Pityriasis Rubra Pilaris

Pityriasis rubra pilaris (PRP) is a psoriasiform dermatosis characterized by widespread scaly plaques involving the scalp, trunk, extremities, palms, and soles with follicular involvement and islands of skin that are spared.[93] Patients with PRP and HIV may develop explosive cystic acne vulgaris in association with the follicular abnormality. Therapy with oral 13-cis-retinoic acid may be effective.

Photodermatitis

Photodermatitis has been described in individuals with HIV[94] as a consequence of drugs that lead to phototoxic reactions or of exposures to substances that result in photoallergic contact dermatitis. Reddish-brown plaques develop on sun-exposed areas such as the back of the neck and dorsa of the hands. The action spectrum is usually ultraviolet A.

Porphyria cutanea tarda has also been described in individuals with HIV.[95,96] Patients develop blisters on sun-exposed areas prone to trauma, such as the dorsa of the hands and sides of the fingers, as well as temporal hypertrichosis and hyperpigmentation. The cause is related to abnormal hepatic uroporphyrinogen decarboxylase activity secondary to either HIV or another infectious agent. Patients have increased circulating uroporphyrins and coproporphyrins ranging from 3,000 to 9,000 IU.[97] Most patients are also relatively immunocompromised, having CD4+ cell counts ranging from 300 to 400 cells/mm^3. Since patients with HIV are often anemic, treatment with hydroxychloroquine (Plaquenil) at a low dosage, 25 to 100 mg one to two times weekly by mouth, is often effective.

Morbilliform Drug Eruption

Widespread pruritic, pink-to-red macules and papules, many often urticarial, frequently develop following the administration of certain drugs in patients with HIV infection. This is an especially likely complication of treatment with trimethoprim-sulfamethoxazole (Bactrim), commonly used for prophylaxis of *P. carinii* pneumonia. Up to 60% of patients with AIDS develop an eruption following the administration of this medication.[98] The eruption may persist for weeks or months after the drug has been discontinued. Treatment consists of the combined use of antihistamines, cool compresses, emollients, and topical corticosteroid preparations. Patients should also be monitored for the development of toxic epidermal ne-

crolysis, which may supervene.[99]

Other reactions to drugs reported in patients with HIV include toxic epidermal necrolysis induced by thiacetazone, chlormezanone, clarithromycin, dilantin, and fluoxitine; morbilliform eruptions induced by pyrimethamine, recombinant CD4, and dapsone; lichenoid eruptions, nail and mucosal pigmentation and dermatomyositis-like periarticular erythema caused by zidovudine; painful erythematous dermal nodules and plaques secondary to granulocyte-macrophage colony-stimulating factor; and genital and oral ulcers induced by foscarnet.[100–105] Dapsone is related chemically to other sulfonamides, such as sulfamethoxazole, so that cross-reactions between these two drugs are common.[106–107] Allergic contact dermatitis and acute anaphylactoid reactions to latex have been described in patients with HIV.[108]

Papular Urticaria

Papular urticaria is an eruption of itchy, red-to-pink, urticarial, dome-shaped papules with a widespread distribution over the trunk and extremities.[109] Lesions may resemble insect bites. Patients complain of severe pruritus and, as with certain other conditions found in patients with HIV, the symptoms as well as the eruption are not readily responsive to conventional treatment. The eruption may persist for months. Treatment consists of topical antipruritic emollient lotions, such as menthol- and phenol-containing preparations, and pramosone; systemic antihistamines, such as doxepin;

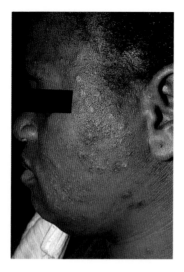

Fig 7-7. Eosinophilic folliculitis is also commonly found in individuals with HIV and advanced immunosuppression. The condition is usually severely pruritic.

and in refractory cases, exposure to low-level ultraviolet B irradiation.[110]

Eosinophilic Pustular Folliculitis

Eosinophilic pustular folliculitis is an acneiform, papular eruption usually associated with severe pruritus that develops in individuals with HIV usually when CD4+ cell counts are at or below 250 cells/mm³.[111,112] Lesions are distributed on the trunk, head, neck, and face (Fig 7-7). Microscopic examination of biopsy specimens shows numerous eosinophils within the infundibula of hair follicles. The condition may be difficult to control with topical medications and oral antihistamines, although therapy with ultraviolet B irradiation as well as Itraconazole 200 mg twice daily for several months

has been shown to relieve the pruritus and resolve the process.[113]

Erythema Elevatum Diutinum

Erythema elevatum diutinum, an unusual form of chronic leukocytolytic vasculitis that progresses to indurated plaques and nodules most commonly over joints, has recently been observed in patients with HIV.[114,115] Erythema elevatum diutinum in immunocompetent hosts has been postulated to occur as a consequence of an infectious process leading to chronic B-cell stimulation. In patients with HIV, either the HIV infection or a co-existing infection could be responsible for the development of this unusual condition.

Calciphylaxis

Widespread systemic and cutaneous calcification may develop in patients with HIV infection and concomitant renal disease.[116] Patients prone to develop this process suffer from chronic renal insufficiency and hyperparathyroidism. Parathyroid hormone sensitizes the tissues to the deposition of calcium and when an insult such as an infection supervenes, marked widespread precipitation of calcium and phosphorous salts occurs. Blood vessel walls are involved, leading to thrombosis and secondary ischemic necrosis of widespread areas of the skin. This in turn leads to ulceration and sepsis that usually proves fatal.

Vascular Abnormalities

A number of vascular abnormalities that involve blood vessels may develop in patients with HIV infection. Extensive leukocytolytic vasculitis caused by drugs, connective tissue diseases, or infectious processes may be seen.[117,118] This may be manifest as petechiae that evolve to purpuric papules, which may become bullous, pustular, and ulcerative.

Widespread telangiectasias of the chest, neck, and face have been observed in patients with HIV.[119] The cause of this process is not known, although it may be related to a circulating vascular proliferation factor. Some patients have had coexisting Kaposi's sarcoma (KS).

A vascular disorder known as hyperalgesic pseudothrombophlebitis has been described in several patients with AIDS. This syndrome is characterized by induration, erythema, and edema of the calf accompanied by severe pain and exquisite tenderness of the overlying skin.[120] The majority of patients with this disorder have cutaneous and/or systemic KS. Whether it is a complication of KS or due to a systemic medication is yet to be determined.

Pigmentary Disorders

Abnormalities of pigmentation may develop in patients with HIV infection and AIDS. Diffuse hyperpigmentation of the face with features similar to those in melasma has been seen in patients with advanced AIDS.[121] Usu-

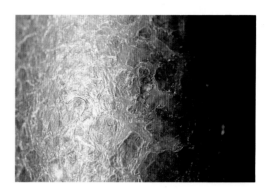

Fig 7-8. Severe widespread xerosis is especially common in patients with end-stage AIDS. The condition may be refractory to treatment with many different emollient regimens.

ally patients have associated xerosis (Fig 7-8). Diffuse pigmentation of the nail beds with grayish-brown longitudinal streaks and macular brown to gray-brown pigmentation of the lips and buccal mucosa have been associated with zidovudine administration.[122,123] Histopathologic findings show slight epidermal hyperpigmentation with an increase in the number of melanophages in the dermis.

Cytomegalovirus adrenalitis may lead to increased secretion of adrenocorticotropic hormone, manifest in the skin as an unusual suntan-like condition that has been observed in up to 56% of patients with CMV infection.[124] Other pigmentation disorders include hyperpigmented erythroderma and vitiligo.[125]

Pruritus

Patients with HIV infection may experience severe pruritus. Occasionally patients may develop idiopathic pruritus as a presenting sign of HIV disease.[126] Insect bite reactions may be severe, leading to bullae and pseudolymphomatous reactions. When pruritus is chronic, patients scratch vigorously, eventually developing excoriations and prurigo nodularis. These lesions may be the sources of secondary skin and soft tissue infections.

Grover's Disease

Grover's disease or transient acantholytic dermatosisis is a widespread pruritic papular eruption characterized by scaly, crusted erythematous papules distributed on the trunk and extremities. It usually develops in middle-aged to elderly individuals and resolves without incident. In patients with HIV, younger individuals may be affected and the condition may be persistent.[127] Histologic evaluation reveals focal acantholytic dyskeratosis within the epidermis.

Poorly Defined Inflammatory Dermatoses

In addition to the specific conditions mentioned, poorly defined inflammatory dermatoses may develop in patients with HIV. Most patients are profoundly immunocompromised when such eruptions develop with CD4+ cell counts less than 150 to 200 cells/mm³.[128] Eruptions with features similar to those in atopic dermatitis and other psoriasiform disorders have been described.[109] Often these disorders do not appear identical to classi-

cal inflammatory dermatoses probably as a consequence of abnormal immunity. Histopathologic findings characteristically include an infiltrate of plasma cells, eosinophils, and an interface dermatitis with individually necrotic keratinocytes bearing similarity to cutaneous graft-vs-host disease.[129] It is important when finding an eruption that does not show correlation between histopathologic and clinical findings to consider the possible diagnosis of HIV disease.

Cutaneous eruptions may flare and be worse than expected in immunocompetent individuals. Atopic dermatitis may be severe; granuloma annulare may be widespread and disseminated[130]; and xerosis may be extensive, leading to severe asteatotic dermatitis with eczema craquele.

Nutritional Disorders

As patients survive longer with HIV infection and AIDS as a consequence of improved prophylaxis, malnutrition has become a serious problem. Cutaneous manifestations of malnutrition may be encountered in patients with AIDS, especially those with advanced AIDS. Follicular hyperkeratosis, a sign of vitamin A deficiency, presents as pilaris-like papules. Acrodermatitis enteropathica leads to circumoral and acral erythema with crusting and develops as a consequence of hypozincemia.[131,132] Scurvy and pellagra are manifest as perifollicular petechiae and photosensitivity dermatitis, respectively.

Disorders of the Hair

Patients with HIV infection may experience pronounced growth of the eyelashes, known as trichomegaly of the eyelashes.[133,134] The reason for the development of this condition is unclear.

Patients with AIDS may develop a diffuse, fine, downy alopecia that may or may not be associated with slight scaling of the scalp.[135] Histologically, there is a perifollicular inflammatory cell infiltrate consisting of lymphocytes, plasma cells, and histiocytes with a decreased number of follicles in anagen. The alopecia may be progressive.

Cutaneous Neoplasms

Multiple basal cell carcinomas, metastatic basal cell carcinoma, and multiple primary malignant melanomas have been described in patients with HIV infection and AIDS.[136–138] All patients with HIV disease should be examined carefully for the presence of cutaneous neoplasms, especially if there is a history of prolonged sun exposure. Malignant melanoma in particular may be very aggressive in patients with HIV.[138]

Other malignant neoplasms that have been reported in patients with HIV include lymphomatoid granulomatosis (angiocentric peripheral T-cell lymphoma), metastatic poorly differentiated lymphoma, and cutaneous T-cell lymphoma manifest by erythroderma and lymphadenopathy.[139,140]

Kaposi's Sarcoma

At the beginning of the AIDS epidemic, KS was observed in over 50% of male homosexual patients with AIDS in San Francisco.[141] The incidence of KS has dropped; with HIV now it is reported in approximately 20% of patients with HIV in San Francisco, almost all of them homosexual men.[142] Recently, KS has been observed in homosexual men with risk factors for HIV infection who have repeatedly tested negative for HIV.[28] Kaposi's sarcoma occurs at all stages of HIV disease, and its severity is not strictly correlated with the degree of immunosuppression. It has recently been suggested that KS may be caused by a sexually transmitted organism such as HPV.[143] According to this theory, the decline in KS incidence may have occurred because of the use of safer sexual practices by homosexual men. Furthermore, recent reports have identified HPV type 16 DNA sequences in KS lesions, a finding that corroborates this theory.[27]

One third of patients with HIV have KS tumors on the legs and feet in a distribution similar to that of classic KS.[141] Lesions are more likely to develop elsewhere on the skin, including the mucous membranes and scalp. Lesions may occur singly or in groups. Individual tumors may also coalesce, forming larger lesions.

Clinically, cutaneous KS lesions may be pink, red, brown, or purple macules, patches, or plaques (Fig 7-9). In early stages, lesions may be overlooked by the patient and physician. In time, lesions darken and become scaly.

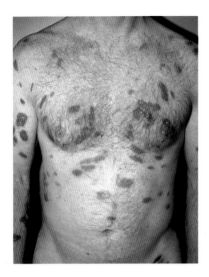

Fig 7-9. Plaque-stage AIDS-associated Kaposi's sarcoma, manifest as patches, plaques, nodules, or tumors. Lesions may be numerous and widespread.

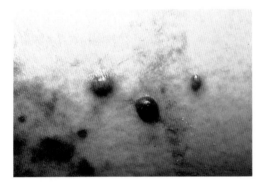

Fig 7-10. Nodular-stage KS. This neoplasm has recently been shown to be associated with HPV type 16, a finding that correlates with its epidemiology.

Some evolve into raised plaques, papules, or nodules that may be mistaken for other malignant, infectious, noninfectious, and inflammatory conditions, including purpura, hemangiomata, bacillary angiomatosis, dermatofibromata, lichen planus, pityriasis rosea, mycosis fungoides, malignant melanoma, cutaneous lymphoma, and secondary syphilis[144,145] (Fig 7-10).

Internal organ involvement often supervenes in patients with KS. As a general rule, approximately one internal lesion develops for every five skin lesions. Gastrointestinal lesions are common but are dangerous only if they cause blockage or hemorrhage. Kaposi's sarcoma of the liver and spleen is less common. Facial, extremity, or genital edema develops when KS involves the lymphatic system. The intraoral lesions of KS are discussed in Chapter 8.

The implications of an incorrect diagnosis of KS are serious. A skin biopsy is recommended whenever KS is a possibility and any clinical doubt about the diagnosis exists.

Treatment of cutaneous KS is essentially undertaken for cosmetic reasons only. Liquid nitrogen cryotherapy is usually the first therapeutic option; radiation therapy may be used in selected instances. Radiation therapy should be used with caution for oral lesions because of the potential for radiation-associated mucosal ulcers. Intralesional injections of 0.2 to 0.4 mg of vinblastine sulfate (Velban) at 2-week intervals is an effective method but may be associated with pain on injection. Other reported methods include intralesional injections with sodium tetradecylsulfate (Sotradecol), which produce a good clinical response without the associated pain and ulcerations noticed with intralesional vinblastine injection.[146]

Systemic chemotherapy is usually avoided since KS is rarely life-threatening. In severe cases, systemic treatment with agents such as vinblastine, etoposide (VePesid), bleomycin sulfate (Blenoxane), vincristine sulfate (Oncovin, Vincasar), or doxorubicin hydrochloride (Adriamycin) may be administered.[145] Systemic interferon alpha-2b and liposomal encapsulated doxorubicin are also effective for widespread disease. Referral to an oncologist experienced in treating AIDS-related malignancies is recommended if the need for systemic chemotherapy arises.

References

1. Tindall B, Barker S, Donovan B, et al. Characterization of the acute clinical illness associated with human immunodeficiency virus infection. Arch Intern Med 1988;148:945–949.

2. Sinicco A, Palestro G, Caramello P, et al. Acute HIV-1 infection: Clinical and biologic study of 12 patients. J Acquired Immune Deficiency Syndrome 1990;3: 260–265.

3. Ciesielski C, Metler R, Hammett T, Ward J, Berkelman R. National surveillance for occupationally acquired HIV infections in the United States. Poster presentation, VIII International Conference on AIDS, Amsterdam, July 19–24, 1992.

4. Kinlock S, de Saussure Ph, Vanhems Ph, Hirshel B, Perrin L. Primary HIV infection: a prospective and retrospective study. Poster presentation, VIII International Conference on AIDS, Amsterdam, July 19-24, 1992.

5. Clark S, Campbell-Hill S, Chopra P, et al. Quantitative assessment of viral replication in acute and early chronic HIV-1 infection: implications for natural history and intervention. Poster presentation, VIII International Conference on AIDS, Amsterdam, July 19–24, 1992.

6. Klatt EC, Shibata D. Cytomegalovirus infection in the acquired immunodeficiency syndrome. Arch Pathol Lab Med 1988;112:540–544.

7. Lin CS, Pinha PD, Krishnan MN, et al. Cytomegalic inclusion disease of the skin. Arch Dermatol 1981;117:282–284.

8. Feldman PS, Walker AN, Baker R. Cutaneous lesions heralding disseminated cytomegalovirus infections. J Am Acad Dermatol 1982;7:545–548.

9. Muehler-Stamou A, Sen HJ, Emodi G. Epidermolysis in a case of severe cytomegalovirus infection. Br Med J 1974;3: 609–611.

10. Medearis DN Jr. Cytomegalic inclusion disease: an analysis of the clinical features based on the literature in six additional cases. Pediatrics 1957;19:467–480.

11. Minars N, Silverman JF, Escobar NR, et al. Fatal cytomegalic inclusion disease: associated skin manifestations in a renal transplant patient. Arch Dermatol 1977;113: 1569–1571.

12. Horn TD, Hood AF. Cytomegalovirus is predictably present in perineal ulcers from immunosuppressed patients. Arch Dermatol 1990;126:642–644.

13. Collaborative DHPG treatment study group. Treatment of serious cytomegalovirus infections with 9-(1,3-dihydroxy-2-propoxymethyl) guanine in patients with AIDS and other immunodefiencies. N Engl J Med 1986;314:801–805.

14. Cockerell CJ. Cutaneous signs of AIDS other than Kaposi's sarcoma. In Friedman-Kien AE (ed): Color Atlas of AIDS. Philadelphia: WB Saunders; 1989:96.

15. Kwan TH, Kaufman HW. Acid fast bacilli with cytomegalovirus and herpes virus inclusions in the skin of an AIDS patient. Am J Clin Pathol 1986;85:236–238.

16. Friedman-Kein AE, LaFleur FL, Gendler E, et al. Herpes zoster: A possible early clinical sign for development of acquired immunodeficiency syndrome in high risk individuals. J Am Acad Dermatol 1986;14:1023–1028.

17. Siegal FP, Lopez C, Hammer GS, et al. Severe acquired immunodeficiency in male homosexuals, manifested by chronic perianal ulcerative herpes simplex lesions. N Engl J Med 1981;305:1439–1444.

18. Hardy WD. Foscarnet treatment of acyclovir-resistant herpes simplex virus infection in patients with acquired immunodeficiency syndrome: preliminary results of a controlled, randomized, regimen-comparative trial. Am J Med 1992;92:30–35.

19. Chatis PA, Miller CH, Schrager LE, Crumpacker CS. Successful treatment with foscarnet of an acyclovir-resistant mucocutaneous infection with herpes simplex virus in a patient with acquired immunodeficiency syndrome. N Engl J Med 1989;320:297–300.

20. Katzman M, Carey JT, Elmets CA, Jacobs GH, Lederman MM. Molluscum contagiosum and AIDS: clinical and immunologic details of two cases. Br J Dermatol 1987;116:131–138.

21. Smith KJ, Skelton HG, Yeager J, James WD, Wagner KF. Molluscum contagiosum. Ultrastructure evidence for its presence in skin adjacent to clinical lesions in patients infected with human immunodeficiency virus type 1. Arch Dermatol 1992;128:223–227.

22. Doherty R, Tanskanen E, Churchill MJ, Deacon NJ. Interactions between human immunodeficiency virus and human papillomavirus. Poster presentation, VIII International Conference on AIDS, Amsterdam, July 19–24, 1992.

23. Tornesello ML, Buonaguro FM, Galloway DA, Beth-Giraldo E, et al. HIV and HPV interaction: transactivation of HPV long control region by HIV-tat protein. Poster presentation, VIII International Conference on AIDS, Amsterdam, July 19–24, 1992.

24. Berger TG, Sawchuk WS, Leonardi C, Langenberg A, Tappero J, Leboit PE. Epidermodysplasia verruciformis-associated papillomavirus infection complicating human immunodeficiency virus disease. Br J Dermatol 1991;126:79–83.

25. Palefsky JM, Gonzales J, Greenblatt RM, Ahn DK, Hollander K. Anal intraepithelial neoplasia and anal papillomavirus infection among homosexual males with group IV HIV disease. JAMA 1990;263:2911–2916.

26. Nelson AM, Mvula M, St Louis M, et al. Increased rates of cervical dysplasia associated with clinical and immunological evidence of immunodeficiency. Poster presentation, VIII International Conference on AIDS, Amsterdam, July 19–24, 1992.

27. Huang YQ, Li JJ, Rush MG, Poiesz BJ, et al. HPV-16-related DNA sequences in Kaposi's sarcoma. Lancet 1992;339:515–518.

28. Friedman-Kien AE, Saltzman BR, Cao YZ, et al. Kaposi's sarcoma in HIV-negative homosexual men. Lancet 1990;335:168–169.

29. Torok TJ. Parvovirus and human disease. Adv Intern Med 1992;37:431–435.

30. Coldiron BM, Freeman RG, Beaudoing DL. Isolation of adenovirus from a granuloma annulare-like lesion in the acquired immunodeficiency syndrome-related complex. J Arch Dermatol 1988;124:654–655.

31. Kimura S, Goto M, Teramura M, et al. Decreased function of granulocytes in patients with HIV infection. Poster presentation, VIII International Conference on AIDS, Amsterdam, July 19–24, 1992.

32. Scully M, Berger TG. Pruritus, *Staphylococcus aureus,* and HIV infection (letter). Arch Dermatol 1990;126:684–685.

33. Gaut P, Wong PK, Meyer RD. Pyomyositis in a patient with the acquired immunodeficiency syndrome. Arch Intern Med 1988;148:1608–1610.

34. Cone LA, Woodard DR, Byrd RG, Schulz K, Kopp SM, Schlievert PM. A recalcitrant, erythematous, desquamating disorder associated with toxin-producing staphylococci in patients with AIDS. J Infect Dis 1992;165:638–643.

35. Janssen F, Zelinsky-Gurung A, Caumes E, Decazed JM. Group A streptococcal cellulitis-adenitis in a patient with the acquired immunodeficiency syndrome. J Am Acad Dermatol 1991;24:363–365.

36. el Baze P, Thyss A, Vinti H, Deville A, Dellamonica P, Ortonne JP. A study of nineteen immunocompromised patients with extensive skin lesions caused by *Pseudomonas aeruginosa* with and without bacteremia. Acta Derm Venereol 1991;71: 411–415.

37. Kielhofner M, Atmar RL, Hamill RF, Musher DM. Life-threatening *Pseudomonas aeruginosa* infections in patients with human immunodeficiency virus infection. Clin Infect Dis 1992;14:403–411.

38. Patterson JW, Kitces EN, Neafie RC. Cutaneous botryomycosis in a patient with acquired immunodeficiency syndrome. J Am Acad Dermatol 1987;16:238–242.

39. Raiteri R, Pippione M, Picciotto L, Martinetto P, Sinicco A. Job's-like syndrome in HIV-1 infection. Abstract, VIII International Conference on AIDS, Amsterdam, July 19–24, 1992.

40. Paganelli R, Scala E, Mezzaraom I, Ansotaque IJ, D'Offizi GP, et al. sCD23 levels in human immunodeficiency virus (HIV) infection with hyperIgE and chronic dermatitis. Poster presentation, VIII International Conference on AIDS, Amsterdam, July 19–24, 1992.

41. Patey O, Halioua B, Casciani JP, Emond A, et al. *Corynebacterium diphtheriae* septicemia in an AIDS patient. Abstract, VIII International Conference on AIDS, Amsterdam, July 19–24, 1992.

42. Johns DR, Tierney M, Felsenstein D. Alteration of the natural history of neurosyphilis by concurrent infection with the human immunodeficiency virus. N Engl J Med 1987; 316:1569–1572.

43. Gregory N, Sanchez M, Buchness MR. The spectrum of syphilis in patients with human immunodeficiency virus infection. J Am Acad Dermatol 1990;22:1061–1067.

44. Glover RA, Piaquadio DJ, Kern S, Cockerell CJ. An unusual presentation of secondary syphilis in a patient with human immunodeficiency virus infection. A case report and review of the literature. Arch Dermatol 1992;128:530–534.

45. Tikjb G, Russel M, Petersen CS, Gerstoft J, Kobayasi T. Seronegative secondary syphilis in a patient with AIDS: identification of *Treponema pallidum* in biopsy specimen. J Am Acad Dermatol 1991;24:506–508.

46. Hicks CB. Seronegative secondary syphilis in a patient infected with the acquired immunodeficiency virus (HIV) with Kaposi's sarcoma. Ann Intern Med 1987; 107:492.

47. Barbaro DJ, Orcutt VL, Coldiron BM. *Mycobacterium avium-intracellulare* infection limited to the skin and lymph nodes in patients with AIDS. Rev Infect Dis 1989;11:625–628.

48. Boudes P, Sobel A, Deforges L, Leblic E. Disseminated *Mycobacterium bovis* infection from BCG vaccination and HIV infection (letter). JAMA 1989;262:2386.

49. Rogers PL, Walker RE, Lane HC, et al. Disseminated *Mycobacterium haemophilium* infection in two patients with AIDS. Am J Med 1988;84:640–642.

50. Rohatgi PK, Palazzolo JV, Saini NB. Acute miliary tuberculosis of the skin in acquired immunodeficiency syndrome. J Am Acad Dermatol 1992;26:285–287.

51. Holton J, Nye P, Miller R. *Mycobacterium haemophilium* infection in a patient with AIDS. J Infect 1991;23:303–306.

52. Piketty C, Lons Danic D, Weiss L, Bu Hoi A, Kazatchkine MD. Atypical sporotrichosis-like infection caused by *Mycobacterium avium* in AIDS. Abstract, VIII International Conference on AIDS, Amsterdam, July 19–24, 1992.

53. Roth C, Theodore C, Aitkin C, Shaw E, et al. Presumed disseminated *Mycobacterium tuberculosis* infection presenting with cutaneous lesions in a patient with AIDS. Abstract, VIII International Conference on AIDS, Amsterdam, July 19–24, 1992.

54. Cockerell CJ, Whitlow MA, Webster GF, Friedman-Kien AE. Epithelioid angiomatosis: a distinct vascular disorder in patients with acquired immunodeficiency syndrome or AIDS-related complex. Lancet 1987;329:654–656.

55. LeBoit PE, Berger TG, Egbert BM, Beckstead JH, Yen TS, Stoler MH. Bacillary angiomatosis. The histopathology and differential diagnosis of a pseudoneoplastic infection in patients with human immunodeficiency virus disease. Am J Surg Pathol 1989;13:909–920.

56. Cockerell CJ, LeBoit PE. Bacillary angiomatosis: a novel pseudoneoplastic, infectious vascular disorder. J Am Acad Dermatol 1990;22:501–519.

57. Welch DF, Pickett DA, Slater LN, Steigerwalt AG, Brenner DJ. *Rochalimaea henselae* sp. nov., a cause of septicemia, bacillary angiomatosis and parenchymal bacillary Peliosis. J Clin Microbiol 1992;30:275–280.

58. Regnery RL, Anderson BE, Clarridge JE, Rodriguez-Barradas MC, Jones DC, Carr JH. Characterization of a novel *Rochalimaea* species, *R. henselae* sp. nov., isolated from blood of a febrile, human immunodeficiency virus-positive patient. J Clin Microbiol 1992;30:265–274.

59. Koehler JE, Quinn FD, Berger TG, LeBoit PE, Tappero JW. Isolation of rochalimaea species from cutaneous and osseous lesions of bacillary angiomatosis. N Engl J Med 1992; 327:1625–1631.

60. Perkins BA, Swaminathan B, Jackson LA, et al. Case 22-1992—Pathogenesis of cat scratch disease (letter). N Engl J Med 1992;327:1599–1600.

61. Torssander J, Karlsson A, Morfeldt-Manson L, Putkonen PO, Wasserman J. Dermatophytosis and HIV infection. A study in homosexual men. Acta Derm Venereol (Stockholm) 1988;68:53–56.

62. Manrique P, Mayo J, Alvarez JA, Ganchegua X, Zabalza I, Ilones M. Polymorphous cutaneous cryptococcosis: nodular, herpes-like and molluscum-like lesions in a patient with acquired immunodeficiency syndrome. J Am Acad Dermatol 1992;26:122–124.

63. Mares M, Sartori MT, Carretta M, Bertaggia A, Girolami A. Rhinophyma-like cryptococcal infection as an early manifestation of AIDS in a hemophilia B patient. Acta Haematol 1990;84:101–103.

64. Rico NJ, Penneys NS. Cutaneous cryptococcosis resembling molluscum contagiosum in a patient with AIDS. Arch Dermatol 1985;121:901–902.

65. Hazelhurst JA, Vismer JF. Histoplasmosis presenting with unusual skin lesions in acquired immunodeficiency syndrome (AIDS). Br J Dermatol 1985;113:345–348.

66. Wheat LJ, Conolly-Stringfield PA, Baker RL, et al. Disseminated histoplasmosis in the acquired immunodeficiency syndrome: clinical findings, diagnosis and treatment, and review of the literature. Medicine 1990;69:361–374.

67. Kalter DC, Tschen JA, Klima M. Maculopapular rash in a patient with acquired immunodeficiency syndrome. Arch Dermatol 1985;121:1455–1456.

68. Lindgren AM, Fallon JD, Horan RF. Psoriasiform papules in the acquired immunodeficiency syndrome. Disseminated histoplasmosis in AIDS. Arch Dermatol 1991;127:722–723, 725–726.

69. Cole MC, Cohen PR, Satra KH, Grossman ME. The concurrent presence of systemic disease pathogens and cutaneous Kaposi's sarcoma in the same lesion: *Histoplasma capsulatum* and Kaposi's sarcoma coexisting in a single skin lesion in a patient with AIDS. J Am Acad Dermatol 1992;26:285–287.

70. Chaker MB, Cockerell CJ. Concomitant psoriasis, seborrheic dermatitis and disseminated histoplasmosis in an HIV infected patient: an example of clinical mimicry with potentially serious consequences. J Am Acad Dermatol 1993;29:311–313.

71. Altarac D, Salomon N, Saltzman BR, Efremov MH, Katchen BR. Histoplasmosis in AIDS: unusual findings. Abstract VIII International Conference on AIDS, Amsterdam, July 19–24, 1992.

72. Supparatpinyo K, Chiewchanvit S, Hirunsri P, et al. *Penicillium marneffei* in patients infected with HIV. Poster presentation, VIII International Conference on AIDS, Amsterdam, July 19–24, 1992.

73. Shaw JC, Levinson W, Montanaro A. Sporotrichosis in the acquired immunodeficiency syndrome. J Am Acad Dermatol 1989;21:1145–1147.

74. Wood GM, McCormack JG, Muir DB, Ellis DH, Ridley MF, Protchard R. Clinical features of human infection with *Scedosporium inflatum*. Clin Infect Dis 1992;14:1027–1033.

75. Scherr GR, Evans SG, Kiyabu MT, Klatt EC. *Pseudallescheria boydii* in the acquired immunodeficiency syndrome. Arch Pathol Lab Med 1992;116:535–536.

76. Hevia O, Kligman D, Penneys NS. Non-scalp hair infection caused by *Microsporum canis* in a patient with acquired immunodeficiency syndrome. J Am Acad Dermatol 1991;24:789–790.

77. Sachot LJ, Hadderingh RJ, Devriese PP. Facial palsy and HIV infection. Abstract, VIII International Conference on AIDS, Amsterdam, July 19–24, 1992.

78. Sadick N, Kaplan MH, Pahwa SG, Sarngadharan MG. Unusual features of scabies complicating human T-lymphotrophic virus type III infection. J Am Acad Dermatol 1986;15:482–486.

79. Skinner SM, DeVillez RL. Sepsis associated with Norwegian scabies in patients with acquired immunodeficiency syndrome. Arch Dermatol 1992;50:213–216.

80. Dominey A, Roen R, Tschen J. Papulonodular demodicidosis associated with acquired immunodeficiency syndrome. J Am Acad Dermatol 1989;20:197–201.

81. Girault C, Borsa-Lebas F, Humbert G. Papulo-nodular demodicidosis: a new opportunistic infection in AIDS. Poster presentation, VIII International Conference on AIDS, Amsterdam, July 19–24, 1992.

82. Gherman CR, Ward RR, Bassis ML. Pneumocystis carinii otitis media and mastoiditis as the initial manifestation of the acquired immunodeficiency syndrome. Am J Med 1991;127:250–252.

83. Hennessey NP, Parro EL, Cockerell CJ. Cutaneous *Pneumocystis carinii* infection in patients with acquired immunodeficiency syndrome. Arch Dermatol 1991;127:1699–1701.

84. Litwin MA, Williams CM. Cutaneous *Pneumocystis carinii* infection mimicking Kaposi's sarcoma. Ann Intern Med 1992;117:48–49.

85. Hirschman JV, Chu AC. Skin lesions with disseminated toxoplasmosis in a patient with the acquired immunodeficiency syndrome. Arch Dermatol 1988;124:1446–1447.

86. Portnoy BL, Micheletti GA. Acanthamoeba infection of skin and sinuses in an AIDS patient: diagnosis and treatment. Abstract, VIII International Conference on AIDS, Amsterdam, July 19–24, 1992.

87. Da-Cruz AM, Machado ES, Menezes JA, et al. Cellular immune responses in a case of American cutaneous leishmaniasis and HIV-associated infection. Abstract, VIII International Conference on AIDS, Amsterdam, July 19–24, 1992.

88. Glezerov V, Masci JR. Disseminated strongyloidiasis and other selected unusual infections in patients with acquired immunodeficiency syndrome. Prog AIDS Pathol 1990;2:137–142.

89. Soeprono FF, Schinella RA, Cockerell CJ, Comite SL. Seborrheic-like dermatitis of acquired immunodeficiency syndrome. J Am Acad Dermatol 1986;14:242–248.

90. Mathes BM, Douglass MC. Seborrheic dermatitis in patients with acquired immunodeficiency syndrome. J Am Acad Dermatol 1985;13:947–951.

91. Duvic M, Johnson TM, Rapini RP, Freese T, Brewton G, Rios A. Acquired immunodeficiency syndrome-associated psoriasis and Reiter's syndrome. Arch Dermatol 1987;123:1622–1623.

92. Winchester R, Bernstein DH, Fischer HD, Enlow R, Solomon G. The co-occurrence of Reiter's syndrome and acquired immunodeficiency. Ann Intern Med 1987;106:19–26.

93. Martin AG, Weaver CC, Cockerell CJ, Berger TG. Pityriasis rubra pilaris in the setting of HIV infection: clinical behaviour and association with explosive cystic acne. Br J Dermatol 1992;126:617–620.

94. Toback AC, Longley J, Cardullo AC, Doddy U, Romagnoli M, DeLeo VA. Severe chronic photosensitivity in association with acquired immunodeficiency syndrome. Arch Dermatol 1986;15:2056–2057.

95. Lobato MN, Berger TG. Porphyria cutanea tarda associated with the acquired immunodeficiency syndrome. Arch Dermatol 1988;124:1009–1010.

96. Herranz MT, el Amrani A, Aranegui P, Jimenez-Alonse JF, Rodenas JM, Vivaldi RM. Porphyria cutanea tarda and acquired immunodeficiency syndrome: pathogenetic mechanisms. Arch Dermatol 1991;12:1585–1586.

97. Picard C, Crickx B, Fegueuz S, Carbon C, et al. Porphyria cutanea tarda in HIV infection. Poster presentation, VII International Conference on AIDS, Florence, Italy, June 16–21, 1991.

98. Gordin FM, Simon GL, Wofsy CD, Mills J. Adverse reactions to trimethoprim sulfamethoxozole in patients with the acquired immunodeficiency syndrome. Ann Intern Med 1984; 100:495–499.

99. Raviglione MC, Dinan WA, Pablo-Mendez A, Palagiano A, Sabatini MT. Fatal toxic epidermal necrolysis during prophylaxis with pyrimethamine and sulfadoxinie in a human immunodeficiency virus-infected person. Arch Intern Med 1988;148:2683–2685.

100. Nunn P, Wasunna K, Kwanyah G, et al. Cutaneous hypersensitivity reactions to thiacetazone among HIV-1 seropositive tuberculosis patients in Nairobi. Poster presentation, VII International Conference on AIDS, Florence, Italy, June 16–21, 1991.

101. Rosenthal E, Pesce H, Vinti RM, et al. Two original observations of chlormezanone and fluoxetine induced toxic epidermal necrolysis in HIV-infected patients. Poster presentation, VII International Conference on AIDS, Florence, Italy, June 16–21, 1991.

102. Blanshard C. Generalized cutaneous rash associated with foscarnet usage in AIDS. J Infect 1991;23:336–337.

103. Picard C, Weiss L, Fegueux S, Belaich S. Cutaneous reactions to pyrimethamine in patients with HIV infection. Abstract, VIII International Conference on AIDS, Amsterdam, July 19–24, 1992.

104. Davey RT, Davey V, Metcalf J, et al. Recombinant human CD4-immunoglobulin in patients with HIV-1 infection. Poster presentation, VII International Conference on AIDS, Florence, Italy, June 16–21, 1991.

105. Gaglioti D, Ficarra G, Adler-Storthz K, et al. Zidovudine-related oral lichenoid reactions. Poster presentation, VII International Conference on AIDS, Florence, Italy, June 16–21, 1991.

106. Mohle-Boetani J, Akula S, Holodny M, Katzenstein D, Garcia G. The sulfone syndrome during dapsone treatment for *Pneumocystis carinii* pneumonia prophylaxis. Poster presentation, VII International Conference on AIDS, Florence, Italy, June 16–21, 1991.

107. Jorde UP, Horowitz HW, Wormser GP. Limitations of dapsone as PCP prophylaxis in HIV-infected patients intolerant of trimethoprim/sulfamethoxazole. Poster presentation, VIII International Conference on AIDS, Amsterdam, July 19–24, 1992.

108. Fisher AA. Condom conundrums. Cutis 1991;48:359–360.

109. James WD, Redfield RR, Lupton GP, et al. A papular eruption associated with T-cell lymphotrophic virus type III disease. J Am Acad Dermatol 1985;13:563–566.

110. Pardo RJ, Bogaert MA, Penneys NS, Byrne GE, Ruiz P. OUVB phototherapy of the pruritic papular eruption of the acquired immunodeficiency syndrome. J Am Acad Dermatol 1992; 26:423–427.

111. Soeprono FF, Scchinella RA. Eosinophilic pustular folliculitis in patients with acquired immunodeficiency syndrome. J Am Acad Dermatol 1986;14:1020–1022.

112. Rosenthal D, LeBoit PE, Klumpp L, Berger TG. Human immunodeficiency virus-associated eosinophilic folliculitis: a unique dermatitis associated with advanced human immunodeficiency virus infection. Arch Dermatol 1991;127:206–209.

113. Buchness MR, Lim HW, Hatcher VA, et al. Eosinophilic pustular folliculitis in the acquired immunodeficiency syndrome. N Engl J Med 1988;318:1183–1186.

114. LeBoit PE, Cockerell CJ. Nodular lesions of erythema elevatum diutinum in patients with human immunodeficiency infection. J Am Acad Dermatol 1993;28: 919–922.

115. de Cunha Bang F, Weismann K, Ralfkiaer E, Pallesen G, Lange Wantzin G. Erythema elevatum diutinum and pre-AIDS. Acta Dermatovenereol (Stockholm) 1986; 66:272–274.

116. Cockerell CJ, Dolan ET. Widespread cutaneous and systemic calcification (calciphylaxis) in patients with acquired immunodeficiency syndrome and renal disease. J Am Acad Dermatol 1992;26: 559–562.

117. Chren MM, Silverman RA, Sorensen RU, Elmets CA. Leukocytoclastic vasculitis in a patient infected with HIV. J Am Acad Dermatol 1989;21:1161–1164.

118. Raffi F, Testa A, Magadur G, Barrier JH. Shonlein-Henoch purpura and glomerulonephritis as the initial manifestation of HIV infection. Presented at the VII International Conference on AIDS, Florence, Italy, June 16–21, 1991.

119. Fallon T Jr, Abell E, Kingsley L, et al. Telangiectasis of the anterior chest in homosexual men. Ann Intern Med 1986;105:679–682.

120. Abramson SB, Odajnyk CM, Grieco AJ, Weismann G, Rosenstein E. Hyperalgesic pseudothrombophlebitis: new syndrome in male homosexuals. Am J Med 1985;78: 317–320.

121. Gallais V, Lacour JP, Perrin C, Ghanem G, Bodokh I, Ortonne JP. Acral hyperpigmented macules and longitudinal melanonychia in AIDS patients. Br J Dermatol 1992;126:387–391.

122. Greenberg RG, Berger TG. Nail and mucocutaneous hyperpigmentation with azidothymidine therapy. J Am Acad Dermatol 1990;22:327–330.

123. Cohen LM, Callen JP. Oral and labial melanotic macules in a patient infected with human immunodeficiency. J Am Acad Dermatol 1992;26:653–654.

124. Grutzmeir S, Bratt G, Sandstrom E. Adrenal insufficiency is an important cause of fatigue and anorexia in AIDS patients with CMV infection. Poster presentation, VIII International Conference on AIDS, Amsterdam, July 19–24, 1992.

125. Tojo N, Yoshimura N, Yoshizawa M, et al. Vitiligo and chronic photosensitivity in human immunodeficiency virus infection. Jpn J Med 1991;30:255–259.

126. Liautaud B, Pape JW, DeHovitz JA, et al. Pruritic skin lesions: a common initial presentation of acquired immunodeficiency syndrome. Arch Dermatol 1989; 125:629–632.

127. Cockerell CJ. Pruritus in HIV infected hosts. In Bernhard JD (ed): Itch: mechanism and management. Philadelphia: WB Saunders; 1993:221–235.

128. Rao BK, Cockerell CJ. Histologic findings in inflammatory skin diseases in patients with AIDS. Poster presentation, VII International Conference on AIDS, Florence, Italy, June 16–21, 1991.

129. Habeshaw J, Hounsell E, Dalgleish A. Does the HIV envelope induce a chronic graft-versus-host-like disease? Immunol Today 1992;13:207–210.

130. Ghadially R, Sibbald RG, Walter JB, Haberman HF. Granuloma annulare in patients with human immunodeficiency syndrome. Arch Dermatol 1989;20:232–235.

131. Karter DL, Karter AJ, Yarrish R, et al. Vitamin A deficiency in patients with AIDS. Poster presentation, VIII International Conference on AIDS, Amsterdam, July 19–24, 1992.

132. Reichel M, Mauro TM, Ziboh VA, Huntley AC, Fletcher MP. Acrodermatitis enteropathica in a patient with the acquired immunodeficiency syndrome. Arch Dermatol 1992;128:415–417.

133. Casanova JM, Puig T, Rubio M. Hypertrichosis of the eyelashes in acquired immunodeficiency syndrome. Arch Dermatol 1987;123:1599–1601.

134. Foon KA, Dougher G. Increased growth of eyelashes in a patient given leukocyte A interferon (Letter). N Engl J Med 1984; 311:1259.

135. Leonidas JR. Hair alteration in black patients with acquired immunodeficiency syndrome. Cutis 1987;39:537–538.

136. Sitz KZ, Kepden M, Johnson DF. Metastatic basal cell carcinoma in acquired immunodeficiency syndrome-related complex. JAMA 1987;257:340–342.

137. Tindall B, Finlayson R, Mutimer K, Billson FA, Munro VF, Cooper DA. Malignant melanoma with human immunodeficiency virus infection in three homosexual men. J Am Acad Dermatol 1989; 20:587-591.

138. McGregor J, Newell ME, Kirkham N, et al. Malignant melanoma in HIV-disease: a report of three cases. Poster presentation, VII International Conference on AIDS, Florence, Italy, June 16–21, 1991.

139. Cadafalch J, Altes A, Brunet J, et al. Peripheral T-cell lymphoma and HTLV-1 infection in AIDS. Poster presentation, VIII International Conference on AIDS, Amsterdam, July 19–24, 1992.

140. Crane GA, Variakojis D, Rosen ST, Sands AM, Roenigk HH Jr. Cutaneous T-cell lymphoma in patients with human immunodeficiency virus infection. Arch Dermatol 1991;127:984–989.

141. Krigel RL, Friedman-Kien AE. Epidemic Kaposi's sarcoma. Semin Oncol 1990;17: 350–360.

142. Rutherford GW, Payne SF, Lemp GF, et al. The epidemiology of AIDS-related Kaposi's sarcoma in San Francisco. J Acquired Immune Deficiency Syndrome 1990; 3:4–7.

143. Beral V, Peterman TA, Berkelman RL, et al. Kaposi's sarcoma among persons with AIDS: A sexually transmitted infection? Lancet 1990;335:123–128.

144. Friedman-Kien AE, Saltzman BR. Clinical manifestations of classical endemic African, and epidemic AIDS-associated Kaposi's sarcoma. J Am Acad Dermatol 1990; 22:1237–1250.

145. Kovacs JA, Deyton L, Davey R, et al. Combined zidovudine and interferon-alpha therapy in patients with Kaposi's sarcoma and the acquired immunodeficiency syndrome (AIDS). Ann Intern Med 1989; 111:280–287.

146. Muzyka BC, Glick M. Sclerotherapy for the treatment of nodular intraoral Kaposi's sarcoma in patients with AIDS. N Engl J Med 1993;328:210–211.

8

Intraoral Manifestations Associated with HIV Disease

Michael Glick

For the dental practitioner, the significance of intraoral manifestations associated with HIV disease cannot be overstated. Many initial clinical signs of HIV infection and AIDS occur in the oral cavity and may serve as markers for early immune deterioration and disease progression.[1] As intraoral manifestations become readily apparent,[2,3] communication of this information to the patient's primary health-care provider will enhance overall care. This chapter surveys the intraoral manifestations common to persons with HIV disease, emphasizing the clinical appearance of the lesions, the significance of the lesions as markers for immune deterioration and disease progression, and treatment modalities for these lesions (Table 8-1).

Intraoral manifestations can be recognized by clinical appearance, histologic characteristics, and causative pathogens. Their clinical appearance provides a presumptive diagnosis that in many instances is sufficient to initiate therapy. Yet, because almost every lesion found in HIV-infected patients can also be found in other immunosuppressed individuals, very few, if any, lesions are truly specific to HIV disease. For lesions to be considered specific to HIV disease, they need to appear more frequently, manifest more severely, or respond differently to therapy compared to other patient populations. For a definitive diagnosis,

Table 8-1. Oral Manifestations Associated with HIV Disease

Lesion	Clinical Appearance	Treatment	Significance
Superficial fungal infections			
Erythematous (atrophic) candidiasis	Red macular patches found on mucosal surfaces; depapillated areas may appear on the dorsal surface of the tongue	Topical antifungal medications	Associated with early stages of HIV disease
Pseudomembranous (thrush) candidiasis	Yellow-white removable plaques found on any oral surface	Topical antifungal medications for patients with CD4+ cell counts above 150–200 cells/mm^3. Oral antifungal medications for patients with CD4+ cell counts below 150–200 cells/mm^3	Associated with initial and progressive immune deterioration and HIV disease progression
Hyperplastic (chronic) candidiasis	Long-standing non-removable confluent white-yellowish plaques that may be stained by food	Oral or intravenous antifungal medications	Associated with severe immune deterioration
Angular cheilitis	Red radiating fissures or linear ulcers at commissures of the mouth. Sometimes covered with a pseudomembrane	Topical antifungal medications	Can be detected during all stages of HIV disease
Deep-seated fungal infections			
Cryptococcosis	Ulceration, nodular	Intravenous antifungal medications, usually amphotericin B	Sign of disseminated disease
Histoplasmosis	Ulceration, nodular	Intravenous antifungal medications, usually amphotericin B	Sign of disseminated disease
Geotrichosis	Pseudomembrane	Intravenous antifungal medications, usually amphotericin B	Sign of disseminated disease

Table 8-1. *(continued)*

Lesion	Clinical Appearance	Treatment	Significance
Aspergillosis	Ulceration, necrosis	Intravenous antifungal medications, usually amphotericin B	Sign of disseminated disease

Viral infections

Lesion	Clinical Appearance	Treatment	Significance
Herpes simplex virus	Intraoral: solitary, multiple or confluent vesicles and ulcerations on keratinized mucosa. Perioral: single or multiple vesicles or ulcers with crusting on the vermillion portion of the lip	Oral acyclovir	Increased frequency and increased severity during progression of HIV disease. Resistance to acyclovir more common during severe immune deterioration
Cytomegalovirus	Nonspecific nonhealing large painful ulceration on any oral mucosal surface	High doses of oral acyclovir may resolve the oral lesion but intravenous ganciclovir must be instituted to treat the disseminated infection	Associated with severe immune suppression with CD4 counts below 100 cells/mm^3. May be an early indication of disseminated CMV infection
Oral hairy leukoplakia	Vertically corrugated slightly elevated white surface alteration usually seen on lateral or ventral margins of the tongue but can also be found on buccal mucosa and floor of the mouth	Oral acyclovir, maintenance dose usually required	An early marker for immune suppression when CD4+ cell counts drop below 300 cells/mm^3. More common among homosexual/bisexual men
Human papilloma virus	White or pink nodules with a cauliflower-like surface, commonly found on the gingiva and tongue	Surgical excision or podophyllin resin; will usually reappear	May be a marker for HIV disease in patients with unknown HIV status

Table 8-1. *(continued)*

Lesion	Clinical Appearance	Treatment	Significance
Bacterial infections			
Bacillary epithelioid angiomatosis	Bluish-red macular-to-nodular lesion with a similar clinical appearance to KS	Oral erythromycin	Associated with severe immune deterioration
Necrotizing ulcerative periodontitis	Rapidly progressive non-self-healing loss of periodontal attachment and bone; deep seated pain and spontaneous bleeding may also be present	Scaling, metronidazole or tetracycline, and an antibacterial mouthrinse	Associated with severe immune suppression with CD4+ cell counts below 100 cells/mm^3. More common in MSM
Linear gingival erythema	Erythematous gingival marginal band that may extend into adjacent and attached mucosa	Scaling, metronidazole or tetracycline, and an antibacterial mouthrinse	Associated with increased immune suppression
Syphilis	Ulcerations, mucous patches, or gummas	Intramuscular injections of penicillin	Lesions are very contagious
Neoplasms			
Kaposi's sarcoma	Red, bluish, or purplish macular or nodular lesion most commonly found on the hard and soft palate. Some lesions may be associated with ulcerations	Radiation therapy, or intralesional injections with vinblastine or sodium tetradecyl sulfate	Represents an AIDS diagnosis. Oral lesions may the first sign of this neoplasm. Associated with CD4+ cell counts below 200 cells/mm^3. More common in MSM
Non-Hodgkin's lymphoma	Ulcerative or exophytic lesions on any mucosal surface	Surgical excision, multiple drug chemotherapy in conjunction with radiation therapy	Found in a younger age bracket among individuals with HIV than among individuals without HIV

Table 8-1. *(continued)*

Lesion	Clinical Appearance	Treatment	Significance
Squamous cell carcinoma	Ulcerative, exophytic, red and white lesion more commonly found on the posterior part of the tongue and the floor of the mouth	Surgical excision, multiple drug chemotherapy in conjunction with radiation therapy	Found in a younger age bracket among individuals with HIV than among individuals without HIV
Miscellaneous lesions			
Hyperpigmentation	Blue, red macular lesions on any mucosal surface	Not indicated	May be an early sign of adrenal insufficiency or secondary to medications
Minor aphthous ulcer	Self-healing, shallow ulceration. More common on nonkeratinized mucosa. Will sometimes lack the characteristic surrounding red halo	Symptomatic relief, topical corticosteroids may be instituted	Not more commonly found in patients with HIV
Major aphthous ulcer	Large (> 10 mm) painful nonhealing deep-seated ulcerations without an associated etiologic pathogen	Topical, mouthrinse, or oral corticosteroid therapy	Associated with severe immune suppression with CD4+ cell counts below 200 cells/mm^3
Necrotizing stomatitis	Rapid localized destruction of alveolar bone accompanied by necrosis of overlying tissues, not necessarily painful initially	Topical or oral metronidazole or tetracycline. Topical, mouthrinse, or oral corticosteroid therapy. Protect lesion with a mouthguard	Associated with severe immune suppression with CD4+ cell counts below 100 cells/mm^3

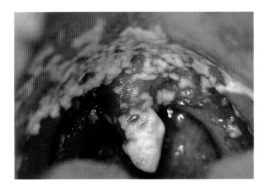

Fig 8-4. Chronic candidiasis, or hyperplastic candidiasis, covering the uvula and soft palate.

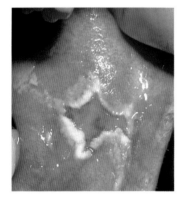

Fig 8-5. Long-standing candidiasis causing mucosal ulceration.

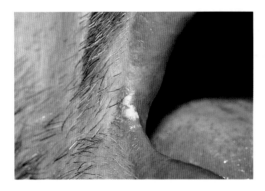

Fig 8-6. Angular candidiasis with pseudomembrane coverage.

underlying mucosa. Long-standing infections, as well as frequent recurrence of this lesion, are associated with a poor HIV disease prognosis. When pseudomembranous candidiasis starts to invade the more keratinized oral tissues, increased immune deterioration can be expected.

Chronic or hyperplastic candidiasis presents as larger areas of coalesced white or discolored plaques (Fig 8-4). This lesion cannot be mechanically wiped off since the candidal hyphae are anchored deep in the mucosa. Long-standing lesions can be associated with the development of painful ulcerations (Fig 8-5). This type of Candida infection is only observed among severely immunosuppressed individuals, many already with a clinical AIDS diagnosis.

Angular cheilitis, secondary to Candida infection, appears as red fissures radiating from the corners of the mouth. It is sometimes covered with a white membranous material that cannot always be wiped off (Fig 8-6). This type of candidiasis usually presents with concurrent intraoral candidiasis.

Severe and long-standing cases of candidiasis may be associated with dysphagia and dysgeusia. In such instances, symptomatic treatment needs to be instituted with antifungal medications. Treatment for oral candidiasis consists of antifungal agents in the form of topical mouthrinses, troches, ointments and creams, and systemic oral or intravenous medications (Table 8-2). Every patient needs to be evaluated for the most appropriate treatment modality, but in general, topical agents can be used for erythe-

Table 8-1. *(continued)*

Lesion	Clinical Appearance	Treatment	Significance
Squamous cell carcinoma	Ulcerative, exophytic, red and white lesion more commonly found on the posterior part of the tongue and the floor of the mouth	Surgical excision, multiple drug chemotherapy in conjunction with radiation therapy	Found in a younger age bracket among individuals with HIV than among individuals without HIV
Miscellaneous lesions			
Hyperpigmentation	Blue, red macular lesions on any mucosal surface	Not indicated	May be an early sign of adrenal insufficiency or secondary to medications
Minor aphthous ulcer	Self-healing, shallow ulceration. More common on nonkeratinized mucosa. Will sometimes lack the characteristic surrounding red halo	Symptomatic relief, topical corticosteroids may be instituted	Not more commonly found in patients with HIV
Major aphthous ulcer	Large (> 10 mm) painful nonhealing deep-seated ulcerations without an associated etiologic pathogen	Topical, mouthrinse, or oral corticosteroid therapy	Associated with severe immune suppression with CD4+ cell counts below 200 cells/mm^3
Necrotizing stomatitis	Rapid localized destruction of alveolar bone accompanied by necrosis of overlying tissues, not necessarily painful initially	Topical or oral metronidazole or tetracycline. Topical, mouthrinse, or oral corticosteroid therapy. Protect lesion with a mouthguard	Associated with severe immune suppression with CD4+ cell counts below 100 cells/mm^3

criteria distinct from clinical appearance, such as the demonstration of a causative pathogen, need to be established. This is especially important in individuals who are not aware of their HIV status since some of these lesions are indicative of HIV infection, and in cases in which oral lesions establish a diagnosis of AIDS, such as with suspected intraoral Kaposi's sarcoma.

Attempts have been made, by experts from both the United States and Europe, to reach a consensus on the classification and diagnostic criteria of the lesions found in HIV-infected patients. The criteria used to describe lesions in this chapter are based on established standards.[4,5] The presence of HIV-associated oral lesions is strongly associated with immune deterioration. When the peripheral CD4+ cell count level drops below 400 cells/mm³, one type of oral lesion may appear. When more than one type of lesion is present concurrently, a patient's CD4+ cell count is usually below 200 cells/mm³.[6] Thus, an increased number of concurrent intraoral lesions in patients with HIV disease suggests progressive immune deterioration. However, many patients take prophylactic medications for systemic and local infections that will influence the clinical emergence of oral manifestations. It is therefore difficult to establish true prevalence data for oral lesions during the natural progression of HIV disease. It is also important to realize that information concerning clinical manifestations associated with HIV disease is gained from large cohorts and case reports, which do not necessarily apply to individual cases. For instance, if the median CD4+ cell count for the emergence of a specific lesion is 150 cells/mm³, the lesion may be found in individuals with CD4+ cell counts ranging from 10 cells/mm³ to 1,000 cells/mm³.

Superficial Fungal Infections: Candidiasis

The most common intraoral lesion among individuals with HIV is oral candidiasis or candidosis, a localized fungal infection predominantly caused by *Candida albicans*.[7] The prevalence of clinical candidiasis in adults infected with HIV has been reported to be over 95%[8]; however, candidiasis is not pathognomonic for HIV disease. Although up to 60% of healthy, nonhospitalized individuals may harbor this pathogen,[9,10] the presence of a clinical infection should alert the practitioner to possible underlying medical conditions, such as the ingestion of broad spectrum antibiotics or corticosteroids, specific nutritional deficiencies and malnutrition, endocrine disorders, malignancies, or other immune deficiency diseases. Oral candidiasis is also more common in elderly patients, infants, denture wearers, and in individuals with xerostomia.

Klein and coworkers showed that unexplained oral candidiasis in healthy adults at risk for HIV infection was a predictor for the development of clinical signs of AIDS in 59% of these patients within three months.[11]

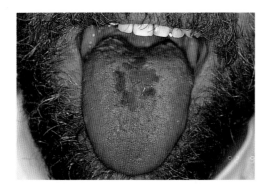

Fig 8-1. Erythematous candidiasis, or atrophic candidiasis, appearing as red patches on the dorsal surface of the tongue.

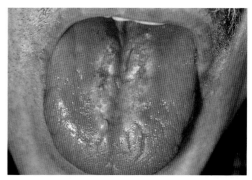

Fig 8-2. Long-standing erythematous candidiasis, or atrophic candidiasis, with ulcerations on the dorsum of the tongue, caused by abrasions from sucking on antifungal troches.

Among the individuals with more severe immunosuppression in this cohort, AIDS developed in 80% within 3 months. In another study of individuals with HIV, the presence of candidiasis was strongly associated with both xerostomia and HIV disease progression.[12] In a large retrospective study of 700 HIV-infected patients, 70% of individuals with oral candidiasis had CD4+ cell counts below 200 cells/mm³ (range, 3 cells/mm³ to 1,005 cells/mm³).[6] The presence and frequency of oral candidiasis in HIV disease are strongly associated with progressive immune deterioration,[13] but local factors such as xerostomia can contribute to an even higher incidence rate.

Four distinct clinical appearances of oral candidiasis have been described. Erythematous or atrophic candidiasis presents as red patches on any oral mucosal surface, but most commonly on the hard and soft palate and the dorsal surface of the tongue (Fig 8-1). Depapillated areas of the dorsum of the tongue, secondary to candidal infections, may cause severe discom-

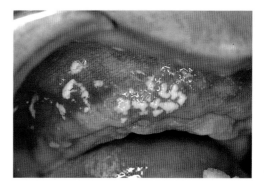

Fig 8-3. Pseudomembranous candidiasis, or thrush, on the anterior endentulous alveolar ridge.

fort and pain if not treated appropriately. Long-standing lesions may even result in ulcerations (Fig 8-2).

Pseudomembranous candidiasis or thrush was described in the initial reported cases of AIDS[14] and has since been incorporated into the Centers for Disease Control and Prevention clinical classification of HIV disease (see Tables 6-1 and 6-2). This lesion presents as white or yellowish plaques on any oral mucosal surface (Fig 8-3). These plaques can easily be wiped off, sometimes leaving an erythematous

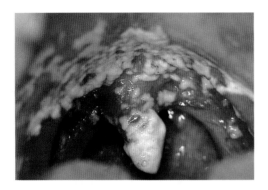

Fig 8-4. Chronic candidiasis, or hyperplastic candidiasis, covering the uvula and soft palate.

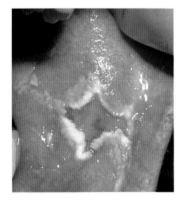

Fig 8-5. Long-standing candidiasis causing mucosal ulceration.

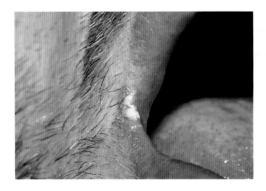

Fig 8-6. Angular candidiasis with pseudomembrane coverage.

underlying mucosa. Long-standing infections, as well as frequent recurrence of this lesion, are associated with a poor HIV disease prognosis. When pseudomembranous candidiasis starts to invade the more keratinized oral tissues, increased immune deterioration can be expected.

Chronic or hyperplastic candidiasis presents as larger areas of coalesced white or discolored plaques (Fig 8-4). This lesion cannot be mechanically wiped off since the candidal hyphae are anchored deep in the mucosa. Long-standing lesions can be associated with the development of painful ulcerations (Fig 8-5). This type of Candida infection is only observed among severely immunosuppressed individuals, many already with a clinical AIDS diagnosis.

Angular cheilitis, secondary to Candida infection, appears as red fissures radiating from the corners of the mouth. It is sometimes covered with a white membranous material that cannot always be wiped off (Fig 8-6). This type of candidiasis usually presents with concurrent intraoral candidiasis.

Severe and long-standing cases of candidiasis may be associated with dysphagia and dysgeusia. In such instances, symptomatic treatment needs to be instituted with antifungal medications. Treatment for oral candidiasis consists of antifungal agents in the form of topical mouthrinses, troches, ointments and creams, and systemic oral or intravenous medications (Table 8-2). Every patient needs to be evaluated for the most appropriate treatment modality, but in general, topical agents can be used for erythe-

Table 8-2. Treatment Modalities for Oral Candidiasis

- Topical therapy

    Clotrimazole (oral troches), 10 mg; 50 troches; dissolve 1 troche 5 times per day

    Nystatin (oral pastilles), 200,000 U; 50 pastilles; dissolve 1 pastille 4–5 times per day

    Nystatin (oral susp), 500,000 U/5 mL; 200 mL; rinse with 1 tsp 4 times per day for 2 min then swallow

    Nystatin (vaginal troches), 100,000 U; 70 troches; dissolve 1 troche 6–8 times per day

    Clotrimazole cream 1%, miconazole cream 2%, ketoconazole cream 2%, or nystatin ointment, 100,000 U/g; one tube (15 mg); apply to infected tissue 4 times per day

- Systemic Therapy

    Ketoconazole tabs, 200 mg; 14 tablets; 2 tabs the first day, subsequently 1 tab per day

    Fluconazole tabs, 100 mg; 14 tablets; 2 tabs the first day, subsequently 1 tab per day

matous, pseudomembranous, and angular cheilitis in patients with CD4+ cell counts above 200 cells/mm³. Oral systemic medications should be instituted for more resistant and refractory cases of pseudomembranous candidiasis as well as in patients with CD4+ cell counts below 200 cells/mm³. Refractory cases of candidiasis may also result from poor absorption of the antifungal medication. Ketoconazole is a commonly used oral antifungal medication that requires gastric acid for absorption. However, gastric hypochlorhydria may be present in patients with AIDS, which reduces the bioavailability of ketoconazole.[15] In such instances, this medication can be dissolved in a carbonated soft drink prior to ingestion. Chronic candidiasis usually does not respond to oral therapy, and intravenous delivery of antifungal medications should be considered. Oral troches should be avoided in patients with xerostomia. Since the troches will not dissolve efficiently and may even cause mucosal abrasions. In such cases, oral suspensions are more comfortable for the patients. Most of the available topical antifungal medications contain carbohydrates to improve the taste of the drug. However, these medications are cariogenic and should be avoided for long-term use in patients with poor oral hygiene or with xerostomia. Vaginal troches dissolved in the mouth are viable alternatives, although the compliance rate may be poor because of the taste of these medications.

In resistant cases, oral rinse with amphotericin B solution may be useful before systemic medications are used. This oral rinse consists of 50 mg of amphotericin B injection diluted in 500 mL of sterile water, resulting in a concentration of 0.1 mg/mL. Patients are instructed to use 15 mL and to swish and expectorate four times per day.[16]

The diagnosis of oral candidiasis is usually based on clinical appearance. However, histologic verification with KOH-, periodic acid-Schiff–, or gram-stained preparations supports the clinical impression. Intraoral candidiasis may have a similar appearance to oral hairy leukoplakia, but oral hairy leukoplakia is most commonly found on the tongue, cannot be removed by scraping, and does not respond to antifungal therapy.

Deep-Seated Fungal Infections: Cryptococcosis, Histoplasmosis, Geotrichosis, and Aspergillosis

Intraoral manifestations of systemic fungal infections, such as cryptococcosis, histoplasmosis, geotrichosis, and aspergillosis, are rare but have been described. These lesions are caused by *Cryptococcus neoformans,*[17] *Histoplasma capsulatum,*[18] *Geotrichum candidum,*[19] and *Aspergillus spp.*[20] and are always signs of disseminated disease. In some cases, the oral lesion may appear before any other manifestation of these infections. Cryptococcosis, histoplasmosis, and aspergillosis have been described as intraoral ulcerations, nodules, or necroses, while geotrichosis may manifest as a pseudomembrane-like lesion. Recognition of such a lesion results in early prevention and treatment. An accurate diagnosis can be established only after histologic verification of the causative pathogen.

Treatment consists of the intravenous administration of antifungal medications such as amphotericin B. Some patients with a history of cryptococcosis and low CD4+ cell counts may be taking a prophylactic regimen with fluconazole.

Viral Infections

Most of the intraoral viral infections in HIV-infected individuals are caused by various types of herpesvirus infections. Such infections can be expected, since this particular family of viruses is associated with periods of latency and reactivation, associated with clinical manifestations, that appear during periods of stress, trauma, or situations associated with immune deterioration and dysfunction. Other intraoral viral infections may be caused by various types of human papilloma viruses.

Herpes Simplex Virus

Reactivation of herpes simplex virus (HSV) infections primarily manifest as labial "cold sores" in immunocompetent individuals. These ulcerations heal within 7 to 10 days and will normally not require therapy. Although HSV infection is not more common among individuals with HIV, reactivation is accompanied by multiple, large, coalesced, painful, long-standing ulcerations that are in turn associated with a high degree of morbidity affecting the labial, palatal, and buccal mucosa (Fig 8-7).[21] The accompanying pain may cause affected individuals to cease oral nutritional intake, resulting in rapid weight loss. In severely immunocompromised individuals with HIV, reactivation of HSV may resemble primary herpetic gingivostomatitis which is usually seen only in patients with primary HSV infections. The HSV-associated ulcerations usually respond well to oral antiviral therapy,

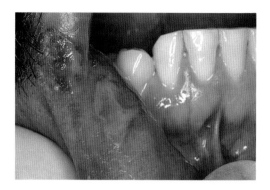

Fig 8-7. Confluent, large ulcerations caused by HSV.

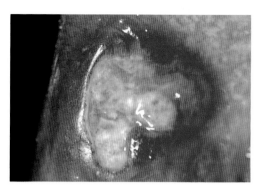

Fig 8-8. Cytomegalovirus-associated ulceration on the buccal mucosa.

such as acyclovir (200 mg orally four times a day), but acyclovir-resistant cases have been described.[22] Lesions caused by HSV Type 2 have a higher incidence of recurrence and are more common in resistant cases. Acyclovir-resistant cases have been successfully treated with intravenous foscarnet therapy.

Cytomegalovirus

Intraoral ulcerations associated with cytomegalovirus (CMV) infection have been reported in individuals with HIV (Fig 8-8).[23–25] Recognition of these lesions is important since they are early signs of disseminated CMV infection. However, CMV-associated ulcerations have a similar appearance to other viral-associated ulcers as well as to major aphthous ulcerations, necessitating histologic verification for a definitive diagnosis.

Cytomegalovirus infection may lead to CMV retinitis, which is the most common occular complication of AIDS.[26] Without treatment, this infec-

tion leads to blindness and death. One detailed necropsy study documented evidence of CMV infection in one or more organs among as many as 90% of AIDS patients.[27] Cytomegalovirus infections among HIV-infected individuals are associated with severe immune suppression; usually the CD4+ cell count is below 100 cells/mm^3.[28] The same relationship exists with intraoral manifestations associated with this infection, which appear only during severe immune deterioration.[6] Administration of intravenous ganciclovir is the most common treatment modality for disseminated CMV infections, but high doses of acyclovir (800 mg orally four times a day) may result in resolution of intraoral ulcerations.

Oral Hairy Leukoplakia

A novel oral lesion, oral hairy leukoplakia (OHL), was first reported in 1984 by Greenspan and coworkers in a cohort of 37 homosexual men from San Francisco.[29] This lesion was ini-

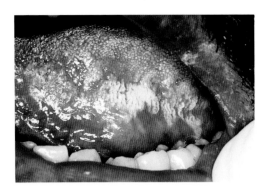

Fig 8-9. Oral hairy leukoplakia on the lateral border of the tongue.

tially described as being asymptomatic, with white vertically corrugated (resembling hair) hyperkeratotic-like projections that appear on the lateral borders of the tongue (Fig 8-9). The lesion can extend from a few millimeters on the lateral border(s) to the entire dorsal surface of the tongue, together with other mucosal surfaces.[30] Extralingual sites as well as sublingual surfaces are usually whitish and plaque-like, without the characteristic corrugated surface. Although the clinical appearance of the lesion is typical, hypertrophic candidiasis must be included in a differential diagnosis. Interestingly, approximately 50% of the lesions contain candidal hyphae,[31] indicating an association with immune suppression. Although original reports postulated that this lesion may be pathognomonic for HIV disease, subsequent studies have documented the presence of this lesion in patients with other types of immune suppression,[32] as well as in an immunocompetent individual.[33]

Since oral hairy leukoplakia is associated with a localized Epstein-Barr virus (EBV) infection, the appearance of this lesion is predictive of immune deterioration and HIV disease progression. In one study, OHL was documented in a median time of 24 months prior to an AIDS diagnosis and 41 months prior to death.[34] An average CD4+/CD8+ ratio of 0.24 (range, 0.04 to 1.0) and an average absolute CD4+ cell count of 149 cells/mm³ (range, 10 to 470 cells/mm³) were also reported in another study among a cohort of 95 HIV-infected individuals.[35] This is consistent with a recent study showing a mean CD4+ cell count of less than 150 cells/mm³ among a representative cohort of individuals with HIV presenting with OHL.[6] Interestingly, this lesion is significantly more common among homosexual/bisexual men than among other groups at risk for HIV infection.

For a definitive diagnosis of OHL, demonstration of EBV in the lesion is advantageous but not essential. In patients of unknown HIV status, a biopsy is indicated to verify a definitive diagnosis. This is important because of the high association between OHL and HIV infection. In patients with HIV, lack of response to antifungal therapy suggests a presumptive diagnosis of OHL.

Although this lesion has been reported to undergo spontaneous regression or disappear during antiretroviral therapy, treatment may be instituted because of patient complaints. Primary treatment consists of oral administration of acyclovir (800 mg orally four times per day).[36] Other systemic antiviral medications, such as

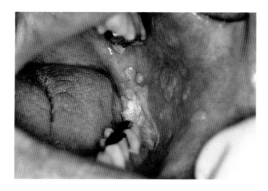

Fig 8-10. Focal epithelial hyperplasia of the retromolar area and the alveolar ridge caused by HPV.

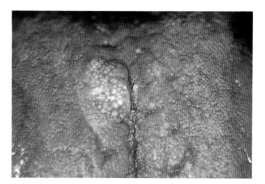

Fig 8-11. Large condyloma on the dorsum of the tongue.

desiclovir and ganciclovir[37]; topical application of podophyllum resin[38] and retinoids[39]; and surgical interventions[40] have also been successful in resolving the lesion. Cessation of therapy is usually associated with recurrence of the lesion and maintenance dose may be needed (acyclovir, 200 mg orally four times per day).

Human Papilloma Virus

Oral lesions associated with human papilloma virus (HPV) present as focal epithelial hyperplasia, oral papillomas, and condylomata (Figs 8-10 and 8-11).[21] Histologic verification is necessary since the clinical appearance may be nonspecific. The most common genotypes found in the oral mucosa in individuals without HIV are 2, 6, 11, 13, 16, and 32; but in patients with HIV, genotype 7 has also been reported.[41] Many treatment modalities have been suggested, but surgical excision and topical application of podophyllin resin have the highest success rate. The recurrence rate, however, is extremely high.

Bacterial Infections

Intraoral lesions associated with opportunistic bacterial infections have been reported to occur in HIV-infected individuals, but they appear to be rare. It is not always possible to ascertain if these lesions are caused primarily by the bacterial pathogens or if the presence of the pathogen is due to a secondary infection. Intraoral ulcerations associated with *Mycobacterium avium intracellulare* have been reported in a patient with disseminated AIDS.[42] Other infections, presumably caused by *Klebsiella pneumoniae*,[43] *Enterobacter cloacae*,[43] *Actinomyces israelii*,[44] and *Escherichia coli*,[45] have also been reported.

Bacillary Epithelioid Angiomatosis

An interesting new bacterial lesion, bacillary epithelioid angiomatosis (BEA), has been reported to occur cutaneously[46] and intraorally.[47] This lesion can easily be clinically misdiagnosed as Kaposi's sarcoma, which will

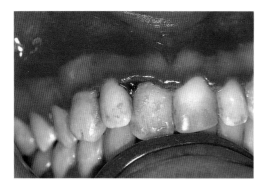

Fig 8-14a. Necrotizing ulcerative periodontitis before treatment.

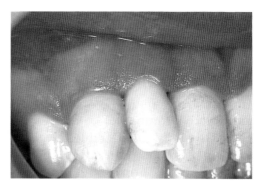

Fig 8-14b. Necrotizing ulcerative periodontitis (NUP) after 3 weeks of treatment.

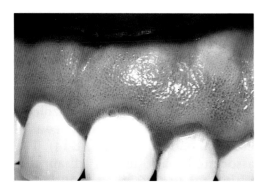

Fig 8–15. Linear gingival erythema. Note the linear erythematous marginal gingiva and the petechiae-like patches on the attached gingiva.

responds poorly to conventional periodontal therapy.

Syphilis

The vast majority of cases of syphilis in the United States before the HIV epidemic were among homosexual/bisexual men. However, very few reports of intraoral syphilis have been described among individuals with HIV. Intraoral manifestations of syphilis are well characterized and usually do not differ in individuals with HIV.[61] These oral lesions may be long-standing, nonhealing ulcerations, similar to gummatous lesions.[62] However, during severe immune deterioration, other manifestations of syphilis, including oral ulcerations, may be present.[63]

Neoplasms

Kaposi's Sarcoma

Kaposi's sarcoma (KS) is by far the most common intraoral neoplasm found in HIV-infected individuals.[64] Findings of intraoral KS are important since the first manifestation of the disease may occur in the oral cavity in 20% to 70% of cases,[6,65] making this lesion a diagnostic criterion for AIDS. Initial lesions are macular; red, purple or blue; and resemble physiologic pigmentation (Fig 8-16). Long-standing lesions may become nodular and

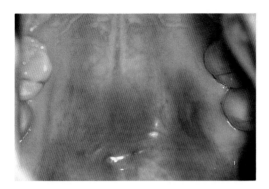

Fig 8-16. Macular KS lesion appearing as bluish, purplish areas on the soft palate.

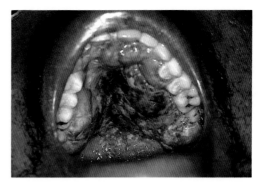

Fig 8-17. Nodular KS lesion covering the entire hard palate.

cover large areas of the palate and gingiva, and progress more rapidly (Fig 8-17). Painful ulcerations associated with KS have also been noted, especially in easily traumatized areas. Kaposi's sarcoma usually only involves soft tissue in the oral cavity, but intraosseous KS lesions have been suggested.[66] Although the clinical features of KS are usually distinguishable from other oral lesions found in HIV-infected patients, a definitive diagnosis with histopathologic confirmation is necessary to establish an AIDS diagnosis and to initiate appropriate therapy. Bacillary epithelioid angiomatosis may clinically resemble KS but can be differentiated with specific histologic stains.[47,67] Intraoral malignant lymphomas may also clinically resemble KS.[68,69]

Over 90% of intraoral AIDS-associated KS lesions appear on the hard or soft palate.[70] The gingiva is the second most common location but usually in conjunction with palatal lesions. However, any intraoral site can be affected, including the tongue and buccal mucosa. Extrapalatal manifestations of intraoral KS may be associated with a more rapid progression and a more aggressive course of the lesion (Fig 8-18).[71] One study of individuals with HIV indicated that oral manifestations of AIDS-associated KS were significantly more common in patients with lower CD4+ lymphocyte counts.[72] A mean CD4+ cell count of less than 70 cells/mm^3 and a predictive value of over 93% of finding this lesion in patients with CD4+ cell counts below 200 cell/mm^3 have also been reported.[6] Even changes in the appearance of the lesion—from flat, macular, to nodular form—may be associated with increased immune suppression.[73]

Intraoral KS has a higher predilection for homosexual/bisexual men compared to other groups at risk for HIV infection and is rarely found among HIV-infected women.[74]

There is no cure for KS, and therapy for intraoral lesions is intended only to reduce the size and number of lesions. Radiation therapy and surgical excision are the more common treatment modalities. Eradication of intraoral lesions can be achieved with low

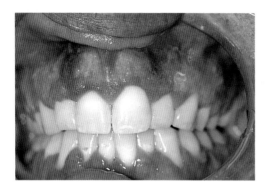

Fig 8-18a. Gingival KS.

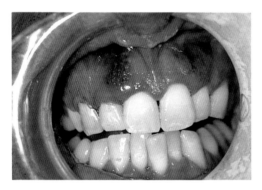

Fig 8-18b. Same gingival KS after 1 month duration.

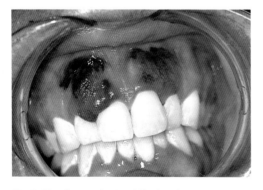

Fig 8-18c. Same gingival KS after 2 months' duration.

doses of radiation (800 to 2,000 rads). However, side effects such as stomatitis and glossitis are common and associated with severe pain and discomfort.[75] An antibacterial mouthrinse, such as chlorhexidine gluconate 0.12% (Peridex, Proctor & Gamble, Cincinnati, OH), used before radiation therapy may reduce the severity of these side effects. During the course of radiation therapy and for the ensuing 7 to 10 days, topical or systemic pain medications may be necessary to enable adequate oral nutritional intake.

Intralesional injections with various chemotherapeutic agents have been used successfully as an alternative treatment to radiation therapy. Injections of vinblastine (vinblastine sulfate, up to 0.1 mg/cm^2) into lesions have been reported to significantly reduce the size of the lesion.[76,77] This type of treatment has been associated with painful ulcerations and necrosis of the affected areas but only for short periods. Two recent reports have described intralesional sclerotherapy, with sodium tetradecyl sulfate (Sotradecol), up to 0.1 mL/cm^2 for the treatment of intraoral KS lesions.[78,79] This type of treatment is rapidly effective and well-tolerated. Few complaints of pain and discomfort were reported by the treated individuals. Long-term use of corticosteroids in patients with KS is contraindicated, since it has been associated with rapid progression of the lesions.[80]

Non-Hodgkin's Lymphoma

Non-Hodgkin's lymphoma (NHL) is the most common lymphoma found in the oral cavity among HIV-infected individuals. It usually presents as a rapidly growing mass involving the palate, maxillary, or mandibular gingiva.[53,81–83] However, macular and ulcerative NHL lesions have also been reported.[69,84] The signs and symptoms of intraoral NHL may present as excessive tooth mobility, intense tooth pain, progressive paresthesia, and widening of the periodontal ligament.[85] Intraoral NHL has been reported to be the initial sign of NHL in HIV-infected patients[86] and may occur with an incidence of between 1.1% and 4.4%.[87,88] One report indicated that 1.1% of 465 HIV-infected patients examined in an oral surgery department presented with a malignant lymphoma of the maxillary sinus or an intraoral lymphoma.[84] All of these patients had CD4+ cell counts below 100 cells/mm³. As with other neoplasms in HIV-infected individuals, NHL presents at a much earlier age than in persons without HIV. Treatment for NHL consists of polychemotherapy, but the mean survival rate is only 5 to 7 months.

Squamous Cell Carcinoma

Intraoral squamous cell carcinoma has been reported in patients with HIV,[89–90] but recent studies have shown that this oral carcinoma does not occur more frequently in this particular cohort.[91,92] It can, however, manifest at a younger age among individuals with HIV than that seen in patients without HIV.

Nonspecific Lesions

Hyperpigmentation

Oral hyperpigmentation secondary to medications such as zidovudine, clofazimine, and ketoconazole, as well as adrenal hypofunction, have been reported to occur in patients with HIV.[93,94] These brownish macular lesions are asymptomatic, but they may cause concern because of their clinically similar appearance to initial macular KS lesions. No treatment is necessary, and the lesions usually resolve spontaneously on cessation of the causative medication or after treatment for adrenal hypofunction.

Ulcerations Not Otherwise Specified

Nonspecific ulcerations in the oral cavity in HIV-infected patients are a diagnostic challenge to the clinician. Such ulcerations have been associated with the acute retroviral syndrome,[95] and use of specific medications, such as foscarnet,[96] interferon,[97] and dideoxycytidine (ddC)[98] but they are mainly categorized as ulcerations of unknown cause or ulcerations not otherwise specified.[5]

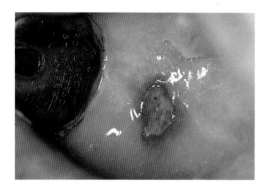

Fig 8-19. Minor aphthous ulceration without the surrounding classic red halo.

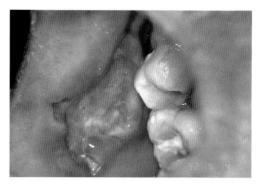

Fig 8-20. Major aphthous ulceration of the right buccal mucosa.

Minor Aphthous Ulcerations

Minor aphthous ulcerations are not more common among individuals with HIV[64] but they may last longer and be more severe in nature. These types of ulcers may also lack the characteristic red halo surrounding the ulceration because of the lack of an inflammatory response (Fig 8-19). Treatment is usually not indicated, but topical corticosteroid therapy may reduce the time of the acute phase. Analgesic mouthrinses could also be instituted for patient comfort.

Major Aphthous Ulcerations

Major aphthous ulcerations are associated with a high degree of morbidity but are not common among individuals with HIV, showing a prevalence of approximately 1% to 3%.[6,99,100] These lesions are classically defined as painful ulcerations with a diameter of greater than or equal to 10 mm, crateriform with a deeply eroded base that rarely undergoes spontaneous

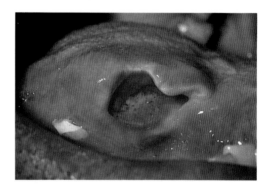

Fig 8-21a. Major aphthous ulceration before treatment.

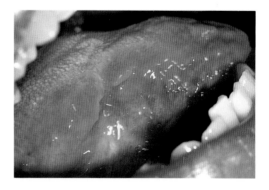

Fig 8-21b. Same major aphthous ulceration after 3 weeks of treatment. Note the scarring.

healing, and they are present for at least 3 weeks (Fig 8-20). Treatment of these ulcers is usually associated with scarring of the affected site (Fig 8-21). Major aphthous ulcerations have not been associated with any specific pathogen, but because of the long period of the acute phase, bacterial superinfections are not uncommon. This type of ulceration is associated with severe immune suppression. One study indicated that the median CD4+ cell counts among patients with major aphthous ulcerations was below 37 cells/mm^3.[100]

Treatment for major aphthous ulcerations usually consists of topical or systemic administration of glucocorticosteroids. However, long-term use of glucocorticosteroids may enhance a patient's immune suppression since these lesions usually appear only when the CD4+ cell count drops below 100 cells/mm^3.[100] Furthermore, one study has indicated that long-term corticosteroid use in patients with HIV and CD4+ cell counts below 50 cells/mm^3 increases the risk of developing clinical CMV disease.[101] As previously mentioned, an association between long-term glucocorticosteroid therapy and more rapid progression as well as the development of KS has been reported.[80] It appears that continuous glucocorticosteroid use for 2 weeks or intermittent use for 30 days affects progression of KS lesions. Regression of the glucocorticosteroid-induced KS lesions is noted on withdrawal of the steroids. Resolution of major aphthous ulcerations has also been accomplished with various antibacterial-antifungal-glucocortico-

Table 8-3. Treatment Modalities for Major Aphthous Ulcerations

- Mile's mixture (84 mg tetracycline, 84,000 U nystatin, 1.04 mg hydrocortisone per 5 mL); 280 mL; swish and expectorate 4 times per day

- Dexamethasone elixir, 0.5 mg/5 mL; 360 mL; rinse and swallow 1 tbs (15 mL) 4 times per day for 4 days, 2 tsp (10 mL) 3 times per day for 3 days, 1 tsp (5 mL) twice a day for 3 days

- Prednisone tabs, 5 mg; 72 tablets; 3 tabs 4 times per day for 4 days, 2 tabs 3 times per day for 3 days, 1 tab twice a day for 3 days

- Levamisole, 50 mg tabs; 27 tablets; 1 tab 3 times per day for 3 days followed by an 11-day latent period; repeat this cycle 3 times

steroid mouthrinses.[102] In refractory cases, levamisole therapy has been beneficial[102] (Table 8-3).

Treatment with thalidomide (200 mg twice a day for 5 days followed by 200 mg once daily) is also effective,[103,104] but this drug is not approved by the Food and Drug Administration and can be obtained only for compassionate use. Colchicine, an antichemotactic agent, also resolves recurrent aphthous ulcerations (0.6 mg two to three times a day) and could be used in patients who do not tolerate corticosteroid therapy or with glucocorticosteroids to reduce the dose of corticosteroids.[105]

Necrotizing Stomatitis

Necrotizing stomatitis (NS) is characterized as a localized acute painful ulceronecrotic lesion that exposes underlying bone and penetrates or

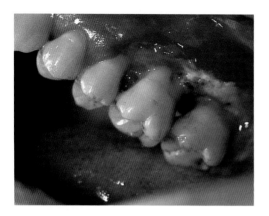

Fig 8-22. Necrotizing stomatitis affecting an area surrounding the upper left first and second molar.

extends into contiguous tissues (Fig 8-22).[106] During the initial stages of this lesion, only mild pain is present. However, intense pain is associated with more long-standing lesions and rapid alveolar bone loss. Similar to major aphthous ulcerations, no specific causative agent has been identified. The histopathologic features of NS and major aphthous ulcerations are also similar. It is possible that these two lesions are the same, with the location of the lesions being the only distinct feature. This lesion may also be a variant of periodontal disease and associated bacteria. Necrotizing stomatitis appears on mucosal tissue overlying osseous areas, while major aphthous ulcerations appear in soft mucosal tissue without underlying osseous structure.

Treatment consists of local and/or systemic antibacterial and corticosteroid therapy and, when anatomically feasible, construction of a mouthguard to protect the area from trauma and superinfections from the oral flora. This mouthguard also serves as a vehicle to deliver topical medications.[107]

Cause and Management of Intraoral Pain

Painful conditions in the oral cavity are associated with a high degree of morbidity, interfering with normal oral functions such as talking, mastication, and swallowing. Failure to treat pain associated with the oral cavity also results in decreased oral nutritional intake and subsequent weight loss, disruption of oral medication, and an impaired quality of life. Consequently, rapid intervention enables the patient to regain essential life functions.

Establishment of a diagnosis is the most important step in the management of oral pain. The pain can be tooth-related, associated with periapical pathologic states, secondary to various periodontal conditions, or as a sequela to dental therapy. These conditions are usually acute but readily treated by general dentists. Treatment for pain of odontogenic origin usually responds better to nonsteroidal anti-inflammatory drugs than to narcotics.[108]

Pain of neurologic and/or myofascial origin is more chronic in nature, is usually caused by a multitude of factors, and can be difficult to diagnose.

Cranial nerves V, VII, and VIII have been affected in patients with HIV, resulting in sensory and motor loss.[109] Conditions causing pain along the

Table 8-4. Causes and Treatment of Oral Pain

- Cause
  - Odontogenic
    - Tooth-related
      - Periapical
      - Periodontal
        - Pericoronitis
    - Dental therapy
      - Endodontic flare-ups
      - Alveolar osteitis
  - Neurologic/myofascial
    - Temporomandibular joint disorders
    - Myofascial pain
    - Trigeminal neuralgia
    - Postherpetic neuralgia
    - Trigeminal and facial neuropathy of unknown origin
  - Ulcerative lesions
    - Fungal
      - Aspergillosis
      - Candidiasis
      - Cryptococcosis
      - Histoplasmosis
    - Viral
      - Cytomegalovirus
      - Herpes simplex virus
      - Varicella-zoster
    - Bacterial
      - Enterobacteriae
      - Mycobacterial
      - Necrotizing ulcerative periodontitis
      - Syphilitic
    - Neoplastic
      - Kaposi's sarcoma
      - Non-Hodgkin's lymphoma
    - Nonspecific
      - Aphthous ulcerations
      - Necrotizing stomatitis
  - Nonulcerative lesions
    - Mucositis
      - Associated with candidiasis
      - Bacterial superinfections of other usually asymptomatic lesions such as oral hairy leukoplakia
      - Secondary to radiation therapy
    - Xerostomia
    - Nutritional deficiencies
- Treatment
  - Disease-specific
  - Symptomatic
  - Nutritional supplement

trigeminal nerve have been reported to be associated with progressive multifocal leukoencephalopathy[110] or lymphoblastic leukemia.[111]

Oral pain is a common complaint during the course of HIV disease. In a retrospective study of 96 hospitalized individuals with HIV, 8% of patients complained of oral pain on admission, while 11% of all patients had complaints of oral pain during their hospital stay.[112] Both odontogenic and neurologic pain associated with the oral cavity are usually not more common or severe among individuals with HIV. However, most painful oral conditions in patients with HIV are associated with oral lesions (Table 8-4).

Symptomatic relief for painful conditions in the oral cavity can be accomplished with analgesic mouthrinses. Mucosal protectives are sometimes used to enhance the effect of the analgesic. Very few, if any, side effects have been associated with such medications (Table 8-5).

Xerostomia

Dry mouth or xerostomia is a common complaint among individuals with HIV. This may be a sign of parotid gland disease,[113,114] but it is also associated with side effects from various medications commonly used by HIV-infected patients. These medications include zidovudine, ddI, foscarnet, antianxiety agents, antihistamines, anticholinergics, antihypertensives,

Table 8-5. Analgesic Mouthrinses and Pastes

- 2% to 4% viscous lidocaine solution; 280 mL; swish and expectorate as needed for pain

- 1% dyclonine and diphenhydramine elixir (1:1 ratio); 280 mL; swish and expectorate as needed for pain

- Other solutions and pastes (mostly as ointments or gels)

    2%–5% lidocaine

    4%–6% cocaine

    0.5%–2% tetracaine

    0.25%–1% dibucaine

    30% benzocaine

- Mucosal protective

    Kaopectate solution; 280 mL; swish and expectorate

decongestants, diuretics, narcotic analgesics (meperidine), and tricyclic antidepressants.[115] Radiation therapy to the head and neck region can also cause xerostomia. Decreased salivary flow enhances the growth of candidal infections in the oral cavity and may contribute to abrasions of the oral mucosa when antifungal troches are dissolving.

Relief from oral dryness can be accomplished by encouraging the patient to continuously sip water during the day or suck on crushed ice. The use of humidifiers at night and application of vaseline to the lips also reduce discomfort. Patients should also avoid any liquids containing caffeine or alcohol, since these compounds act as diuretics.

Conservative therapy also includes the stimulation of salivary flow by chewing sugarless gum or sucking on sugarless candies. Decreased salivary flow promotes the rate of tooth decay; thus, only sugarless stimulants should be used.

Commercial over-the-counter artificial saliva substitutes may be instituted to achieve temporary relief from severe dryness (Sali-Synt, Moi—Stir, Orex, V.A. Dralube, Xero-Lube).[116]

The use of pilocarpine to stimulate salivary flow has also been studied with various degrees of success.[117] A low starting dose should be gradually increased to achieve an individual therapeutic beneficial response without causing side effects (2.5 mg three times per day to 7.5 mg three times per day as tablets or solution). Patients on this type of medication must be followed up by their physician for side effects, including excessive sweating and cardiovascular symptoms. Discontinuation or change of xerostomia-causing drugs is a viable solution prior to treatment for this condition. This should be done in accordance with the patient's physicians.

Nutritional Deficiencies

Nutritional deficiencies, such as vitamin B_{12} deficiency, present with a fiery red, painful tongue, loss of taste sensation, and sometimes loss of muscle tone of the tongue. The mucosa may take on a yellowish-green color and may be so sore that denture wearers cannot use their dentures.

Oral manifestations of folate deficiency are similar to those of vitamin B_{12} deficiency, but angular cheilitis, ulcerations of the mucosa and periodontal tissue, and pharyngitis may be present.

Alleviation of pain can be accomplished with analgesic mouthrinses, but the underlying vitamin B_{12} and folate deficiencies must be corrected. In general, mouthrinses with high alcohol content should be avoided in patients with ulcerations and mucositis, since these compounds may exacerbate the pain. Adjunct therapy with mucosal protectives, such as Kaopectate, is not associated with any side effects and will benefit patients. Furthermore, it is of the utmost importance that patients experiencing oral pain continue their oral nutritional intake. Additional nutritional supplements should be used in all patients with impaired oral functions.

References

1. Glick M. Evaluation of prognosis and survival of HIV infected patients. Oral Surg Oral Med Oral Pathol 1992;74:386–392.

2. Scully C, Laskaris G, Pindborg J, Porter SR, Reichart P. Oral manifestations of HIV infection and their management. I. More common lesions. Oral Surg Oral Med Oral Pathol 1991;71:158–166.

3. Scully C, Laskaris G, Pindborg J, Porter SR, Reichert P. Oral manifestations of HIV infection and their management. II. Less common lesions. Oral Surg Oral Med Oral Pathol 1991;71:167–171.

4. Greenspan JS, Barr CE, Sciubba JJ, Winkler JR, USA Oral AIDS Collaborative Group. Oral manifestations of HIV infection: definitions, diagnostic criteria and principles of therapy. Oral Surg Oral Med Oral Pathol 1992;73:142–144.

5. EC-Clearinghouse on Oral Problems Related to HIV Infection and WHO Collaborating Centre on Oral Manifestations of the Immunodeficiency Virus. Classification and diagnostic criteria for oral lesions in HIV infection. J Oral Pathol Med 1993;22:289–291.

6. Glick M, Muzyka BC, Lurie D, Salkin LM. Oral manifestations associated with HIV disease as markers for immune suppression and AIDS. Oral Surg Oral Med Oral Pathol 1994;77:344–349.

7. Franker CK, Lucartorto FM, Johnson BS, Jacobsen JJ. Characterization of the mycoflora from oral mucosal surfaces of some HIV-infected patients. Oral Surg Oral Med Oral Pathol 1990; 69:683–687.

8. Samaranayake LP. Oral mycoses in HIV infection. Oral Surg Oral Med Oral Pathol 1992;73:171–180.

9. Brawner DL, Cutler JE. Oral *Candida albicans* isolates from nonhospitalized normal carriers, immunocompetent hospitalized patients, and immunocompromised patients with or without acquired immunodeficiency syndrome. J Clin Microbiol 1989;27:1335–1341.

10. Fotos PG, Vincent SD, Hellstein JW. Oral candidosis. Oral Surg Oral Med Oral Pathol 1992;74:41–49.

11. Klein RS, Harris CA, Butkus Small C, Moll B, Lesser M, Friedland GH. Oral candidiasis in high-risk patients as the initial manifestation of the acquired immunodeficiency syndrome. N Engl J Med 1984; 311:354–358.

12. McCarthy GM, Mackie ID, Koval J, Sandhu HS, Daley TD. Factors associated with increased frequency of HIV-related oral candidiasis. J Oral Pathol Med 1991; 20:332–336.

13. Korting HC, Ollert M, Georgii A, Froschl M. In vitro susceptibilities and biotypes of *Candida albicans* isolates from the oral cavities of patients infected with human immunodeficiency virus. J Clin Microbiol 1989;26:2626–2631.

14. Gottlieb MS, Schanker HM, Fan PT, Saxon A, Weisman JO, Pozalski I. Pneumocystis pneumonia—Los Angeles. MMWR 1981;30:250–251.

15. Lake-Bakaar G, Tom W, Lake-Bakaar D, Gupta N, Beidas S, Elsakr M, Straus E. Gastropathy and ketoconazole malabsorption in the acquired immunodeficiency syndrome (AIDS). Ann Intern Med 1988;109:471–473.

16. Branfell R, Chase SL, Cohn JR. Treatment of oral candidiasis with amphotericin B solution. Clin Pharmacol 1988;7:70–72.

17. Glick M, Cohen SG, Cheney RT, Crooks GW, Greenberg MS. Oral manifestations of disseminated *cryptococcus neoformans* in a patient with acquired immunodeficiency syndrome. Oral Surg Oral Med Oral Pathol 1987;64:454–459.

18. Heinic GS, Greenspan D, MacPhail LA, et al. Oral *Histoplasma capsulatum* infection in association with HIV infection: a case report. J Oral Pathol Med 1992;21:85–89.

19. Heinic GS, Greenspan D, MacPhail LA, Greenspan JS. Oral *Geotrichum candidum* infection associated with HIV infection. Oral Surg Oral Med Oral Pathol 1992;73:726–728.

20. Rubin MM, Jui V, Sadoff RS. Oral aspergillosis in a patient with acquired immunodeficiency syndrome. J Oral Maxillofac Surg 1990;48:997–999.

21. Eversole LR. Viral infections of the head and neck among HIV-seropositive patients. Oral Surg Oral Med Oral Pathol 1992;73:155–163.

22. MacPhail LA, Greenspan D, Schiodt M, Drennan DP, Mills J. Acyclovir-resistant, foscarnet-sensitive oral herpes simplex type 2 lesion in a patient with AIDS. Oral Surg Oral Med Oral Pathol 1989;67:427–432.

23. Glick M, Cleveland DB, Salkin LM, Alfaro-Miranda M, Fielding AF. Intraoral cytomegalovirus lesion and HIV-associated periodontitis in a patient with acquired immunodeficiency syndrome. Oral Surg Oral Med Oral Pathol 1991;72:716–720.

24. Jones AC, Freedman PD, Phelan JA, Baughman RA, Kerpel SM. Cytomegalovirus infections of the oral cavity. A report of six cases and review of the literature. Oral Surg Oral Med Oral Pathol 1993;75:76–85.

25. Dodd CL, Winkler JR, Heinic GS, Daniels TE, Yee K, Greenspan D. Cytomegalovirus infection presenting as acute periodontal infection in a patient infected with the human immunodeficiency virus. J Clin Periodontol 1993;20:282–285.

26. Pertel P, Hirschtick R, Phair J, Chmiel J, Poggensee L, Murphy R. Risk of developing cytomegalovirus retinitis in persons infected with the human immunodeficiency virus. J Acquired Immune Deficiency Syndrome 1992;5:1069–1074.

27. Drew WL, Sweet ES, Miner RC, Mocarski ES. Multiple infections by cytomegalovirus in patients with acquired immunodeficiency syndrome: documentation with Southern blot hybridization. J Infect Dis 1984;150:952–953.

28. Crowe SM, Carlin JB, Stewart KI, Lucas CR, Hoy JF. Predictive value of CD4 lymphocyte numbers for the development of opportunistic infections and malignancies in HIV-infected persons. J Acquired Immune Deficiency Syndrome 1991;4:770–776.

29. Greenspan D, Greenspan JS, Conant M, Petersen V, Silverman Jr S, de Souza Y. Oral "hairy" leucoplakia in male homosexuals: evidence of association with papillomavirus and a herpes-group virus. Lancet 1984;2:831–834.

30. Kabani S, Greenspan D, deSouza Y, Greenspan JS, Cataldo E. Oral hairy leukoplakia with extensive oral mucosal involvement. Oral Surg Oral Med Oral Pathol 1989;67:411–415.

31. Kanas RJ, Abrams AM, Jensen JL, Wuerker RB, Handlers JP. Oral hairy leukoplakia: ultrastructural observations. Oral Surg Oral Med Oral Pathol 1988;65:333–338.

32. Syrjanen S, Laine P, Happonen R-P, Niemela M. Oral hairy leukoplakia is not a specific sign of HIV-infection but related to immunosuppression in general. J Oral Pathol Med 1989;18:28–31.

33. Felix DH, Watret K, Wray D, Southam JC. Hairy leukoplakia in an HIV-negative, nonimmunosuppressed patient. Oral Surg Oral Med Oral Pathol 1992;74:563–566.

34. Greenspan D, Greenspan JS, Overby G, et al. Risk factors for rapid progression from hairy leukoplakia to AIDS: a nested case-control study. J Acquired Immune Deficiency Syndrome 1991;4:652–658.

35. Reichart PA, Langford A, Gelderblom HR, Pohle HD, Becker J, Wolf H. Oral hairy leukoplakia: observations in 95 cases and review of the literature. J Oral Pathol Med 1989;18:410–415.

36. Glick M, Pliskin ME. Regression of oral hairy leukoplakia after oral administration of acyclovir. Gen Dent 1990;38:374–375.

37. Greenspan JS, Greenspan D. Oral hairy leukoplakia: diagnosis and management. Oral Surg Oral Med Oral Pathol 1989;67:396–403.

38. Lozada-Nur F. Podophyllin resin 25% for treatment of oral hairy leukoplakia: an old treatment for a new lesion. J Acquired Immune Deficiency Syndrome 1991;4:543–546.

39. Lozada-Nur F. Common early oral markers: clinical presentation, diagnostic techniques and management of early oral markers of HIV infection. J Calif Dent Assoc 1989;17:36–45.

40. Herbst JS, Morgan J, Raab-Traub N, Resnick L. Comparison of the efficacy of surgery and acyclovir therapy in oral hairy leukoplakia. J Am Acad Dermatol 1989;21:753–756.

41. Greenspan D, deVilliers EM, Greenspan JS, deSouza YG, zur Hausen H. Unusual HPV types in oral warts in association with HIV infection. J Oral Pathol 1988;17:482–487.

42. Volpe F, Schwimmer A, Barr C. Oral manifestation of disseminated *Mycobacterium avium intracellulare* in a patient with AIDS. Oral Surg Oral Med Oral Pathol 1985;60:567–570.

43. Greenspan D, Greenspan JS, Pindborg JJ, Schiodt M. AIDS and the dental team. Copenhagen: Munksgaard, 1986.

44. Yeager BA, Hoxie J, Weisman RA, Greenberg MS, Bilaniuk LT. Actinomycosis in the acquired immunodeficiency syndrome-related complex. Arch Otolaryngol Head Neck Surg 1986;112:1293–1295.

45. Silverman Jr, S. AIDS update: oral findings, diagnosis, and precautions. J Am Dent Assoc 1987;115:559–563.

46. Cockerell CJ, Whitlow MA, Webster GF, Friedman-Kien AE. Epithelioid angiomatosis: a distinct vascular disorder in patients with the acquired immunodeficiency syndrome or AIDS-related complex. Lancet 1987;2:654–656.

47. Glick M, Cleveland DB. Oral mucosal bacillary (epithelioid) angiomatosis in a patient with AIDS associated with rapid alveolar bone loss—Report of a case. J Oral Pathol Med 1993;22:235–239.

48. Koehler JE, Tappero JW. Bacillary angiomatosis in patients infected with human immunodeficiency virus. Clin Infect Dis 1993;17:612–624.

49. Yeung SCH, Stewart GJ, Cooper DA, Sindhusake D. Progression of periodontal disease in HIV seropositive patients. J Periodontol 1993;64:651–657.

50. Lucht E, Heimdahl A, Nord CE. Periodontal disease in HIV-infected patients in relation to lymphocyte subsets and specific micro-organisms. J Clin Periodontol 1991;18:252–256.

51. Yeung SCH, Stewart GJ, Cooper DA, Sindhusake D. Progression of periodontal disease in HIV seropositive patients. J Periodontol 1993;64:651–657.

52. Moore LVH, Moore WEC, Riley C, Brooks CN, Burmeister JA, Smibert RM. Periodontal microflora of HIV positive subjects with gingivitis or adult periodontitis. J Periodontol 1993;64:48–56.

53. Groot RH, van Merkesteyn JPR, Bras J. Oral manifestations of non-Hodgkin's lymphoma in HIV-infected patients. Int J Oral Maxillofac Surg 1990;19:194–196.

54. Palmer GD, Morgan PR, Challacombe SJ. T-cell lymphoma associated with periodontal disease and HIV infection. J Clin Periodontol 1993;20:378–380.

55. Zambon JJ, Reynolds HS, Genco RJ. Studies of the subgingival microflora in patients with acquired immunodeficiency syndrome. J Periodontol 1990;61:699–704.

56. Weiss SJ. Tissue destruction by neutrophils. N Engl J Med 1989;320:365–376.

57. Winkler JR, Murray PA, Grassi M, Hammerle C. Diagnosis and management of HIV-associated periodontal lesions. J Am Dent Ass 1989;119(suppl):25–34.

58. Glick M, Muzyka BC, Salkin LM, Lurie D. Necrotizing ulcerative periodontitis: a marker for immune deterioration and a predictor for the diagnosis of AIDS. J Periodontol 1994;65:393–397.

59. Masouredis CM, Katz MH, Greenspan D, et al. Prevalence of HIV-associated periodontitis and gingivitis in HIV-infected patients attending an AIDS clinic. J Acquir Immune Deficiency Syndrome 1992;5:479–483.

60. Glick M, Pliskin ME, Weiss RC. The clinical and histologic appearance of HIV-associated gingivitis. Oral Surg Oral Med Oral Pathol 1990;69:395–398.

61. Regezi JA, Sciubba JJ. Oral pathology: clinical pathologic correlations. Philadelphia: WB Saunders; 1989:34–37.

62. Kearns G, Pogrel MA, Honda G. Intraoral syphilis (gumma) in a human immunodeficiency virus-positive man: a case report. J Oral Maxillofac Surg 1993;51:85–88.

63. Ficarra G, Zaragoza AM, Stendardi L, Parri F, Cockerell CJ. Early oral presentation of lues maligna in a patient with HIV infection. Oral Surg Oral Med Oral Pathol 1993;75:728–732.

64. Epstein JB, Silverman Jr S. Head and neck malignancies associated with HIV infection. Oral Surg Oral Med Oral Pathol 1992;73:193–200.

65. Ficarra G, Berson AM, Silverman Jr S, et al. Kaposi's sarcoma of the oral cavity: a study of 134 patients with a review of the pathogenesis, epidemiology, clinical aspects, and treatment. Oral Surg Oral Med Oral Pathol 1988;66:543–560.

66. Langford A, Pohle H-D, Reichart P. Primary intraosseous AIDS-associated Kaposi's sarcoma. Int J Maxillofac Surg 1991;20:366–368.

67. Regezi JA, MacPhail LA, Daniels TE, et al. Oral Kaposi's sarcoma: a 10-year retrospective histopathologic study. J Oral Pathol Med 1993;22:292–297.

68. Reichart PA, Schiodt M. Non-pigmented oral Kaposi's sarcoma. Int J Oral Maxillofac Surg 1989;18:197–199.

69. Dodd CL, Greenspan D, Schiodt M, et al. Unusual oral presentation of non-Hodgkin's lymphoma in association with HIV infection. Oral Surg Oral Med Oral Pathol 1992;73:603–608.

70. Epstein JB, Scully C. HIV infection: clinical features and treatment of thirty-three homosexual men with Kaposi's sarcoma. Oral Surg Oral Med Oral Pathol 1991;71:38–41.

71. Chaudhry AP, Chachoua A, Saltzman BR, et al. AIDS-associated Kaposi's sarcoma. J Am Dent Assoc 1987;115:824–825.

72. Feigal DW, Katz MH, Greenspan D, et al. The prevalence of oral lesions in HIV-infected homosexual and bisexual men: three San Francisco epidemiological cohorts. AIDS 1991;5:519–525.

73. Petit JC, Ripamonti U, Hille J. Progressive changes of Kaposi's sarcoma of the gingiva and palate. J Periodontol 1986;57:159–163.

74. Dodd CL, Greenspan D, Greenspan JS. Oral Kaposi's sarcoma in a woman as a first indication of HIV infection. J Am Dent Assoc 1991;122:61–63.

75. Cooper S, Fried PR. Toxicity of oral radiotherapy in patients with acquired immunodeficiency syndrome. Arch Otolaryngol Head Neck Surg 1987;113:327–328.

76. Epstein JB, Lozada-Nur F, McLeod WA, et al. Oral Kaposi's sarcoma in acquired immunodeficiency syndrome. Review of management and report of the efficacy of intralesional vinblastine. Cancer 1989;64:2424–2430.

77. Nichols MC, Flaitz CM, Hicks MJ. Treating Kaposi's sarcoma lesions in HIV-infected patients. J Am Dent Assoc 1993;124:78–84.

78. Muzyka BC, Glick M. Sclerotherapy for the treatment of nodular intraoral Kaposi's sarcoma in patients with AIDS. N Engl J Med 1993;328:210–211.

79. Lucatorto FM, Sapp JP. Treatment of oral Kaposi's sarcoma with sclerosing agent in AIDS patients. Oral Surg Oral Med Oral Pathol 1993;75:192–198.

80. Gill PS, Lourerio C, Bernstein-Singer M, Rarick MU, Sattler F, Levine AM. Clinical effect of glucocorticosteroids on Kaposi's sarcoma related to the acquired immunodeficiency syndrome (AIDS). Ann Intern Med 1989;110:937–940.

81. Kaugars GE, Burns JC. Non-Hodgkin's lymphoma of the oral cavity associated with AIDS. Oral Surg Oral Med Oral Pathol 1989;67:433–436.

82. Brahim JS, Katz RW, Roberts MW. Non-Hodgkin's lymphoma of the hard palate mucosa and buccal gingiva associated with AIDS. J Oral Maxillofac Surg 1988; 46:328–330.

83. Green TL, Eversole LR. Oral lymphomas in HIV-infected patients: association with Epstein-Barr virus DNA. Oral Surg Oral Med Oral Pathol 1989;67:437–442.

84. Langford A, Dienemann D, Schurman D, et al. Oral manifestations of AIDS-associated non-Hodgkin's lymphomas. Int J Oral Maxillofac Surg 1991;20:136–141.

85. Vallejo GH, Garcia MD, Lopez A, Mendieta C, Moskow BS. Unusual periodontal findings in an AIDS patient with Burkitt's lymphoma. J Periodontol 1989;60:723–727.

86. Colmenero C, Gamallo G, Pintado V, Patron M, Sierra I, Valencia E. AIDS-related lymphoma of the oral cavity. Int J Oral Maxillofac Surg 1991;20:2–6.

87. Kaplan LD, Abrams DI, Feigal E, et al. AIDS-associated non-Hodgkin's lymphoma in San Francisco. JAMA 1989;26:719–724.

88. Ziegler JL, Beckstead JA, Volberding PA, et al. Non-Hodgkin's lymphoma in 90 homosexual men: relation to generalized lymphadenopathy and the acquired immunodeficiency syndrome. N Engl J Med 1984;311:565–570.

89. Silverman S Jr, Migliorati CA, Lozada-Nur F, Greenspan D, Conant M. Oral findings in people with or at high risk for AIDS: a study of 375 homosexual males. J Am Dent Assoc 1986;112:187–192.

90. Tenzer JA, Sugarman M, Britton JC. Squamous cell carcinoma of the gingiva found in a patient with AIDS. J Am Dent Assoc 1992;123:65–67.

91. Biggar RJ, Burnett W, Mikl J, Nasca P. Cancer among New York men at risk of acquired immune deficiency syndrome. Int J Cancer 1989;43:979–985.

92. Monfardini S, Vaccher E, Pizzocara G, et al. Unusual malignant tumors in 49 patients with HIV infection. AIDS 1989;3:449–452.

93. Langford A, Pohle H-D, Gelderblom H, Zhang X, Reichart PA. Oral hyperpigmentation in HIV-infected patients. Oral Surg Oral Med Oral Pathol 1989;67:301–307.

94. Porter SR, Glover S, Scully C. Oral hyperpigmentation and adrenocortical hypofunction in a patient with acquired immunodeficiency syndrome. Oral Surg Oral Med Oral Pathol 1990;70:59–60.

95. Tindall B, Cooper DA. Primary HIV infection: host response and intervention strategies. AIDS 1991;5:1–14.

96. Gilquin J, Weiss L, Kazatchkine MD. Genital and oral erosions induced by foscarnet. Lancet 1990;335:287.

97. Penneys NS, Hick B. Unusual cutaneous lesions associated with acquired immune deficiency syndrome. J Am Acad Dermatol 1985;13:845–852.

98. McNeeley MC, Yarchoan R, Broder S, Lawley TJ. Dermatologic complications associated with administration of 2',3'-dideoxycytidine in patients with human immunodeficiency virus infection. J Am Acad Dermatol 1989;21:1213–1217.

99. Phelan JA, Eisig S, Freedman PD, Newsome N, Klein RS. Major aphthous-like ulcers in patients with AIDS. Oral Surg Oral Med Oral Pathol 1991;71:68–72.

100. Muzyka BC, Glick M. Major oral ulcerations in HIV disease. Oral Surg Oral Med Oral Pathol 1994;77:116–120.

101. Nelson MR, Erskine D, Hawkins DA, Gazzard BG. Treatment with corticosteroids—a risk factor for development of clinical cytomegalovirus disease in AIDS. AIDS 1993;7:375–378.

102. Glick M, Muzyka BC. Alternate treatment for major aphthous ulcerations in patients with AIDS. J Am Dent Assoc 1992;123:61–65.

pound through laboratory and animal studies. Approval for investigational new drug (IND) status by the FDA depends on the preclinical testing results. An integral part of IND approval is the manufacturer's specific stated purpose for the proposed use of the drug.

The human testing stage is initiated only after a drug has an approved IND status. This stage is divided into three clinical phases.

In phase I, 20 to 80 healthy volunteers are tested for less than a year to determine the drug's pharmacologic action, safe dose range, absorption, distribution, metabolism and excretion, and the duration of action. In phase II, the drug is administered to 100 to 300 patient volunteers for approximately 2 years to assess the drug's effectiveness and safety. These individuals can have different stages of the disease, depending on the purpose of the drug. During phase III, 1,000 to 3,000 patient volunteers are used to confirm efficacy and identify adverse reactions to the drug from long-term use. This phase continues for about 3 years. If all three clinical phases are successful, a new drug application (NDA) is submitted to the FDA. The NDA review process and final approval by the FDA may take an additional 2 to 3 years. Only after NDA approval can a drug manufacturer begin to market and distribute the drug.

Because of lobbying from HIV-infected persons and other concerned individuals, some exceptions to this process have been granted. Certain drugs that show promising results during phase I and that are intended for serious and life-threatening diseases can be processed with an *expedited review*. This may reduce the time for Phase II and Phase III by 2 to 3 years. Furthermore, a physician can obtain approval, under special circumstances, to use a drug for a purpose not described in an IND protocol. This falls under the category of *compassionate use*.

Much discussion has focused on which parameter should be used to assess both beneficial response and end points for clinical trials. The FDA has accepted CD4+ T-helper lymphocyte counts as a marker for the effectiveness of anti-HIV therapy. However, other markers have also been proposed: p24 antigenemia, HIV viremia, presence of proviral DNA, neopterin levels, and ß$_2$-microglobulin levels. On the basis of present knowledge, the CD4+ cell count remains the most reliable standard.[2]

By the end of 1993, the Pharmaceutical Manufacturers Association indicated that 103 drugs and a larger number of drug combinations were being developed for use in HIV disease. Only 21 drugs have been approved by the FDA for the treatment of AIDS and AIDS-related conditions, compared to 1 in 1987 (Tables 9-1 and 9-2).[3]

Therapeutic and Prophylactic Modalities

The management of HIV disease can arbitrarily be divided into a preventive

Table 9-1. Approved AIDS Medications*

Generic Drug Name	Trade Name	Indication
Acyclovir	Zovirax†	Herpes zoster and herpes simplex virus
Atovaquone	Mepron†	Treatment of PCP in patients not tolerating trimethoprim-sulfamethoxazole
Didanosine (ddI)	Videx‡	Patients with HIV not tolerating, or not showing clinical progress with, zidovudine therapy
Dronarinol	Marinol§	Treatment of anorexia associated with weight loss in patients with AIDS
Epoetin alfa	Procrit‖	Anemia in patients receiving zidovudine
Fluconazole	Diflucan¶	Cryptococcal meningitis, candidiasis
Foscarnet sodium	Foscavir#	CMV retinitis
Ganciclovir	Cytovene**	CMV retinitis
Interferon alpha-2a	Roferon-A††	Kaposi's sarcoma
Interferon alpha-2b	Intron A‡‡	Kaposi's sarcoma
Itraconazole	Sporanox§§	Histoplasmosis, blastomycosis
Ketoconazole	Nizoral§§	Histoplasmosis, blastomycosis, candidiasis
Megestrol acetate (oral suspension)	Megace‡	Treatment of anorexia and cachexia associated with AIDS
Pentamidine isethionate, aerosol	NebuPent‖‖	PCP prophylaxis
Pentamidine isethionate, IM and IV	Pentam 300‖‖	PCP treatment
Pyrimethamine	Daraprim†	Toxoplasmosis treatment
Rifabutin	Mycobutin¶¶	MAC prophylaxis
stavudine or d4T	Zerit‡	Patients with HIV who have shown no benefit or have become intolerant to other antiretroviral drugs

Table 9-1. *(continued)*

Generic Drug Name	Trade Name	Indication
Trimethoprim-sulfamethoxazole	Bactrim[††], Septra[†]	PCP treatment
Zalcitabine (ddC)	HIVID[††]	In combination with zidovudine in patients with CD4+ cell counts less than or equal to 300 cells/mm³
Zidovudine (AZT)	Retrovir[†]	Asymptomatic and symptomatic patients with CD4+ cell counts below 500 cells/mm³

*Adapted from AIDS Medicines in Development. Washington DC: Pharmaceutical Manufacturers Association; 1993.
[†]Burroughs Wellcome, Research Triangle Park, NC.
[‡]Bristol-Myers Squibb, New York, NY.
[§]Unimed, Buffalo Grove, IL.
[||]Ortho Biotech, Raritan, NJ.
[¶]Pfizer, New York, NY.

[#]Astra Pharmaceutical, Westborough, MA.
[**]Syntex, Palo Alto, CA.
[††]Hoffman-La Roche, Nutley, NJ.
[‡‡]Schering-Plough, Madison, NJ.
[§§]Janssen Pharmaceutica, Titusville, NJ.
[||||]Fujisawa, Deerfield, IL.
[¶¶]Adria Laboratories, Columbus, OH.

and a treatment branch. Each branch includes anti-retrovirals to prevent further infection and slow down the replication of HIV, cytokines to offset cell depletion often associated with anti-retroviral therapy, immune modulators to improve the existing immune response, and anti-infectives for opportunistic infections.

Most patients are treated with combinations of different medications. Such an approach is becoming increasingly common and has many advantages over single drug therapy: it may extend the duration of effectiveness beyond that of a single drug; it has the potential for synergistic activity; it may diminish the development of resistant viral strains; and it may reduce the level of side effects from a single agent by decreasing dosages.

Anti-Retroviral Therapy

The ideal drug for HIV treatment must be easy to administer, preferably orally with a good oral bioavailability profile to penetrate the blood-brain barrier, and must not create resistant viral strains after long-term administration. This optimum agent is yet to be found.

Several different approaches have been applied to prevent or slow HIV infectivity and replication (Fig 9-1). The most common, and the only FDA-approved, anti-retroviral therapy in-

Table 9-2. Common Drugs Used in HIV Disease and Their Indications*

Name of Drug†	Indications‡
acyclovir (Zovirax) caps, tabs, susp . . .	Antiherpetic
Adriamycin (*see* doxorubicin)	
alprazolam (Xanax) tabs	Antianxiety
Amgen (*see* filgrastim)	
amikacin (Amikin) IM	Antibacterial (MAC)
Amikin (*see* amikacin)	
amitriptyline (Elavil) tabs, IM hydrochloride	Tricyclic antidepressant
amphotericin B (Fungizone) IV, cream . . .	Antifungal
Ativan (*see* lorazepam)	Anti-PCP
atovaquone (Mepron)	Anti-PCP
azithromycin (Zithromax) tabs .	Antibacterial (MAC)
AZT (*see* zidovudine)	
Bactrim (*see* trimethoprim and sulfamethoxazole)	
Biaxin (*see* clarithromycin)	
Benadryl (*see* diphenhydramine)	
Blenoxane (*see* bleomycin)	
bleomycin (Blenoxane) IM, IV	Antineoplastic
BuSpar (*see* buspirone)	
buspirone (BuSpar) tabs	Antianxiety
ciprofloxacin (Cipro) tabs, IV . .	Antibacterial (MAC)
Cipro (*see* ciprofloxacin)	
chlorhexidine gluconate 0.12% mouth rinse (Peridex)	Antibacterial
clarithromycin (Biaxin) tabs . . .	Antibacterial (MAC)
clofazimine (Lamprene) caps . .	Antibacterial (MAC)
clotrimazole (Mycelex) tabs, lozenge	Antifungal
cycloserine (Seromycin) caps	Anti-TB
cytovene (*see* ganciclovir)	
dapsone (Dapsone) tabs	Anti-PCP
Daraprim (*see* pyrimethamine)	
ddC (*see* dideoxycytidine)	
ddI (*see* dideoxyinosine)	
Desyrel (*see* trazodone)	
Dexamethasone (*see* glucocorticosteroids)	
d4T (*see* stavudine)	
dideoxyinosine (Videx, ddI) powder, tabs	Antiretroviral
dideoxycytidine (HIVID, ddC) caps, syrup	Antiretroviral
Diflucan (*see* fluconazole)	
diphenhydramine (Benadryl) caps . . .	Antihistamine

Name of Drug†	Indications‡
diphenoxylate hydrochloride (Lomotil) tabs	Antidiarrheal
Dolophine (*see* methadone)	
doxorubicin (Adriamycin) IV	Antineoplastic
dronarinol (Marinol) caps . .	Antiemetic, antianorexic
Elavil (*see* amitriptyline hydrochloride)	
Epogen (*see* erythropoietin)	
erythropoietin (Procrit, Epogen) IV . . .	Hematopoietic stimulant
ethambutol (Myambutol) tabs	Anti-TB
ethionamide (Trecator-SC) tabs	Anti-TB
Fansidar (sulfadoxine and pyrimethamine) tabs	Antioxoplasmosis
filgrastim (G-CSF, Neupogen, Amgen) IV, SC	Neutrophil stimulant
fluconazole (Diflucan) tabs	Antifungal
Floxin (*see* ofloxacin)	
fluoxetine (Prozac) caps, liquid	Antidepressant
foscarnet (Foscavir) IV . . .	Anti-CMV, Resistant HSV
Foscavir (*see* foscarnet)	
ganciclovir (Cytovene) IV	Anti-CMV
G-CSF (*see* filgrastim)	
GM-CSF (*see* sargramostim)	
glucocorticosteroids (Prednisone, Dexamathasone) tabs, susp	Anti-inflammatory, immune suppressive
Halcion (*see* triazolam)	
HIVID (*see* dideoxycytidine)	
Humatin (*see* paromomycin)	
Immunex (*see* sargramostim)	
Imodium (*see* loperamide)	
INH (*see* isoniazid)	
interferon alpha (Roferon A) IV, SC . .	Antineoplastic
isoniazid (INH) tabs	Anti-TB
itraconazole (Sporanox) caps	Antifungal
kanamycin (Kantrex) IM, caps	Antibacterial
ketoconazole (Nizoral) tabs	Antifungal
Lamprene (*see* clofazimine)	
leucovorin (Leucovorin) tabs	Hematopoietic stimulant
Leukine (*see* GM-CSF)	
Lomotil (*see* diphenoxylate hydrochloride)	
loperamide (Imodium) caps	Antidiarrheal

Table 9-2. *(continued)*

Name of Drug†	Indications‡	Name of Drug†	Indications‡
lorazepam (Ativan) tab . . . . Antianxiety		Retrovir (*see* zidovudine)	
Marinol (*see* dronarinol)		Rifamate (*see* rifampin *and* isoniazid) caps	
Megace (*see* megestrol)		Rifadin (*see* rifampin)	
megestrol (Megace) tabs		rifampin (Rifadin) IV, caps . . . . Anti-TB	
Mellaril (*see* thioridazine)		Ritalin (*see* methylphenidate hydrochloride)	
Mepron (*see* atovaquone)		Roferon A (*see* interferon alpha)	
methadone (Methadone, Dolophine) tabs, sol, amp . . . . Detoxificant		Sandostatin (*see* octreotide)	
methylphenidate hydrochloride (Ritalin) tabs . . . . Psychostimulant		sargramostim (GM-CSF, Prokine, Leukine, Immunex) IV, SC. . . . . Neutrophil and monocyte stimulant	
Myabutol (*see* ethambutol)		Septra (*see* trimethoprim and sulfamethoxazole)	
Mycelex (*see* clotrimazole)		spiramycin tabs. . . . . Anticryptosporidosis	
Neupogen (*see* filgrastim)		Sporanox (*see* itraconazole)	
Nizoral (*see* ketoconazole)		stavudine or d4T (Zerit). . . . . Antiretroviral	
nystatin (Nystatin, Mycostatin) pastilles, tabs, susp . . . . Antifungal		streptomycin tabs . . . . Anti-MDR TB	
nortriptyline (Pamelor) caps. Tricyclic antidepressant		sulfadiazine or sulfadoxine (*see* Fansidar) tabs . . . . Antitoxoplasmosis	
octreotide (Sandostatin) IM. . . . . Antidiarrheal		thioridazine (Mellaril) tabs, susp . . . Antidepressant	
ofloxacin (Floxin) tabs. . . . . . . Antibacterial (MAC)		triazolam (Halcion) tabs. . . . . Anti-insomnia	
Oncovin (*see* vincristine)		trazodone (Desyrel) tabs . . . . Antidepressant	
Pamelor (*see* nortriptyline)		Trecator-SC (*see* ethionamide)	
para aminosalicylic acid (PAS) tabs . . Anti-MDR TB		trimethoprim and sulfamethoxazole (TMP/SMX, Bactrim, Septra) tabs . . . . Anti-PCP	
paromomycin (Humatin) caps. . . . . Antigastrointestinal infections		trimetrexate tabs . . . . Anti-PCP	
Peridex (*see* chlorhexidine gluconate 0.12%)		Velban (*see* vinblastine)	
Pentam (*see* pentamidine)		Videx (*see* dideoxyinosine)	
pentamidine (Pentam) IV, aerosolized . . . . Anti-PCP		vinblastine (Velban) IV. . . . . Antineoplastic	
piritrexim tabs . . . . Anti-PCP		vincristine (Oncovin) IV. . . . . Antineoplastic	
Prednisone (*see* glucocorticosteroids)		Xanax (*see* alprazolam)	
primaquine tabs. Anti-PCP		zalcitabine (*see* dideoxycytodine)	
Procrit (*see* erythropoietin)		zidovudine (AZT, Retrovir, ZDV) caps . . . Antiretroviral	
Prokine (*see* GM-CSF)		Zithromax (*see* azithromycin)	
Prozac (*see* fluoxetine)		Zovirax (*see* acyclovir)	
pyrazinamide (Pyrazinamide) tabs . . . . Anti-TB			
pyrimethamine (Daraprim, Fansidar) tabs. . . . . Antitoxoplasmosis			

*This list is not conclusive and should be used only as an indicator for any patient's medical conditions presently being treated.

†Trade names capitalized. caps = capsules; tabs = tablets; IM = intramuscular; IV = intravenous; SC = subcutaneous; susp = suspension.

‡MAC = *M. avium* complex; TB = tuberculosis; PCP = *Pneumocystis carinii* pneumonia; CMV = cytomegalovirus; HSV = herpes simplex virus; MDR TB = multiple drug resistant tuberculosis.

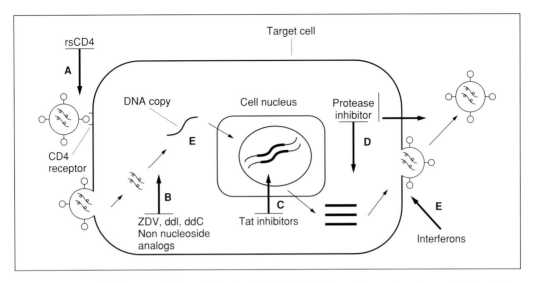

Fig 9-1. Antiretroviral therapy. **A**, Recombinant soluble CD4 (rsCD4) can be used as decoys attaching to the gp120 receptor of the virus, preventing virus attachment to the naturally occuring CD4 receptor of the target cell. **B**, Inhibition of reverse transcriptase prevents transcription of HIV RNA into HIV proviral DNA. Zidovudine (ZDV), didanosine (ddI), and zalcitabine (ddC) competitively inhibit reverse transcriptase and cause chain termination of the proviral DNA (see Fig 9-2). The non-nucleoside analogs also inhibit reverse transcriptase but do not cause chain termination. **C**, Tat inhibitors prevent activation of the tat gene. This reduces the stimulation for viral replication. **D**, Protease inhibitors prevent cleavage of long viral proteins, which are created during stimulation of viral genome, into smaller useful viral structural components. These longer proteins cannot be used to assemble infectious viruses. **E**, Interferons can stabilize the host cell's membrane, preventing budding of the virus.

hibits HIV replication with the help of nucleoside analogs. These compounds have a dual action: they act as competitive inhibitors of the reverse transcriptase, and they prematurely terminate proviral DNA synthesis (Fig 9-2).[4] The four anti-retroviral nucleoside analogs approved for use in the United States are zidovudine (AZT, azidothymidine, Retrovir, ZDV), ddI (dideoxyinosine, Videx, didanosine), ddC (dideoxycytidine, HIVID, zalcitabine), and stavudine or d4T (Zerit).

Other approaches are also being investigated, such as recombinant soluble CD4 molecules, tat inhibitors,

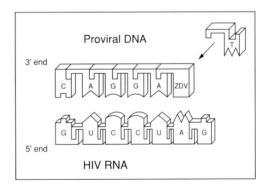

Fig 9-2. Chain termination by nucleoside analogs. The proviral DNA chain is terminated by incorporating nucleoside analogs, such as zidovudine (ZDV), in place of the appropriate nucleoside.

and protease inhibitors. Clinical trials are being conducted with recombinant soluble CD4 (rCD4) molecules as decoys for the HIV membrane-bound gp120.[5] In vitro studies show rCD4 binding to gp120, blocking HIV interaction with CD4 receptors of target cells.[6] In vitro studies also show that the drug prevents the fusion of HIV-infected cells with uninfected CD4+ lymphocytes.[7] A lack of clinical success with this drug is attributed to the lower affinity between rCD4 and gp120, compared to the affinity between the naturally occurring CD4 receptor and gp120. Furthermore, such therapy entails numerous daily injections of rCD4 to competitively compete with naturally occurring CD4 receptors.

Tat inhibitors offer a new approach that prevents activation of a specific HIV gene (tat). When this transactivating gene is stimulated, enhanced viral replication occurs.[8] In vitro results show great promise, and clinical trials were started in 1992.

During viral replication, large polyproteins are produced within the HIV-infected cells. These large precursor proteins need to be cleaved into smaller proteins to become structural components of the final virion. An aspartyl enzyme (a protease) is responsible for facilitating this breakdown. Protease inhibitors have been developed and are used to prevent polyprotein cleavage, resulting in the formation of nonfunctional, noninfectious virions.[9,10] The advantage of protease inhibitors over reverse transcriptase inhibitors is that they can inhibit HIV production from chronically infected cells, whereas reverse transcriptase inhibitors only prevent viral replication during the initial cellular infection.

Nucleoside Analogs

Zidovudine (AZT, azidothymidine, Retrovir®, ZDV) was the first agent approved by the FDA for the treatment of HIV. In 1984 it was discovered that it could inhibit HIV replication.[11] Clinical trials began in 1985, and by 1987 the drug had received FDA approval and became available to HIV-infected patients. Initial dosages of the drug were very high, resulting in severe drug toxicity,[12] but recent clinical trials have established its efficacy and reduced toxicity when used in lower doses in asymptomatic patients with HIV and CD4 counts below 500 cells/mm³ (normal range, 600 to 1,600 cells/mm³).[13,14] The optimum dosage has subsequently been reduced from 800 to 1,200 mg daily to 300 to 600 mg orally in equally divided doses.

The same studies indicate that the early administration of zidovudine delays the progression of the disease from the asymptomatic stage to the more advanced stages. Furthermore, the median survival time was four times longer for patients who took zidovudine compared with those patients not treated with this drug.[15] However, a recent European study has indicated that the survival time over 3 years for patients treated with zidovudine does not differ from that in patients not taking this medication.[16] This last study has brought about changes in the protocol for zidovudine administration. Current recommendations in the United States are to administer 500 to 600 mg zidovudine orally in equally divided daily doses for patients with CD4+ cell counts of 500 cells/mm³ and below, regardless of symptoms. However, in light of recent clinical studies and long-term experiences in the use of zidovudine, this recommendation may change (Table 9-3). Patients without symptoms and with CD4+ cell counts between 200 cells/mm³ and 500 cells/mm³ will either be given zidovudine or alternatively not receive medication but will be followed up for signs of disease progression. In cases of deterioration, zidovudine therapy is recommended.

Table 9-3. National Institute of Allergy and Infectious Diseases HIV Therapy Guidelines*

- CD4+ cell count below 500 cells/mm³:
  Observe with no antiretroviral therapy
- CD4+ cell count between 200–500 cells/mm³:
  If asymptomatic:
  1. Observe with no antiretroviral therapy or,
  2. Start ZDV alone (200 mg po tid) or,
  3. Start ZDV + ddI or,
  4. Start ZDV + ddC
  If symptomatic:
  1. Start ZDV alone or,
  2. Start ZDV + ddI or,
  3. Start ZDV + ddC
  If AZT intolerance develops on ZDV monotherapy, switch to ddI monotherapy
  If clinical progression occurs on ZDV monotherapy:
  1. Switch to ddI monotherapy or,
  2. Switch to ddC monotherapy or,
  3. Add ddI to ZDV regimen or,
  4. Add ddC to ZDV regimen
  If tolerating long-term ZDV monotherapy (approx. 13 months):
  1. If CD4+ cell count is above 300 cells/mm³ , continue ZDV
  2. If CD4+ cell count is below 300 cells/mm³ , switch to ddI

- CD4+ cell count between 50–200 cells/mm³:
  Start antiretroviral therapy as for asymptomatic patients with CD4+ cell counts between 200–500 cells/mm³
  Manage ZDV intolerance as for patients with CD4+ cell counts between 200–500 cells/mm³
  Manage ZDV clinical progression as for patients with CD4+ cell counts between 200–500 cells/mm³
  If tolerating long-term ZDV monotherapy (approx 13 months), switch to ddI monotherapy
- CD4+ cell count below 50 cells/mm³:
  Start antiretroviral therapy as for asymptomatic patients with CD4+ cell counts between 200–500 cells/mm³
  If AZT intolerance develops on ZDV monotherapy:
  1. Switch to ddI monotherapy or,
  2. Switch to ddC monotherapy or,
  3. Stop antiretroviral therapy
  If clinical progression occurs on ZDV monotherapy:
  1. Switch to ddI monotherapy or,
  2. Switch to ddC monotherapy
  If tolerating long-term ZDV monotherapy (approx 13 months):
  Switch to ddI monotherapy

*Adapted from NIAID News Bulletin, NIH, June 25, 1993. ZDV = zidovudine; ddI = dideoxyinosine; ddC = dideoxyctyidine.

Table 9-4. Incidence of Hematologic Side Effects to Zidovudine*

Side Effect/ Zidovudine Dose	Stage of Disease Progression			
	Asymptomatic; CD4+ > 500 cells/mm³	Symptomatic; CD4+ > 200 cells/mm³	Advanced Symptoms; CD4+ > 200 cells/mm³	Advanced Symptoms; CD4+ < 200 cells/mm³
Granulocytopenia (< 750 cells/mm³)				
Zidovudine dose (mg)				
500	1.8%	. . .	. . .	. . .
1200	. . .†	4%	. . .	. . .
1500	6.4%	. . .	10%	47%
Anemia (Hgb < 8 g/dL)				
Zidovudine dose (mg)				
500	1.1%	. . .	. . .	. . .
1200	. . .	4%	. . .	. . .
1500	6.4%	. . .	3%	29%

*Modified from Richman DD, Fischl MA, Grieco MH, et al. N Engl J Med 1987; 317:192–197; Volberding PA, Lagakos SW, Koch MA, et al. N Engl J Med 1990,322.941–949; Sattler FR, Ko R, Antoniskis D, et al. Ann Intern Med 1991;114:937–940.
† . . . = not applicable.

The most common side effects with high-dose zidovudine are associated with myelosuppression and include anemia and neutropenia. However, the incidence of these side effects is reduced with the lower dosage. An increased toxicity with zidovudine is also noted after long-term use, and it becomes more severe and more frequent in the advanced stages of the disease (Table 9-4). Zidovudine-induced neutropenia is most common in persons with CD4+ cell counts below 100 cells/mm³. In addition, concomitant use of zidovudine with other neutropenia-inducing drugs, such as trimethoprim-sulfamethoxazole (Bactrim), pyrimethamine and sulfadiazine (Fansidar), and ganciclovir (Cytovene), may further enhance the neutropenia. Even with the lower regimen, complaints of malaise, headache, and confusion are reported. Other side effects resulting from zidovudine therapy include fatigue, rashes, and myopathy.

The anemia associated with high-dose zidovudine may be severe and may require the administration of blood transfusions. To combat these side effects, cytokines are being used to increase red blood cell and neutrophil counts. Erythropoietin is a human glycoprotein produced by the kidney, liver, macrophages, and other cells and stimulates red blood cell production. Recombinant human erythropoietin, rHuEpo, is used as a treatment IND in AIDS-related anemias. Administration of this drug is beneficial in patients with zidovudine-induced anemia who already have low levels of this cytokine.[17,18] Granulocyte colony stimulating factor (G-CSF) and granulocyte macrophage colony stimulating factor (GM-CSF) are human cytokines that induce proliferation and differentiation of white blood cell precursors in the bone marrow.[19] Both cytokines have been manufactured with recombinant technology. Granulocyte colony stimulating factor (Amgen) acts specifically as a potent neutrophil stimulator, while GM-CSF (Immunex) is used for myelopoiesis in zidovudine-induced bone marrow suppression. Treatment with GM-CSF significantly improves patient tolerance to bone marrow–suppressive AIDS medications.[20] In addition to the effect of ZDV on HIV replication, this medication has also been effective in the amelioration of symptoms associated with AIDS dementia complex.[21]

Patients may develop zidovudine-resistant HIV strains already after 6 months of therapy.[22] HIV zidovudine resistance is the result of mutations in several amino acid residues of the reverse transcriptase gene of HIV. A progressive resistance develops with increased accumulation of these mutations.[23] Consequently, the level of resistance increases during the later stages of the disease, which corresponds with increased viral replication. Cross-resistance among other anti-retroviral drugs exists, but some nucleoside analogs maintain sensitivity.[24]

Drug interactions with zidovudine have been documented, but only a few have been investigated enough to draw definitive conclusions.[25] Concomitant use of acetaminophen and zidovudine had been presumed to enhance toxicity of zidovudine,[12] but recent controlled studies could not determine any detrimental interac-

tions between the two drugs.[26,27] It is possible that the observed higher incidence of neutropenia in patients taking zidovudine and acetaminophen is not caused by the medications; rather, acetaminophen is prescribed to patients with fever where the infection causing the fever also results in neutropenia. No adverse effects have been documented with the combined use of aspirin and zidovudine.[12,28]

An investigation of the effect of concomitant use of ibuprofen and zidovudine in a group of HIV-infected patients and hemophilia showed a 30% increase in bleeding tendencies when the two drugs were used together.[29] Although zidovudine glucuronidation can be inhibited 10% to 30% by naproxen, alterations in the pharmacokinetics of zidovudine have not been documented.[30]

Acyclovir is sometimes used in combination with zidovudine since in vitro tests have indicated a synergistic interaction between these two drugs.[31] A clinical study evaluating the efficacy and safety of zidovudine and acyclovir in a trial including 265 patients for 2 years suggested that the addition of high-dose acyclovir significantly improved the survival time of patients.[32] Since herpesviruses have also been associated with the activation of HIV transcription, the administration of acyclovir may reduce the incidence of herpesvirus activation and consequently reduce stimulation of HIV replication.[33]

Dapsone is a drug used for prophylaxis against *Pneumocystis carinii* pneumonia. This drug, alone and when used in combination with zidovudine, is associated with the development of anemia, neutropenia, and thrombocytopenia.[34,35] The concomitant use of zidovudine and tuberculostatic agents, such as isoniazid, rifampin, ethambutol, and pyrazinamide, has been associated with an increased frequency of marked anemia (hemoglobin less than 9.5g/dL).[36]

The second anti-retroviral drug approved by the FDA was ddI (dideoxyinosine, Videx, didanosine). This drug is administered as chewable tablets or as a powder dissolved in water twice daily. The chewable tablets are buffered to enhance gastric absorption of the drug, but this will interfere with other medications that require an acidic environment for absorption, such as ketoconazole and dapsone. Accordingly, these drugs must be ingested at least 2 hours before the administration of ddI.

The following recommendations are in place for the use of ddI: as initial antiretroviral therapy in combination with zidovudine, or as monotherapy in patients with CD4+ cell counts below 300 cells/mm³, or for patients with CD4+ cell counts below 500 cells/mm³ who are intolerant to zidovudine. The most serious side effects of ddI are pancreatitis and peripheral neuropathy, infrequently anemia or leukopenia, and seizures.[37] Severe xerostomia has also been reported in patients treated with ddI.[38]

The most potent HIV inhibitor in vitro when compared to other nucleoside analogs is ddC (dideoxycytidine, HIVID®, zalcitabine). However, this drug is only approved to be used in combination with zidovudine in patients with HIV and CD4+ cell counts below 300 cells/mm³.

Side effects attributed to this drug include severe, painful peripheral neuropathy, oral ulcerations, fever, and rash. The oral ulcerations can be noted 2 to 6 weeks after initiation of ddC therapy.[39]

The latest nucleoside analog approved by the FDA is stavudine or d4T (Zerit). It is indicated for patients who do not tolerate or who show no benefit to other nucleoside analogs. Side effects include pain, tingling, and numbness in the hands and feet.

Numerous anti-retroviral combination therapy clinical trials are presently being conducted. They include acyclovir with zidovudine, alpha interferon with zidovudine, ddC with zidovudine, interleukin-2 with zidovudine, and interleukin-2 with alpha interferon.

Alpha interferon appears to interfere with assembly of the HIV virion but also inhibits viral replication in macrophages and in T lymphocytes in vitro and may have a synergistic effect with zidovudine.[40,41]

Interleukin-2 is a lymphokine that is responsible for T-lymphocyte activation and proliferation. This human lymphokine is used to stimulate the immunologic reaction against HIV.[42]

Non-Nucleoside Analogs

Other reverse transcriptase inhibitors are also being tested but are not yet approved by the FDA.[43] These compounds are also referred to as non-nucleoside analogs since, although they inhibit reverse transcriptase, they do not terminate DNA synthesis by incorporation during the transcription process. Non-nucleoside analog reverse transcriptase inhibitors include deoxyfluorothymidine (FLT), carbocyclic didehydrodideoxyguanosine (carbovir), 3-thiacytidine (3TC, Lamivadine), foscarnet (Foscavir), nevirapine, and tetrahydroimidazobenzodiazepine (TIBO).

Antiviral Medications

Acyclovir (Zovirax). Acyclovir is an anti-herpetic medication used mainly to treat infections caused by herpes simplex viruses. In dental therapy, acyclovir is also used to treat various intra-oral herpes virus infections, including cytomegalovirus infections[44] and oral hairy leukoplakia.[45] This drug is very well tolerated and only a few side effects have been reported, even with high-dose oral administration.

Ganciclovir (DHPG, Cytovene). Ganciclovir is used for the treatment of cytomegalovirus retinitis in HIV-infected patients. This complication appears during the later stages of HIV disease when patients' CD4 cell counts drop below 100 cells/mm[3]. In vitro studies indicate that ganciclovir can inhibit the anti-retroviral activity of zidovudine and, in combination with zidovudine, add to the cytotoxic effect of both drugs.[46] In particular, neutropenia and thrombocytopenia may occur and require discontinuation of therapy in less than 20% in patients with decreased granulocyte counts and in 5% to 10% of patients with thrombocytopenia.[47] This medication is administered intravenously, usually for the rest of the patient's life.

Foscarnet (trisodium phosphonoformate, PFA, Foscavir). Foscarnet is administered intravenously and is primarily used to treat cytomegalovirus retinitis. Side effects include impaired renal function sometimes resulting in proteinuria. General dryness of the skin and intraoral dryness have been noted in patients taking this medication. Oral ulcerations have also been associated with the administration of foscarnet.[48]

Antineoplastic Agents

Alpha interferon (recombinant alpha interferon, Roferon, Intron A, Alferon-N Injection). This is the first drug approved for the treatment of Kaposi's sarcoma. As previously mentioned, this compound may also have anti-HIV properties and is consequently being tested in combination with zidovudine.[40,41] Naturally occurring alpha interferon is produced in response to viral infections. It exhibits an antiviral activity by inhibition of transcription and/or translation of viral messenger RNA. The drug is a recombinant-produced protein that is administered intramuscularly. Side effects include flulike symptoms and, when high doses are being used, neutropenia.

Antimycobacterial Medications

Amikacin sulfate (Amikin). An aminoglycoside antibiotic used for the treatment of *Mycobacterium avium-intracellulare,* this drug is poorly absorbed orally and is therefore administered intramuscularly.

Azithromycin (Zithromax). This is an oral macrolide antibiotic used for the treatment of *M. avium-intracellulare,* toxoplasmosis, and cryptosporidiosis.

Ciprofloxacin (Cipro). Ciprofloxacin is an oral quinolone antibiotic used for combination treatment of *M. avium intracellulare.* Side effects have been documented,[49] but do not affect dental therapy. However, this antibiotic should not be relied on to reduce the oral flora since it is not effective against anaerobic bacteria. Because sucralfate can significantly reduce the serum concentration of ciprofloxacin, these two drugs should not be used together.[50]

Clarithromycin (Biaxin). An oral macrolide used for the treatment of *M. avium-intracellulare* and in combination for the treatment of toxoplasmosis, this medication is often given to patients with CD4+ cell counts below 100 cells/mm^3 as prohylaxis for mycobacterial infections.

Clofazimine (Lamprene). Clofazimine is used for the treatment for *M. avium-intracellulare.* Few serious side effects have been documented, but cutaneous hyperpigmentation can occur. This side effect is reversible with discontinuation of the drug.

Ethambutol (Myambutol). Ethambutol is used in combination with other medications for the treatment and prophylaxis of tuberculosis and *M. avium-intracellulare.* Few serious side effects have been documented, but optic neuritis and alteration of color perception may be noticed.

Isoniazid (INH). Isoniazid is used for the treatment and prophylaxis of tuberculosis. Hepatotoxicity can occur, but serious side effects are uncommon. Concurrent use of prednisolone or alcohol may increase the metabolism of isoniazid and consequently reduce the efficacy of the drug. There has also been a report of decreased efficacy of ketoconazole when administered with isoniazid.[51]

Para-aminosalicylic acid (PAS). An oral antibiotic used for the treatment of multiple drug–resistant tuberculosis (MDR-TB), it is used to delay the development of resistance to other anti-TB medications.

Pyrazinamide (PZA). An oral antibiotic used for the treatment of TB, it has few side effects.

Rifampin (Rifabutin, Mycobutin). Rifampin is used for treatment and prophylaxis of TB and *M. avium-intracellulare.* An increased incidence of adverse reactions to antituberculoid drugs has been documented among individuals with HIV, when compared to healthy subjects.[52] Rifampin was thought to be the culprit in many of these cases. This drug increases the rate of hepatic drug metabolism by enhancing the hepatic microsomal enzyme system. Reduced bioavailability of fluconazole and ketoconazole have also been reported.[51,53] Some patients may also notice orange staining of urine, sweat, and even tears during rifampin therapy.

Streptomycin. This drug was originally used as a first line medication against TB but is recently used for the treatment of multiple drug–resistant TB. The drug is administered intramuscularly and has numerous toxic side effects.

Antifungal Medications

Amphotericin B (Fungizone). An intravenous medication used for the treatment of progressive, disseminated fungal infections, this drug is usually instituted for individuals with very low CD4+ cell counts. Toxicity includes anemia. Topical preparations are also available for cutaneous Candida infections.

Clotrimazole (Mycelex). An approved medication for treatment of candidiasis; this drug is available as a cream, tablet, or troche. It is the most commonly used oral troche for oral candidiasis.

Fluconazole (Diflucan). Fluconazole is approved for the treatment of candidiasis and as prophylaxis for cryptococcosis. Very few adverse reactions have been documented with the oral administration of this drug[54]; however, concomitant use with rifampin decreases the half-life of fluconazole.[53] In such cases, an increased dosage of fluconazole may be required to achieve an adequate clinical response. This medication has a good compliance rate since it needs to be administered orally only once or twice per day.

Flucytosine (5-FC, Ancobon). This medication is used alone or, more commonly, in combination with amphotericin B for the treatment of cryptococcosis.

Itraconazole (Sporanox). This oral medication is approved for the treatment of blastomycosis and histoplasmosis, but also appears to be effective against candidiasis. It is also being investigated as treatment for cryptococcosis and aspergillosis. Reduced absorption has been documented in patients with AIDS and when taken in combination with antacids and rifampin.

Ketoconazole (Nizoral). Ketoconazole has been approved for the treatment of candidiasis, blastomycosis, and histoplasmosis. This drug needs gastric acid to be properly absorbed. Thus, the concomitant use of antacids, cimetidine, and buffered medications, such as ddI, reduces the bioavailability of this drug. It is advisable to administer this drug at least 2 hours before the use of antacids.

Increased absorption of ketoconazole can be achieved if the drug is administered with acidic fluids like colas. Adverse reactions associated with ketoconazole administration include nausea, anorexia, vomiting, and hepatotoxicity. If this medication is taken with food, tolerance to the drug may improve. Administration of rifampin or isoniazid with ketoconazole can reduce the serum level of ketoconazole by 80%.[51] Consequently, these drugs should not be used together. This drug should also not be given to patients taking wafarin since the anticoagulant effect of warfarin may be enhanced.[55] Cardiac arrhythmia may also occur if ketaconazole is administered with terfenadine or astemizole. Thus, concomitant use of these medications should be avoided.

Nystatin (Mycolog, Mycostatin). This antifungal medication is supplied as tablets, pastilles, ointment, cream, and suspension. It is approved for treatment of candidiasis but is usually only effective in patients with high CD4+ cell counts. This medication has no systemic effect since it is inactivated by gastric acid.

Antiparasitic Agents

Atovaquone (Mepron, BW566c80). Approved for the treatment of *P. carinii pneumonia* (PCP) for individuals who cannot tolerate trimethoprim-sulfamethoxazole, this drug is also being investigated for the treatment of toxoplasmosis, cryptosporidiosis, and microsporidiosis.

Azithromycin (Zithromax). See *Antimycobacterial medications.*

Clarithromycin (Biaxin). See *Antimycobacterial medications.*

Clindamycin (Cleocin). This antibiotic is used in the treatment of PCP and toxoplasmosis. Adverse gastrointestinal reactions such as diarrhea, nausea, and pseudomembranous colitis have been documented in patients taking this medication. Diarrhea may occur in up to 21% of all patients.[56] In one study where clindamycin was used for prophylaxis against toxoplasmosis in patients with HIV and CD4+ cell counts below 200 cells/mm³, 30.8% of patients developed diarrhea and 21.2% exhibited skin rashes.[57]

This medication is effective against *Actinomyces* species and *Bacteroides* and is therefore also used for oral infections. Allergic manifestations to clindamycin may include glossitis and stomatitis.

Corticosteroids. Oral or intravenous glucocorticosteroids are used as an adjuvant for the treatment of PCP. These medications are also used to treat oral ulcerations. The most severe side effect is adrenal suppression, and replacement therapy before dental treatment may be necessary.[58] An increased incidence of Kaposi's sarcoma has been associated with administration of glucocorticosteroids.[59]

Dapsone. Dapsone is another drug used for prophylaxis against PCP. As previously mentioned, concomitant use with this sulfone and zidovudine may result in the development of anemia, neutropenia, and thrombocytopenia.[34,35]

Paromomycin (Humatin). Paromomycin is an oral antibiotic investigated for use against cryptosporidiosis.

Pentamidine (Pentam, NebuPent). This medication, administered intravenously, intramuscularly, or in aerosolized form, is approved for prophylactic treatment of PCP in individuals with CD4+ cell counts below 200 cells/mm³ or with previous bouts of PCP. It is less effective than trimethoprim-sulfamethoxazole for treatment of acute episodes of PCP. No adverse systemic reactions are associated with aerosolized therapy.

Piritrexim. This oral medication has anti-protozoal and anti-neoplastic properties and is used to treat PCP. Side effects include bone marrow suppression.

Primaquine. Primaquine is used for treatment of acute PCP in combination with clindamycin.

Pyrimethamine (Daraprim, Fansidar). An antifolate used in combination with sulfadiazine, this drug combination is used for the treatment of toxoplasma encephalitis. Severe side effects have been reported in 60% to 70% of patients, necessitating discontinuation of therapy in up to 45% of all cases.[60,61]

Spiramycin. Spiramycin is a macrolide antibiotic used to treat cryptosporidiosis.

Sulfadiazine. See pyrimethamine.

Trimethoprim-sulfamethoxazole (TMP/SMX, Co-trimoxazole, Bactrim, Septra). Of all the usual drugs used in patients with AIDS, drug reactions are most commonly noted with TMP/SMX. This drug is used as prophylaxis for PCP in patients with CD4+ cell counts below 200 cells/mm³. Adverse reactions to this drug, such as allergic reactions and bone marrow suppression, are very common in patients with AIDS.[62] One study reported that 57% of patients with AIDS receiving this medication exhibited adverse effects, including skin rash (10%), nausea and vomiting (7%), leukopenia (17%), and elevated liver enzyme levels (20%).[63] These reactions develop within the first 10 to 14 days after therapy. Bone marrow suppression due to zidovudine therapy may be enhanced in patients concurrently taking TMP/SMX.

Trimetrexate. Trimetrexate is an oral antifolate medication used as a second-line treatment for PCP together with leucovorin (folate acid).

Anti-Wasting Syndrome Medication

Dronarinol (Marinol). This is an FDA-approved drug used to stimulate appetite in patients with HIV and anorexia.

Megestrol acetate (Megace). Megestrol acetate is used as an appetite stimulant for malnourished persons.

Cytokines

EPO (Epoetin alfa, Procrit, Epogen). This is a synthetic compound, similar to erythropoietin, that stimulates red blood cell production. Patients with zidovudine-treatment–associated anemia may respond well to this medication.

G-CSF (Filgrastim, Neupogen, Amgen). This is a recombinant protein of the naturally occurring granulocyte colony stimulating factor, which induces proliferation and differentiation of granulocytes. This drug is used for patients with severe neutropenia.

GM-CSF (Sargramostim, Leukine, Immunex). This is a recombinant protein of the naturally occurring granulocyte-macrophage colony stimulating factor, which induces proliferation and differentiation of granulocytes and macrophages. This drug is used to counteract the influence of myelosuppressive drugs, such as ganciclovir, by boosting the white blood cell counts.

Anti-HIV Dementia Medications

Methylphenidate hydrochloride (Ritalin). This drug is used to improve symptoms related to HIV dementia by acting as a central nervous system stimulant.

Miscellaneous

Leucovorin (folic acid). This medication is used with a folic acid antagonist, such as pyrimethamine and trimetrexate, to diminish the toxicity of these drugs. It is also being used in patients with megaloblastic anemia not caused by vitamin B_{12}, and nutritional deficiencies.

Diphenoxylate hydrochloride with atropine sulfate (Lomotil). This medication is related to the narcotic meperidine. It also has an anticholinergic effect and is used for patients with diarrhea.

Loperamide (Imodium). This drug inhibits peristalsis; therefore, it is used as an anti-diarrheal agent.

Drug Hypersensitivity

Drug reactions to antibiotics, such as amoxicillin, clavulanic acid, ciprofloxacin, dicloxacillin, erythromycin, and clindamycin, have been reported.[64]

In one study, 38% of patients with HIV receiving thalidomide for severe oral ulcerations developed extensive erythematous macular exanthem.[65] The use of ampicillin in patients with Epstein-Barr virus infections, such as infectious mononucleosis and mononucleosis caused by cytomegalovirus, has resulted in an increased frequency of cutaneous reactions.[66,67] Most patients with HIV have been exposed to both viruses, which often reactivate during advanced stages of the disease. Amoxicillin has been documented to cause an increased incidence of rashes in HIV-infected patients.[68]

A large number of patients with HIV develop adverse drug reactions. These reactions become more frequent during the progression of disease and increase with a greater number of administered medications.[69]

Few medications impact on the provision of dental care. Instead, medications used in HIV disease often offer the dental professional a good indication of CD4+ cell count, as well as present and past infections. But, some of the medications prescribed by dental practitioners may not be effective because of lack of absorption, bioavailability, or interactions with other drugs. Medications should be prescribed judiciously, especially in patients taking several pharmacologic agents and in those with advanced stages of HIV disease.

References

1. Kessler DA. The regulation of investigational drugs. N Engl J Med 1989;320:281–288.

2. Rathbun RC. Surrogate markers for assessing treatment response in HIV disease. Ann Pharmacother 1993;27:450–455.

3. AIDS Medicines in Development. Washington DC: Pharmaceutical Manufacturers Association; 1993.

4. Yarchoan R, Mitsuya H, Myers CE, Broder S. Clinical pharmacology of 3'-azido-2',3'-dideoxythymidine (zidovudine) and related dideoxynucleosides. N Engl J Med 1989;321:726–738.

5. Schooley RT, Merigan TC, Gaut P, et al. Recombinant soluble CD4 therapy in patients with the acquired immunodeficiency syndrome (AIDS) and AIDS-related complex. Ann Intern Med 1990;112:247–253.

6. Kahn JO, Allan JD, Hodges TL, et al. The safety and pharmacokinetics of recombinant soluble CD4 (rCD4) in subjects with the acquired immunodeficiency syndrome (AIDS) and AIDS-related complex. Ann Intern Med 1990;112:254–261.

7. Siliciano RF, Lawton T, Knall C, et al. Analysis of host-virus interactions in AIDS with anti-gp120 T cell clones: effect of HIV sequence variant and mechanism for CD4+ cell depletion. Cell 1988;54:561–575.

8. Hsu MC, Schutt AD, Holly M, et al. Inhibition of HIV replication in acute and chronic infections in vitro by a tat antagonist. Science 1991;254:1799–1802.

9. Roberts NA, Martin JA, Kinchington D, et al. Rational design of peptide-based HIV proteinase inhibitors. Science 1990;248: 358–361.

10. Johnson VA, Merrill DP, Chou TC, Hirsch MS. Human immunodeficiency virus type-1 (HIV-1) inhibitory interactions between protease inhibitor Ro 31-8959 and zidovudine, 2',3'-deoxycytidine, or recombinant interferon alpha against zidovudine-sensitive or-resistant HIV-1 in vitro. J Infect Dis 1992;166:1143–1146.

11. Mitsuya H, Weinhold KJ, Furman PA, et al. 3'-Azido-3'-deoxythymidine (BW A5090): an antiviral agent that inhibits the infectivity and cytopathic effect of human T-lymphotrophic virus type III/lymphadenopathy-associated virus in vitro. Proc Natl Acad Sci USA 1985;82:7096.

12. Richman DD, Fischl MA, Grieco MH, et al. The toxicity of azidothymidine (AZT) in the treatment of patients with AIDS and AIDS-related complex: a double-blind, placebo-controlled trial. N Engl J Med 1987;317:192–197.

13. Fischl MA, Parker CB, Pettinelli C, et al. A randomized controlled trial of a reduced daily dose of zidovudine in patients with acquired immunodeficiency syndrome. N Engl J Med 1990;323:1009–1014.

14. Volberding PA, Lagakos SW, Koch MA, et al. Zidovudine in asymptomatic human immunodeficiency virus infection. A controlled trial in persons with fewer than 500 CD4-positive cells per cubic millimeter. N Engl J Med 1990;322:941–949.

15. Moore RD, Hidalgo J, Sugland BW. Zidovudine and the natural history of the acquired immunodeficiency syndrome. N Engl J Med 1991;324:1412–1416.

16. Aboulker J-P, Swart AM. Preliminary analysis of the Concorde trial. Lancet 1993;341: 889–890.

17. Henry DH, Beall GN, Benson CA, et al. Recombinant human erythropoietin in the treatment of the anemia associated with human immunodeficiency virus infection and zidovudine therapy: overview of four clinical trials. Ann Intern Med 1992; 117:739–748.

18. Erythropoietin Epo Study Group, Rudnick SA. Human recombinant erythropoietin (rHuepo): a double blind, placebo-controlled study in acquired immunodeficiency syndrome (AIDS) patients with anemia induced by disease and AZT (abstract no. 7, Proc Am Soc Clin Oncol 1989;8:2.

19. Ruef C, Coleman DL. Granulocyte-macrophage colony-stimulating factor: pleiotropic cytokine with potential clinical usefulness. Rev Infect Dis 1990;12:41–62.

20. Groopman JE. Management of the hematologic complications of human immunodeficiency virus infection. Rev Infect Dis 1990;12:931–937.

21. Sidtis JJ, Gatsonis C, Price RW, et al. Zidovudine treatment of the AIDS dementia complex: results of a placebo-controlled trial. Ann Intern Med 1993;33: 343–349.

22. Larder BA, Darby G, Richman DD. HIV with reduced sensitivity to zidovudine (AZT) isolated during prolonged therapy. Science 1989;243:1731–1734.

23. Larder BA, Kemp SD. Multiple mutations in HIV-1 reverse transcriptase confer high-level resistance to zidovudine. Science 1989;246:1155–1158.

24. Larder BA, Chesebro B, Richman DD. Susceptibilities of zidovudine-susceptible and resistant human immunodeficiency virus isolates to antiviral agents determined by using a quantitative plaque reduction assay. Antimicrob Agents Chemother 1990; 34:436–441.

25. Berger DM, Meenhorst PL, Koks CHW, Beijnen JH. Drug interactions with zidovudine. AIDS 1993;7:445–460.

26. Steffe EM, King JH, Inciardi JF, et al. The effect of acetaminophen on zidovudine metabolism in HIV-infected patients. J Acquired Immune Deficiency Syndrome 1990;3:691–694.

27. Sattler FR, Ko R, Antoniskis D, et al. Acetaminophen does not impair clearance of zidovudine. Ann Intern Med 1991;114:937–940.

28. Fischl MA, Richman DD, Grieco MH, et al. The efficacy of azidothymidine (AZT) in the treatment of patients with AIDS and AIDS-related complex: a double-blind, placebo-controlled trial. N Engl J Med 1987;317:185–191.

29. Ragni MV, Miller BJ, Whalen R, Ptachcinski R. Bleeding tendency, platelet function, and pharmacokinetics of ibuprofen and zidovudine in HIV(+) haemophilic men. Am J Haematol 1992;40;176–182.

30. Sahi J, Gallicano K, Conway B, et al. Lack of pharmacokinetic interaction between naproxen (N) and zidovudine (Z) (abstract). Clin Pharmacol Ther 1992;51:184.

31. Mitsuya H, Broder S. Strategies for antiviral therapy in AIDS. Nature 1987;325:773–778.

32. Cooper DA, Pehrson PO, Pedersen C, et al. The efficacy and safety of zidovudine alone or as cotherapy with acyclovir for treatment of patients with AIDS and AIDS-related complex: a double-blind, randomized trial. AIDS 1993;7:197–207.

33. Nabel GJ, Rice SA, Knipe DM, Baltimore D. Alternative mechanisms for activation of human immunodeficiency virus enhancer in T cells. Science 1988;239:1299.

34. Martin MA, Cox PH, Beck K, Styer CM, Beall GN. A comparison of the effectiveness of three regimens in the prevention of *Pneumocystis carinii* pneumonia in human immunodeficiency virus-infected patients. Arch Intern Med 1992;152:523–528.

35. Pinching AJ, Helbert M, Peddle B, et al. Clinical experience with zidovudine in patients with acquired immunodeficiency syndrome and acquired immunodeficiency syndrome-complex. J Infect 1989;18:33–40.

36. Antoniskis D, Easly AC, Espina BM, Davidson PT, Barnes PF. Combined toxicity of zidovudine and tuberculosis chemotherapy. Am Rev Respir Dis 1992;145:430–434.

37. Hirsch MS, D'Aquila RT. Therapy for human immunodeficiency virus infection. N Engl J Med 1993;328:1686–1695.

38. Dodd CL, Greenspan D, Westenhouse JL, Katz MH. Xerostomia associated with didanosine. Lancet 1992;340:790.

39. McNeeley MC, Yarchoan R, Broder S, Lawley TJ. Dermatologic complications associated with administration of 2',3'-dideoxycytidine in patients with human immunodeficiency virus infection. J Am Acad Dermatol 1989;21:1213–1217.

40. Brook MG, Gor D, Forster S, Harris JR, Jeffries DS, Thomas HC. Anti-HIV effects of alpha interferon (Letter). Lancet 1989;1:42.

41. Berglund O, Engman K, Ehrnst A, et al. Combined treatment of symptomatic HIV-1 infection with native interferon-alpha and zidovudine. J Infect Dis 1991;163:710–715.

42. Schwartz DH, Skowrong G, Merigan TC. Safety and effects of interleukin-2 plus zidovudine in asymptomatic individuals infected with human immunodeficiency virus. J Acquired Immune Deficiency Syndrome 1991;4:11–23.

43. Johnston MI, Hoth DF. Present status and future prospects for HIV therapies. Science 1993;260:1286–1293.

44. Glick M, Cleveland DB, Salkin LM, Alfaro-Miranda M, Fielding AF. Intraoral cytomegalovirus lesion and HIV-associated periodontitis in a patient with acquired immunodeficiency syndrome. Oral Surg Oral Med Oral Pathol 1991;72:716–720.

45. Glick M, Pliskin ME. Regression of oral hairy leukoplakia after oral administration of acyclovir. Gen Dent 1990;38:374–375.

46. Medina DJ, Hsuing GD, Mellors JW. Ganciclovir antagonizes the anti-human immunodeficiency virus type 1 activity of zidovudine and didanosine *in vitro*. Antimicrob Agents Chemother 1992;36:1127–1130.

47. The United States Pharmacopeia Drug Information. Drug Information for the Health Care Professional, ed 11. Rockville, MD: The United States Pharmocopeial Convention; 1991.

48. Gilquin J, Weiss L, Kazatchkine MD. Genital and oral erosions induced by foscarnet. Lancet 1990;335:287.

49. Campoli-Richards DM, Monk JP, Price A, Benfield P, Todd PA, Ward A. Ciprofloxacin: a review of its antibacterial activity, pharmacokinetic properties and therapeutic use. Drugs 1988;35:373–447.

50. Garrelts JC, Godley PJ, Peterie JD, Gerlach EH, Yakshe CC. Sucralfate significantly reduces ciprofloxacin concentration in serum. Antimicrob Agents Chemother 1990;34:931–933.

51. Engelhard D, Stutman HR, Marks MI. Interaction of ketoconazole with rifampin and isoniazid. N Engl J Med 1984;311:1681–1683.

52. Small PM, Schechter GF, Goodman PC, Sande MA, Chaisson RE, Hopewell PC. Treatment of tuberculosis in patients with advanced human immunodeficiency virus infection. N Engl J Med 1991;324:289–294.

53. Lazar JD, Wilner KD. Drug interactions with fluconazole. Rev Infect Dis 1990;12:327–333.

54. Grant SM, Clissold SP. Fluconazole. A review of its pharmacodynamics and pharmacokinetic properties, and therapeutic potential in superficial and systemic mycoses. Drugs 1990;39:877–916.

55. Daneshmend TK, Warnock DW. Clinical pharmokinetics of ketoconazole. Clin Pharmacokinet 1988;14:13–34.

56. Kucers A, McK. Bennet N. The Use of Antibiotics: A Comprehensive Review with Clinical Emphasis, ed 4. Philadelphia: JB Lippincott; 1987.

57. Jacobson MA, Besch CL, Child C, et al. Randomized study of clindamycin or pyrimethamine prophylaxis for toxoplasmic encephalitis in patients with advanced HIV disease (abstract no. 298). In: Program and Abstracts of the 31st Interscience Conference on Antimicrobial Agents and Chemotherapy. Washington, DC: American Society for Microbiology; 1991:148.

58. Glick M. Glucocorticosteroid replacement therapy: literature review and suggested replacement therapy. Oral Surg Oral Med Oral Pathol 1989;67:614–620.

59. Gill PS, Lourerio C, Bernstein-Singer M, Rarick MU, Sattler F, Levine AM. Clinical effect of glucocorticosteroids on Kaposi's sarcoma related to the acquired immunodeficiency syndrome (AIDS). Ann Intern Med 1989;110:937–940.

60. Leport C, Raffi F, Matheron S, et al. Treatment of central nervous system toxoplasmosis with pyrimethamine/sulfadiazine combination in 35 patients with acquired immunodeficiency syndrome. Am J Med 1988;84:94–100.

61. Haverkos HO. Assessment of therapy for toxoplasmosis encephalitis. The TE Study Group. Am J Med 1987:82:907–914.

62. Gordin FM, Simon GL, Wofsy CB, Mills J. Adverse reactions to trimethoprim-sulfamethoxazole in patients with acquired immunodeficiency syndrome. Ann Intern Med 1984;100:495–499.

63. Medina I, Mills J, Leoung G, et al. Oral therapy for *Pneumocystis carinii* pneumonia in AIDS: a randomized double blind trial comparing trimethoprim and sulfamethoxazole with dapsone and trimethoprim. N Engl J Med 1990;323:776–782.

64. Bayard PJ, Berger TG, Jacobsen MA. Drug hypersensitivity reactions and human immunodeficiency virus disease. J Acquired Immune Deficiency Syndrome 1992;5:1237–1257.

65. Williams I, Weller IVD, Malni A, Anderson J, Waters MF. Thalidomide hypersensitivity in AIDS. Lancet 1991;337:436–437.

66. Pullen H, Wright N, Murdoch L. Hypersensitivity reactions to antibacterial drugs in infectious mononucleosis. Lancet 1967;2:1176–1178.

67. Klemola E. Hypersensitivity reaction to ampicillin in cytomegalovirus mononucleosis. Scand J Infect Dis 1970;2:29–31.

68. Battegay M, Opravil M, Wuthrich B, Luthy R. Rash with amoxicillin-clavulanate therapy in HIV-infected patients (Letter). Lancet 1989;2:1100.

69. Harb GE, Alldredge BK, Coleman R, Jacobsen MA. Pharmacoepidemiology of adverse drug reactions in hospitalized patients with human immunodeficiency virus disease. J Acquired Immune Deficiency Syndrome 1993;6:919–926.

10

HIV Testing

William J. Kassler and Howard M. Kassler

Many of the estimated one million persons in the United States who are infected with the human immunodeficiency virus (HIV) are unaware of their infection, and dentists probably see a large number of them as patients on a regular basis. Since many asymptomatically infected persons might otherwise have no need to seek health care, HIV testing in the context of dental practice plays an important role in identifying people who are unaware of their infection. Persons who learn that they are infected can then receive appropriate medical care.

Early treatment with antiviral medications and prophylaxis for HIV-related complications is thought to slow the progression of the disease,

delay the onset of complications, preserve immune function (thereby decreasing the frequency and severity of infections), and improve quality of life. Persons who learn that they are infected can also take steps to avoid transmitting infection to others. Preventing the spread of HIV requires that persons at risk of transmitting the infection change their behavior, and knowledge of one's HIV status plays a role in initiating behavioral changes. Prevention counseling targeted at seropositive individuals further assists them in their efforts to avoid infecting others. It is here that dental health-care workers play an instrumental role.

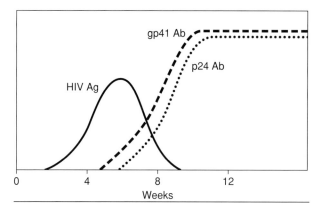

Fig 10-1. HIV serology. Detection of antibodies against HIV can be detected in the blood 4 to 12 weeks after the initial infection. Antibody tests performed before this time may yield negative results, although an infection has occurred. (Reproduction granted with the approval of Abbott Laboratories, all rights reserved by Abbott Laboratories.)

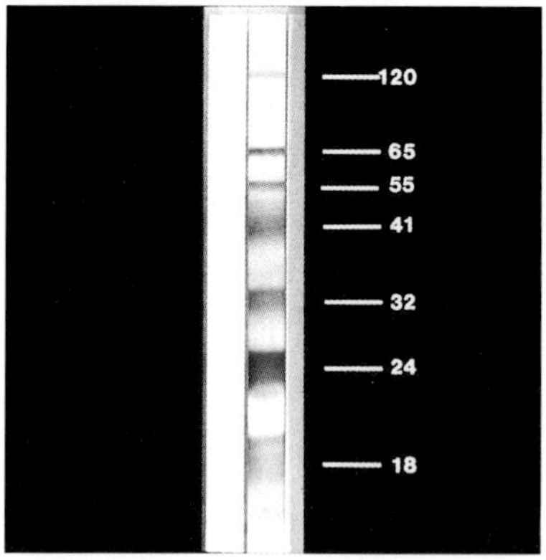

Fig 10-2. Pattern of distinct bands on a cellulose strip indicates the presence of antibodies against specific proteins of the HIV structure. (Reproduction granted with the approval of Abbott Laboratories, all rights reserved by Abbott Laboratories.)

HIV Serologic Testing

HIV serologic tests are used to indirectly detect an HIV infection by testing for the presence of anti-HIV antibodies. These tests are performed to screen asymptomatic persons for evidence of infection and to confirm or eliminate the diagnosis in a person with symptoms.

HIV antibodies may not be detectable in the blood until 4 to 12 weeks after initial infection (Fig 10-1). While some infected persons may take longer than 3 months to seroconvert, 95% do so within 6 months following exposure.[1] HIV infection longer than 6 months following exposure without detectable antibody is uncommon. Therefore, individuals who have been recently exposed to HIV should be retested within 3 to 6 months after their last exposure.

The Testing Process

The antibody test for HIV is a two-component procedure, beginning with a screening test, commonly an enzyme immunoassay (EIA, also known as enzyme linked immunosorbent assay [ELISA]). When the EIA is nonreactive, the HIV test is reported as negative. When the EIA is reactive, it must be confirmed by repeating the EIA on the same sample. If the repeat test is still reactive, another test, usually a Western blot assay, is performed on the sample to validate the EIA (the immunofluorescence assay is sometimes used for confirmation). When both the EIA and the Western blot are reactive, the HIV antibody test is reported as positive.

For a Western blot to be fully reactive, the test must be reactive for all the relevant viral proteins (ie, p24, gp41, and gp160). These proteins appear as a pattern of distinct bands on the cellulose strips of the Western blot (Fig 10-2).

If some but not all of the virus-specific bands are present on the Western blot, the test is considered indeterminate. An indeterminate test result is equivocal; the patient could be uninfected or the patient could be in the process of seroconverting. Persons with indeterminate serologic test results should be interviewed for additional risk information and should be retested to determine true antibody status. Among recently infected persons who have an indeterminate Western blot, a repeat test is commonly positive in 6 months, whereas follow-up tests of uninfected persons with indeterminate results often show no change.[2]

A Western blot is nonreactive only if no virus-specific bands are present. If the EIA is reactive but the Western blot is nonreactive, the test is reported as negative.[2]

Accuracy of the HIV Test

Tests for HIV need to be extremely accurate. They must have a low false-negative rate, because telling an infected person that he or she is negative delays medical treatment and may result in further spread of the disease. Tests for HIV must also have a low false-positive rate, because of the emotional consequences of a person mistakenly believing that he or she has a potentially fatal disease.

The accuracy of HIV tests (like any laboratory test) is determined partially by the test's sensitivity, specificity, and predictive value. Sensitivity is the probability that the test will be positive if the specimen is a true positive; specificity is the probability that a test will be negative if the specimen is a true negative. The positive predictive value is the probability that a person with a positive test is truly positive, and it depends on the level of infection (prevalence) in the population to which the test is applied.

Licensed EIA tests performed in U.S. reference laboratories have excellent performance characteristics, with sensitivity and specificity exceeding 99%. With such accuracy, when the test is used in populations with a high prevalence of HIV infection, the positive predictive value for HIV serology (EIA and Western blot) approaches 99.9%; however, in populations with a low prevalence of HIV infection, the positive predictive value may drop as low as 65%.[3] Thus, when a high-risk person, such as an injecting drug user, is tested, the likelihood of a false-positive test result is less than one in 1,000. However, when a low-risk person, such as a female blood donor with no risk factors, is tested, the likelihood of a false-positive result may be as high as 35%.

This is one reason why screening in low-risk, low-prevalence populations (such as requiring HIV tests for all marriage licenses) is difficult; there may be an unacceptably high number of false-positive test results. Screening programs for HIV are most effective when targeted at specific populations that are at high risk and therefore have a high prevalence of HIV infection.

Indications for HIV Testing

The HIV test can be used as a diagnostic test or a screening test. As a diagnostic test, HIV serology can be used to confirm or rule out HIV infection when a patient's medical history, signs or symptoms suggest the possibility of HIV infection. As a screening test, HIV serology is used to test asymptomatic persons for evidence of disease. Given the relatively low prevalence of HIV in most primary care settings, screening is best targeted toward individuals at high risk for being infected with HIV. Therefore, screening should be considered for sexually active patients who have multiple sex partners; a history of sexually transmitted diseases (STDs); a sex partner with multiple sexual contacts or with a known or suspected STD; or an individual who frequents health-care settings, such as STD clinics, that serve high-risk patients.

A complete and accurate risk assessment helps determine who should be recommended for HIV testing. Through a sexual history, one can determine whether a patient's behaviors place him or her at high risk for HIV infection.[4] A minimal sexual history should include the patient's sexual orientation; whether the patient is sexually active either in an exclusive relationship or with several partners; whether the patient has recently changed sex partners or acquired a new partner; and whether the patient has a history of STDs.[5]

Discussing sexual behavior during the dental visit may be uncomfortable for both dentists and for patients, but if there is significant justification for concern, a way should be found to broach that subject tactfully. The dentist might begin by acknowledging that these are sensitive questions and explaining to the patient why it is important to discuss these issues[6]: "I realize that a person's sexual behavior is a very personal thing, but I need to ask you some questions so we can explore whether you are at risk for certain medical conditions, such as HIV infection."[7] Such discussions are facilitated by clear communication of respect, compassion, and a nonjudgmental attitude. It is also helpful to reassure the patient that treatment will be provided regardless of their lifestyle or HIV status.

Dentists practicing in geographic areas with higher seroprevalence rates should have a lower threshold for recommending HIV testing. In communities where HIV infection is more common, it is more likely that at-risk behaviors will lead to HIV infection; it is therefore appropriate to test for HIV more frequently. Because some people deny risk even after detailed questioning, testing may be appropriate in some areas and for some demographic groups even without a history of at-risk behavior.[7]

While screening asymptomatic patients for HIV may be appropriate in some settings, as a practical matter, HIV testing is most commonly recommended in dental practices when a patient's signs and symptoms suggest the possibility of HIV infection. Testing for HIV may also be recommended as part of a post-exposure protocol (see Chapter 15). The results of the HIV test should never be used to deny dental care to infected patients.

Tests Should Be Voluntary and Confidential

Although HIV testing is compulsory for blood donors, immigrants, military recruits, and some prisoners, routine office testing should always be voluntary.[3,8] Some studies have shown that mandatory HIV testing may inhibit some persons from seeking health care.[9,10]

Confidentiality is crucial to HIV testing to protect the patient from any adverse consequences of unwanted disclosure of test results. Considerable stigma is associated with HIV, and persons infected with the virus can experience discrimination in housing, employment, health care, and insurance. Because of these potential harmful consequences, and because, despite best intentions, strict confidentiality may not always be possible, some patients will not want to be tested in the office. These patients should be referred to an HIV testing site. Some publicly funded HIV testing sites offer the test anonymously, where the patient is identified by number only.

Because anonymity protects against any real or perceived adverse consequence of disclosure, anonymous testing may attract those who otherwise might not be tested. The negative side of anonymous testing is that the health-care system cannot contact HIV-infected persons who do not return for their results. Important services such as medical referral, counseling, and the notification of sex partners and needle-sharing partners cannot take place if the infected person does not return.

As for any other test or procedure that has the potential for harm, patients should give informed consent for the HIV test. Informed consent should include a description of the testing procedure and a discussion of the risks and the benefits of taking the test. For example, if the test result is positive, benefits to the patient can include early access to medical care to prevent early HIV-related morbidity and mortality. The information can also help patients protect their sex partners. Patients should weigh these potential benefits against potential harms before deciding to proceed with the HIV test.

Prevention Counseling for HIV

Counseling associated with HIV testing traditionally has two components. Pre-test counseling takes place when the blood is drawn, and post-test counseling takes place later when the results are provided to the patient. During pre-test counseling, the provider asks for informed consent for the HIV test. The provider also assesses the patient's risk behaviors, helps the patient recognize his or her risk, and helps the patient to develop a plan to reduce those risks. During post-test counseling, the provider informs the patient of the results and discusses the meaning of the test results; a positive test result means that the patient is infected with HIV and is capable of infecting others, and a negative test result means the patient is probably not infected but is still vulnerable unless his or her behavior is changed. In the patient without HIV, the post-test session is a good time to reinforce the steps necessary to avoid becoming infected. In the patient with HIV, the post-test session is used to reinforce the behaviors necessary to avoid transmitting infection, to help make appointments for medical follow-up, and to provide referral for additional services if needed, such as psychological or behavioral counseling, and social services.[11]

Counseling can be considered a primary prevention strategy, distinct from HIV testing, to assist individuals in adopting or maintaining safer behaviors. Counseling referrals should be offered to patients on the basis of their risk for acquiring or transmitting HIV. Minimum ethical requirements at the time of HIV testing are to ensure that patients give informed consent, and to ensure that all patients are aware of the risks of transmission through their future behaviors.[12,13] These requirements constitute the same standard of care as that for testing for any communicable disease.

When the HIV Test Result Is Positive

Informing a patient of a positive test result is usually extremely distressing to the patient and should be done in person. Patients' reactions can span a wide range of emotions, from denial to anger, fear, remorse, and resignation, and the clinician should be prepared to be supportive. Often this simply involves listening to the patients express their feelings.[7]

After allowing time for the patient to react, the clinician should tell the patient what the test result means. A positive test result means that the patient is both infected and infectious. A positive test result does not necessarily mean that the patient has AIDS; the prognosis should be discussed.

Referral of patients with HIV for medical services is important. The initial workup for a patient newly diagnosed with HIV would include T-lymphocyte analysis (CD4+ cell count), complete blood cell count, serologic test for syphilis, and tuberculin skin testing. Referral to psychological counseling, support groups, social service agencies, and other community resources is also important. Referral to the public health department for partner notification should be considered.

Partner notification is an important prevention strategy for breaking the cycle of transmission. Uninfected partners can reduce the risks of acquiring infection by changing their behaviors, and infected partners can receive early medical intervention and avoid transmission of the infection to others. There are two strategies for partner notification: patient referral, where index patients notify partners themselves, and provider referral, where named partners are notified and counseled by health department personnel.[14] While HIV-infected persons have an ethical responsibility to notify the partner with whom they share needles and sex, who may not be aware of their risk for infection, partner notification is often more effective when assisted by the health department.[15]

Cases of HIV should be reported in accordance with local statutory requirements, and as promptly as possible. In every state, AIDS is a reportable disease. Requirements for reporting asymptomatic HIV infection differ from state to state; dentists doing HIV testing should become familiar with local reporting requirements. This information can be obtained from state or local health departments.

New Testing Technology

There have been many recent technological advances in HIV diagnostic testing. Some of the most promising include: the availability of office-based, 10-minute HIV tests, the potential for saliva-based tests, the potential for home-based collection, and eventually home testing. While these technological advances in HIV testing may alter how testing is conducted in the future, and may alter the need for traditional pre- and post-test HIV counseling, the basic elements of informed consent, risk assessment, referral for risk reduction counseling, and referral for additional services will remain the same.

Rapid HIV Tests

The Food and Drug Administration has recently approved a new, easy-to-read, rapid HIV test. The Single Use Diagnostic System (SUDS) HIV-1 test uses EIA technology to obtain results within 10 minutes, and the SUDS test is comparable to a standard EIA. In clinical trials involving 8,588 specimens at 11 sites, the SUDS was shown to have a sensitivity of 99.9% and a specificity of 99.6%. (Murex: Summary basis of approval documents submitted to FDA, 1992.) A negative test result does not require further confirmation; test results can be obtained at the visit, eliminating the need to return for results. A positive test result requires confirmation by Western blot, so patients with a positive test need to return. While the SUDS test is currently the only rapid HIV test available, several others are being developed or are under evaluation for licensure and will probably be available in the near future.

The potential advantages of using a rapid diagnostic test include: patients receive their results sooner, improved patient satisfaction, greater ability to conduct counseling relevant to their HIV-infection status, and provision of negative results at less cost since only one visit is needed. The potential disadvantages of the rapid test include increased expense and the need for laboratory trained personnel on site.

Saliva-Based Tests

Because antibodies to HIV can be detected in the saliva of HIV-infected persons, saliva has been proposed as a noninvasive alternative to serum for HIV testing. Saliva-based tests have the advantage of ease of collection; medically trained personnel are not needed, there is a reduced risk of needle stick injuries, and saliva-based testing may be more acceptable to patients. However, the reliability of the current generation of saliva-based tests is less than that of serum.[16–18] Saliva-based tests can be useful for surveillance and other epidemiologic studies, but more development to improve test performance needs to take place before these tests can be useful clinically.

While there are currently no commercial, FDA approved, saliva-based HIV tests available in the United States, a new generation of saliva tests are available overseas. One of these, the GAC-ELISA, which is the only test developed specifically for oral fluids (the others use modified tests originally designed for serum or plasma), shows promise.

The Dentists' Role in HIV Testing

Unless and until saliva-based HIV testing becomes available, testing for HIV infection by dentists will not be commonplace.[19] However, many dental practitioners are comfortable ordering various laboratory tests for their patients when signs and symptoms indicate such a need. For these dentists, it is certainly reasonable and desirable also to consider HIV testing under appropriate circumstances. Other dentists, when presented with evidence that may indicate systemic disease or increased medical risk, feel more at ease apprising the patient's physician about their concerns and allowing the physician to follow up as necessary. Given that the dentist may be the first and only health-care provider seen by some high-risk or asymptomatically infected patients, the astute practitioner has an opportunity and an obligation to encourage and guide patients in these matters.

References

1. Horsburgh CR, Jason J, Longini I, et al. Duration of human immunodeficiency virus infection before detection of antibody. Lancet 1989;2:637–639.

2. CDC. Update: serologic testing for antibody to human immunodeficiency virus. MMWR 1988;36:833–845.

3. Lo B, Steinbrook RL, Cooke M, Coates TJ, Walters EJ, Hulley SB. Voluntary screening for human immunodeficiency virus (HIV) infection. Ann Intern Med 1989;110:727–733.

4. Siwek J. Taking a sexual history: an individualized approach. Am Fam Physician 1989; 40:83–84.

5. Kassler WJ, Wasserheit JN, Cates W. Sexually transmitted diseases. In Woolf S (ed): Health Promotion and Disease Prevention in Clinical Practice. Philadelphia: Williams & Wilkins; in press.

6. HIV Blood Test Counseling: Physician Guidelines. Chicago: American Medical Association; 1993.

7. Kassler WJ, Wu AW. Addressing HIV in the office practice: assessing risk, counseling, and testing. Primary Care 1992;19:19–33.

8. CDC. 1993 Sexually transmitted diseases treatment guidelines. MMWR 1993;24(RR-14):1–102.

9. Kegeles SM, Catania JA, Coates TJ, Pollack LM, Lo B. Many people who seek anonymous HIV-antibody testing would avoid it under other circumstances. AIDS 1990;4:585–588.

10. Kegeles SM, Coates TJ, Lo B, Catania JA. Mandatory reporting of HIV testing would deter men from being tested. JAMA 1989;261:1275–1276.

11. CDC. Technical guidance on HIV counseling. MMWR 1993;42(RR-2):11–16.

12. CDC. Report from the HIV Strategic Planning Task Force. Atlanta: Division of STD/HIV Prevention; 1993.

13. CDC. Recommendations for HIV testing services for inpatients and outpatients in acute-care hospital settings. MMWR 1993;42(RR-2):1–6.

14. CDC. Partner notification for preventing human immunodeficiency virus (HIV) infection—Colorado, Idaho, South Carolina, Virginia. MMWR 1988;37:393–402.

15. Landis S, Schoenbach V, Weber D, et al. Results of a randomized trial of partner notification in cases of HIV infection in North Carolina. N Engl J Med 1992;326:101–106.

16. Francoise G, Thorstensson R, Luton P, et. al. Multicenter European evaluation of HIV testing on serum and saliva samples. Int Conf AIDS 1993;9:766-PO-C31-3293.

17. Warnecke C, Stark K, Bienzle U, Pauli G. Saliva testing for HIV-specific antibodies is attractive. Int Conf AIDS 1993;9:767-PO-C31-3301.

18. Ichikawa S, Tsukano K, Ito A, Zu G, Kihara M, Soda K. Usefulness of saliva for detecting antibodies to HIV-1. Int Conf AIDS 1993;9:767-PO-C31-3299.

19. Glick M. HIV-testing: more questions than answers. Dent Clin North Am 1990;34:45–54.

11

Laboratory Parameters of HIV Infection

Michael Glick

Medical and dental health-care providers rely on laboratory markers to determine the status and progression of diseases. Because the risk of infections and bleeding tendencies are major concerns for dental-care providers, knowledge of pertinent laboratory parameters associated with HIV disease helps practitioners anticipate and prevent potential complications that may result from dental therapy.

Immunologic and hematologic alterations invariably occur during the progression of HIV disease, resulting in immune dysfunctions that render the body susceptible to infections, anemia, and hemostatic abnormalities that in turn cause increased bleeding and coagulation irregularities (see Appendix A). A more detailed discussion on how the immunologic and hematologic changes affect treatment of patients can be found in Chapter 12. Familiarity with these laboratory parameters can also enhance the dental practitioner's understanding of HIV disease.

The most characteristic immunologic finding in HIV disease is the progressive decline and dysfunction of circulating CD4+ T lymphocytes (See Chapter 5). However, other immunologic abnormalities during the course of HIV disease involve not only T lymphocytes (quantitative and functional decreased CD4+ cell response and an early and sustained increased number of CD8+ cells) but also the B lymphocyte response, monocyte and macrophage abnormalities, and impaired neutrophil response.

T lymphocytes are produced in the thymus, where they mature into different cells that are modified to express characteristic surface proteins, or receptors, called *clusters of differentiation* (or CD). The CD marker plays an important role in recognizing foreign antigens and for cell surface adhesion. Two distinct T-lymphocyte cell lines are recognized: cells expressing CD4 receptors, called CD4+ T-helper lymphocytes; and cells expressing CD8 receptors, called CD8+ T-suppressor lymphocytes or CD8+ T-cytotoxic lymphocytes. Normally, approximately 70% of T lymphocytes are CD4+ cells, and 25% express CD8+ surface proteins.

CD4+ T-lymphocyte Cell Count

CD4+ T-helper lymphocytes are responsible for coordinating many important functions of the immune system. The activation of CD4+ lymphocytes results in the activation of B lymphocytes to produce antibodies, activation of monocytes and macrophages, and activation of cytotoxic T lymphocytes. The overall result of CD4+ T-lymphocyte activation and regulation includes the killing of invading viruses, fungi, parasites, and to a certain extent bacteria and tumor cells. Depletion and dysfunction of CD4+ lymphocytes are reflected in almost all of the immune defects found in individuals with HIV infections. Significantly, the immune response against bacterial infections can be stimulated successfully without CD4+ cell activation. Throughout most of the course of HIV disease, B lymphocytes ward off most opportunistic bacterial infections by producing an appropriate and sufficient antibody response. Antibodies are effective in neutralizing bacterial infections since bacteria, in contrast to viruses, multiply outside of cells (extracellular). An appropriate immune response against bacteria is of importance to dental providers as dissemination of bacteria occurs during dental therapy. An important exception is mycobacterial infections, such as tuberculosis, which proliferate inside cells (intracellular). Antibodies cannot effectively reach these bacteria, and a cytotoxic-mediated immune response by T lymphocytes is required.

CD4+ T-lymphocyte counts are used for a variety of purposes. They serve as indicators for initiating therapeutic interventions and markers for therapeutic trials, and they help monitor immune deterioration and disease progression. They also facilitate differential diagnosis of opportunistic infections, including oral lesions, and help establish Centers for Disease Control (CDC) HIV and AIDS classification and case surveillance definitions. Each of these functions is essential for HIV care.

However, it is important to understand the limitations of using CD4+ T-lymphocyte counts for all of these purposes. First, CD4 counts are measured from blood samples, but only about 2% of all CD4+ cells circulate in the peripheral blood system. Thus, levels of CD4+ cells in the peripheral blood represent only a small portion of the total number of CD4+ cells in the body. Furthermore, a variety of factors influences the percentage of CD4+ cells found in the blood without affecting the total number of T lymphocytes in the body. CD4+ cells are affected by a diurnal rhythm, which is at its lowest level in the morning (8:00 AM to 11:00 AM) and at its highest level in the evening (10:00 PM to 12:00 AM).[1] The change between morning and evening measurements can be substantial; 10% to 16% is not uncommon.[2,3]

Biologic factors directly influence the total number of circulating lymphocytes and the consequent number of measurable CD4+ lymphocytes. Strenuous exercise, nicotine, and the use of glucocorticosteroids decrease the number of circulating lymphocytes, while medications, such as some antibiotics (cephalosporins) and zidovudine, can decrease or increase the number of cells.[4] It is also important to realize that when HIV-infected individuals experience concomitant illnesses, changes in T lymphocyte level will occur. This fluctuation in T-lymphocyte count also occurs in individuals without HIV who suffer from various infections.

CD4 counts are also influenced by the handling and transportation of the blood sample. Blood samples preserved with the anticoagulant ethylenediamine tetraacetic acid (EDTA)—purple-top tubes commonly used for complete blood cell counts—need to be tested within 6 hours. Flow cytometry, a laboratory technique to differ-

entiate between the different lymphocyte subtypes, must be performed within 30 hours. If the blood sample is collected in tubes with heparin as an anticoagulant—green-top tubes—flow cytometry should be performed within 48 hours. After this time, the changes in the proportion of lymphocytes are not valid.[5,6] Error due to the instruments used for CD4+ cell determination can be substantial. Depending on how the test is performed, a CD4 count of 530 cells/mm^3 might represent a true value ranging from 300 to 760 cells/mm^3.[2] The use of trained clinical personnel and an experienced laboratory and reliance on a number of consecutive test results decreases the error associated with handling and laboratory techniques.

The CD4+ cell count is calculated by multiplying the white blood cell count (WBC) by the lymphocyte differential (both measured with automated hematologic instruments) and the CD4 lymphocyte percentage (CD4%), measured with flow cytometry: CD4 count = WBC count × % lymphocytes × CD4%. As previously mentioned, hematologic measurements are subject to considerable variations. These variations may be especially high if manual differentiation is being used. Even in individuals without HIV, the WBC count is associated with an approximate 6% coefficient of variation.[2] The lymphocyte percentage may have a coefficient of variation of 4.1% in patients with HIV while the absolute number of CD4+ T cells can vary 8.4% from normal controls.[4]

Determination of CD4% with flow

cytometry is less subject to error from delayed processing—specimens can be measured up to 48 hours after being collected—and the results are more reproducible. Furthermore, CD4% levels are not dependent on a WBC count and a differential count, making this measurement less prone to accumulated laboratory errors. Compared to absolute CD4+ cell counts, CD4% is less subject to variations on repeat measurement.[7,8] Many experts believe that CD4% more accurately reflects immunologic changes and may even have a slightly better prognostic significance than CD4+ cell count.[8] In that most clinical treatment decisions and therapeutic trials, as well as the CDC's classification of HIV disease, use CD4+ cell counts as guidelines, studies have been conducted to evaluate the relationship between the absolute CD4+ cell count and CD4%. Data from 1,000 consecutive specimens from three different laboratories showed that an individual with a CD4% of less than 14% would have a 82% to 87% chance of having a CD4+ cell count below 200 cells/mm³, and an individual with a CD4% of less than 27% would have a 83% to 95% chance of having a CD4+ cell count below 500 cell/mm³.[9]

A normal CD4+ cell count is estimated to be 544 to 1663 cells/mm³, with a median cell count of 935 cells/mm³. Lymphocyte cell counts in infants and children differ from adult values. A CD4+ cell count of 500 cells/mm³ in an adult corresponds to a CD4+ cell count of 1,750 cells/mm³ in infants less than 12 months old, of 1,000 cells/mm³ in children between 12 months and 24 months of age, of 750 cells/mm³ in children between the age of 2 to 6 years, and equal to adult levels after the age of 6 years. As previously mentioned, a continuous decline of CD4+ lymphocytes is noted during the progression of HIV disease. This has prompted clinicians to institute prophylactic medications both against HIV infection and various opportunistic infections. Anti-retroviral prophylaxis is routinely used in the United States when a patient's CD4+ cell count drops below 500 cells/mm³.[10] This practice may change due to a large European trial that indicated that survival of HIV-infected patients was equivalent regardless of whether zidovudine was instituted early or late in the course of infection.[11]

Prophylactic intervention against *Pneumocystis carinii* pneumonia (PCP) is instituted when patients' CD4+ cell counts fall below 200 cells/mm³.[12] Many clinicians also institute prophylaxis against mycobacterial and fungal infections when patients' CD4+ cell counts are less than 100 cells/mm³.

CD4+ cell counts obviously constitute an important marker for disease progression. Studies have correlated clinical expressions of HIV disease with CD4+ cell counts to predict onset of opportunistic infections. Although it is impossible to apply results from large cohort studies to individual cases, the clinical progression of HIV disease correlates with changes in the CD4+ cell count.[13,14] The CD4+ cell count and clinical markers for HIV disease progression are discussed further in Chapters 5, 6, 8, and 12.

Classification of HIV disease and the definition of AIDS were based solely on clinical signs and symptoms until December 31, 1992.[15] However, as of January 1, 1993, CD4+ cell counts have been included in the definition of AIDS.[16] Accordingly, a person with HIV and a CD4+ cell count below 200 cells/mm^3 is defined as having AIDS, even without the presence of signs and symptoms.

CD8+ Cell Count

CD8+ T-cytotoxic/suppressor lymphocytes kill other cells that are perceived as being infected with foreign pathogens, such as viruses. This is part of what is known as the cell-mediated cytotoxic immune response. These cells are also capable of regulating some of the functions of the immune response. Activation and an increased number of CD8+ lymphocytes have been noted during the early course of HIV disease.[17,18] But the number of CD8+ cells eventually decreases during the more advanced stages of the disease. This subsequent decline has not been associated with a functional impairment or infection with HIV.[19,20] A study of long-term asymptomatic HIV-infected patients showed a significantly higher level of CD8+ cells compared to that in patients with advanced stages of HIV disease.[21] It has been proposed that CD8+ cells are capable of producing a lymphokine that can suppress HIV replication,[22] which would indicate a direct relationship between high levels of this subtype of T lymphocytes and survival. During progression to AIDS, the ability of CD8+ lymphocytes to kill HIV-infected cells diminishes, as does the immune system's ability to suppress HIV replication.[23,24] A normal CD8+ cell count is 272 to 932 cells/mm^3 with a median count of 519 cells/mm^3.

CD4+/CD8+ Ratio

Another way to evaluate immune status is to measure the ratio of CD4+ to CD8+ cells. This measurement bypasses some of the biologic factors associated with CD4+ cell variations. A normal ratio is 0.93 to 4.50, with a median of 1.72. Low ratios are associated with increased immune suppression.

p24 Antigen/Antibody

The p24 antigen represents the core protein of HIV, and detectable serum levels are associated with increased HIV replication and more rapid disease progression.[25,26] Antibodies to this protein are formed shortly after seroconversion and are detectable during the quiescent stages of HIV disease.[27] Approximately 7% of asymptomatic patients with high CD4+ cell counts show very low levels of measurable antigens, while 75% of individuals with CD4+ cell counts below 200 cells/mm^3 show signs of p24 antigenemia.[27]

β-2 Microglobulin

ß-2 microglobulin is the short chain of the class I major histocompatibility complex. A nonspecific marker for cell destruction, increased levels of this protein can be found during seroconversion and during progression of HIV disease.[28] The normal serum concentration, as measured in homosexual men, is equal or less than 254 nmol/L. Measurements of this protein are mainly used for research purposes.

Erythrocyte Sedimentation Rate

An elevated erythrocyte sedimentation rate (ESR) is present in diseases causing an inflammatory response. This marker is not disease-specific and is elevated in many autoimmune disorders. In patients with HIV and CD4+ cell counts below 500 cells/mm³, an elevated ESR, in combination with a decreased CD4+ cell count and an elevated ß-2 microglobulin level is a good predictor for disease progression.[29] Some studies have indicated that an ESR level >35 mm in 1 hour is a significant and relatively early marker for progression to AIDS.[30,31]

Neopterin

Neopterin is produced by macrophages in response to T-cell activation.[32] This protein is a marker for immune stimulation and is there-fore associated with HIV disease progression.[33] Neopterin can be measured in serum and in the urine of individuals with HIV. A normal serum concentration is less than 10 nmol/L.[34] This marker is also mostly used for research purposes. Both ß-2 microglobulin and neopterin are nonspecific markers for HIV infection since they can be elevated in other immune disorders, malignancies, and other viral infections such as that with cytomegalovirus.

Platelet Count

Platelets or thrombocytes help to form the initial hemostatic plug that results in cessation of bleeding. A normal platelet count is 150,000 to 400,000 cells/mm³. The bleeding time is a measurement of both quantitative and qualitative functions of the platelets. A prolonged bleeding time is noticeable when the platelet count has dropped below 100,000 cells/mm³. Spontaneous bleeding usually occurs when the platelet count has fallen below 20,000 cells/mm³. General dental procedures and even simple extractions can be performed in patients with platelet counts above 60,000 cells/mm³. Below this level, special precautions need to be considered. In severe cases, platelet transfusions may be necessary.

Thrombocytopenia is not uncommon in individuals with HIV. One large study of 1,500 infected men indicated that up to 6.7% presented with platelet counts below 150,000 cells/

mm[3] on at least one occasion.[35] An increased incidence of thrombocytopenia may be present among injection drug users. One study showed that 9% of injection drug users with HIV had platelet counts below 100,000 cells/mm[3] vs only 3% of homosexual men.[36] The origin of thrombocytopenia in HIV disease is not clear, but many cases have been attributed to HIV-related immune thrombocytopenic purpura (ITP).[37] Interestingly, one study found ITP to be most common early in HIV disease, when a patient's CD4+ cell counts are between 600 cells/mm[3] and 300 cells/mm[3].[36] In cases of ITP, a bleeding time will help assess patient's bleeding tendencies. Other studies suggest that after patients manifested signs and symptoms of disease, thrombocytopenia becomes more common during the more advanced stages.[38] It is possible that HIV-related ITP is the result of circulating immune complexes deposited on platelets, causing increased platelet clearance and destruction.[39,40] Successful treatment for HIV-related ITP has been accomplished with splenectomies and prednisone therapy.[41] Destruction and decreased production of platelets also occur in individuals with HIV-related thrombocytopenia. While platelets from healthy control subjects survive for 198 ± 15 hours (approximately 8 days), platelets among untreated patients with HIV survive 92 ± 33 hours (approximately 4 days) compared to 129 ± 44 hours (approximately 5 days) in zidovudine-treated individuals.[42]

Bleeding Time

An increased bleeding time will assess both quantitative and qualitative platelet functions. Thus, increased bleeding time (> 0–7 min) in the presence of a normal platelet count indicates abnormal platelet function.

Total WBC Count and Differential WBC Count

Alterations in the bone marrow, which are common in HIV disease, are usually associated with drug therapy but can also be caused directly by HIV infection. The normal total WBC count is approximately 4,500 to 10,000 cells/mm[3]. Leukopenia, a WBC count below 4,500 cells/mm[3] is not uncommon in individuals with HIV. This is caused not only by decreasing numbers of lymphocytes but also suppressed cellular production in the bone marrow, resulting in a decreased number of granulocytes and monocytes. Granulocytopenia mainly results from a reduction in neutrophils (neutropenia). A normal absolute number of neutrophils in the peripheral blood is between 3,000 cells/mm[3] and 6,000 cells/mm[3]. Severe neutropenia is considered when the neutrophil count drops below 500 cells/mm[3].

Neutropenia is of great concern for dental-care providers, since neutrophils provide one of the body's earliest defenses against bacterial pathogens. Thus, patients with neutropenia are more susceptible to bacterial infections. This has been shown in immunocompromised patients who experience a significant increase in bacterial infections when the absolute neutrophil count falls below 500 cells/mm[3].[43]

In one large, multicenter study, less than 1% of asymptomatic patients with HIV and mean CD4+ cell counts above 700 cells/mm[3] presented with granulocytopenia, while over 13% of patients with mean CD4+ cell counts below 250 cells/mm[3] have granulocytopenia.[35] In patients with AIDS, up to 44% have low granulocyte counts.[44] Although antibodies against granulocytes,[35,45] impaired granulopoiesis,[46,47] and infiltrative processes such as infections and malignancies involving the bone marrow have been documented, most cases of clinically relevant granulocytopenia result from drug toxicity.

An initial study of zidovudine reported severe granulocytopenia (less than 500 cells/mm[3]) in 16% of patients receiving the drug.[48] However, there was no reported incidence of increased bacterial infections or sepsis. Subsequent studies with lower doses of zidovudine could not document a higher incidence of bacterial infections or sepsis.[49,50] The lack of bacterial infections in most studies of zidovudine may be due to the discontinuation of therapy or reduction of the dosage when granulocyte counts dropped below 500 cells/mm[3] or 1,000 cells/mm[3]. In a longitudinal study of 30 patients, a significantly higher number of bacterial infections was documented in patients with neutrophil counts below 500 cells/mm[3], compared to patients with neutrophil counts between 500 and 1,000 cells/mm[3].[51] Other drugs such as ganciclovir,[52] trimethoprim-sulfamethoxazole,[53,54] and other myelosuppressive drugs have also been associated with neutropenia but without evidence of an increased incidence of bacterial infections. The myelosuppressive effect of these drugs may be enhanced when combined with zidovudine.[55]

Treatment of granulocytopenia in HIV disease has been successful with myeloid growth factors such as granulocyte-macrophage colony-stimulating factor (GM-CSF).[56] Side effects associated with this type of therapy include fever, facial flushing, skin rash, and phlebitis at the infusion sites.

Hemoglobin

Normal adult hemoglobin levels for men are 14 g/dL to 18 g/dL, and for women, 12 g/dL to 16 g/dL. A decreased hemoglobin level may be due to a reduction of red blood cell production as well as impaired hemoglobin production. A decrease in the red blood cell count is common among individuals with HIV. During the early, asymptomatic stage of HIV disease, 8% of patients not receiving medications that are associated with red blood cell production were found to be anemic.[44] An increased incidence of anemia was found during the progression of disease, where 20% of symptomatic patients and up to 70% of patients with AIDS manifested signs of anemia. In patients with CD4+ cell counts above 700 cells/mm[3], 3.2% of homosexual men with HIV had anemia whereas 20.9% had anemia when CD4+ cell counts dropped below 250 cells/mm³.[35] Some studies have suggested that 70% to 95% of all patients with AIDS have anemia[57–59] with mean hemoglobin levels ranging from 9.7 to 11.7g/dL.[60,61]

The most common cause of anemia in patients with HIV is associated with zidovudine therapy. Initial studies with zidovudine were associated with severe bone marrow suppression, which resulted in 21% of the treated individuals needing multiple blood transfusions due to anemia.[48] Subsequent studies have shown a decreased incidence of anemia when lower doses of zidovudine are used.[49,50]

Anemia in patients with HIV has also been associated with *Mycobacterium avium* complex (MAC) infections.[62] One study showed that patients with positive blood culture results for MAC received blood transfusions more than five times more than patients with negative blood culture results.[63]

Low serum levels of vitamin B_{12} have been reported in up to 20% of individuals with HIV.[64] Since HIV can infect mononuclear cells of the intestinal mucosa directly, possibly as a result of rectal inoculation, this infection may result in malabsorption of vitamin B_{12} from the terminal ileum.[65] However, clinical complications due to vitamin B_{12} deficiency are rare. Since signs of this deficiency can be detected in the oral cavity, dental practitioners need to be aware of this possibility. Patients may present with a fiery red, painful tongue, loss of taste sensation, and loss of muscle tone of the tongue.

Oral candidiasis may also be present due to B_{12} deficiency. Yellow-green, sore mucosa and periodontal tissue may be another oral manifestation. The initial patient complaint may be an inability to wear dentures.

Treatment for HIV-related anemia includes reduction of the dose of zidovudine, administration of recombinant human erythropoietin,[66] and blood transfusions. In cases of vitamin B_{12} deficiency, replacement of the vitamin is sufficient.

General dental procedures can be performed safely at hemoglobin levels above 7.0 g/dL. However, respiratory depressive drugs should not be used with patients with hemoglobin levels below 10 g/dL.

Prothrombin Time and Partial Thromboplastin Time

Prothrombin time (PT) and partial thromboplastin time (PTT) are quantitative measurements of an individual's clotting ability. Increased PT and PTT measurements indicate increased bleeding tendencies. Partial thromboplastin time evaluates clotting factors of the intrinsic and common pathways (all factors except VII and XIII). A normal PTT test result is 25 to 38 seconds, but this can be increased due to heparin.

Prothrombin time identifies defects of the vitamin K-dependent coagulation factors in the extrinsic and common pathways (factor VII, factor X, and factor II) as well as factor V and factor I. A normal PT test is less than 2 seconds deviation from the control (usually 9 seconds to 11 seconds). Increased PT results are present in patients taking oral anticoagulants such as warfarin. Obviously, coagulation deficiencies are present in patients with HIV and hemophilia, but abnormalities of coagulation have been documented secondary to HIV disease. A lupus-like anticoagulant has been found in the sera of individuals with HIV.[67–70] Individuals with this anticoagulant exhibit prolonged PTT and in some cases also prolonged PT. One study[69] indicated a strong correlation between active PCP and the presence of the lupus anticoagulant. None of these studies indicate clinical evidence of bleeding complications. Thus, prolonged PTT in the presence of the lupus anticoagulant in HIV disease may suggest a direct interference with the test instead of a true clinical anticoagulation abnormality. The presence of lupus anticoagulant is therefore not a contraindication for procedures that cause bleeding.

In summary, changes in immunologic and hematologic laboratory parameters are important to recognize since they alert the dental-care provider to the potential complications during the course of an individual's HIV disease.

References

1. Miyawaki T, Taga K, Nagaoki T, Seki H, Suzuki Y, Taniguchi N. Circadian changes of the T lymphocyte subsets in human peripheral blood. Clin Exp Immunol 1984; 54:618–622.

2. Koepke JA, Landay AL. Precision and accuracy of absolute lymphocyte counts. Clin Immunol Immunopathol 1989;52:19–27.

3. Malone JL, Simms TE, Gray GC, Wagner KF, Burge JR, Burke JS. Sources of variability in repeated T-helper lymphocyte counts from human immunodeficiency virus type 1- infected patients: total lymphocyte count fluctuations and diurnal cycle are important. J Acquired Immune Deficiency Syndrome 1990;3:144–151.

4. CDC. Guidelines for the performance CD4+ cell determination in persons with human immunodeficiency virus infection. MMWR 1992;41(RR-8):1–17.

5. Shield CF III, Marlett P, Smith A, Gunter L, Goldstein G. Stability of human leukocyte differentiation antigens when stored in room temperature. J Immunol Methods 1983;62:347–352.

6. Weiblen BJ, Debell K, Giorgio A, Valeri CR. Monoclonal antibody testing of lymphocytes after overnight storage. J Immunol Methods 1984;70:179–183.

7. Kessler HA, Landay A, Pottage JC, Benson CA. Absolute number versus percentage of T-helper lymphocytes in human immunodeficiency virus infection. J Infect Dis 1990;161:356–357.

8. Taylor TMG, Fahey JL, Detels R, Giorgi JV. CD4 percentage, CD4 number, and CD4:CD8 ratio in HIV infection: which to choose and how to use. J Acquired Immune Deficiency Syndrome 1989;2: 114–124.

9. Kidd PG, Cheng S-C, Paxton H, Landay A, Gelman R. Prediction of CD4 count from CD4 percentage: experience from three laboratories. AIDS 1993;7:933–940.

10. Johnston MI, Hoth DF. Present status and future prospects for HIV therapies. Science 1993;260:1286–1293.

11. Aboulker J-P, Swart AM. Preliminary analysis of the Concorde trial. Lancet 1993;341: 889–890.

12. CDC. Guidelines for prophylaxis against *Pneumocystis carinii* pneumonia for persons infected with HIV. MMWR 1989;38:1–9.

13. Stein DS, Korvick JA, Vermund SH. CD4+ lymphocyte cell enumeration for prediction of clinical course of human immunodeficiency virus disease: a review. J Infect Dis 1992;165:352–363.

14. Glick M, Muzyka BC, Lurie D, Salkin LM. Oral manifestations associated with HIV disease as markers for immune suppression and AIDS. Oral Surg Oral Med Oral Pathol 1994;77:344–349.

15. Revision of the CDC surveillance case definition for acquired immunodeficiency syndrome. MMWR 1987;36:1–15.

16. CDC. 1993 revised classification system for HIV infection and expanded surveillance case definition for AIDS among adolescents and adults. MMWR 1992;41(No.RR-17):1–19.

17. Giorgi JV, Nishanian PG, Schmid I, Hultin LE, Cheng HL, Detels R. Selective alterations in immunoregulatory lymphocyte subsets in early HIV (human T-lymphotropic virus type III/lymphadenopathy-associated virus) infection. J Clin Immunol 1987;7:140–150.

18. Gaines H, von Sydow MAE, von Stedingk LV, et al. Immunological changes in primary HIV-1 infection. AIDS 1990;4:995–999.

19. Pantaleo G, DeMaria A, Koenig S, et al. CD8+ T-lymphocytes of patients with AIDS maintain normal broad cytolytic function despite the loss of human immunodeficiency virus-specific cytotoxicity. Proc Natl Acad Sci USA 1990;87:4818–4822.

20. Schnittman SM, Psallidopoulos MC, Lane HC, et al. The reservoir for HIV in human peripheral blood is a T-cell that maintains expression of CD4. Science 1989;245:305–308.

21. Lifson AR, Buchbinder SP, Sheppard HW, et al. Long term human immunodeficiency virus infection in asymptomatic homosexual and bisexual men with normal CD4+ lymphocyte counts: immunologic and virologic characteristics. J Infect Dis 1991;163:959–965.

22. Walker CM, Levy JA. A diffuse lymphokine produced by CD8+ T lymphocytes suppresses HIV replication. Immunology 1989;66:628–630.

23. Hoffenbach A, Langlade-Demoyen P, Dadaglio G, et al. Unusually high frequencies of HIV-specific cytotoxic T-lymphocytes in humans. J Immunol 1989;142:452–462.

24. Joly P, Guillon J, Mayaud C, et al. Cell-mediated suppression of HIV-specific cytotoxic T-lymphocytes. J Immunol 1989;143:2193–2201.

25. Allain JP, Laurian Y, Paul DA, et al. Long term evaluation of HIV antigen and antibodies to p24 and gp41 in patients with hemophilia. N Engl J Med 1987;317:1114–1121.

26. MacDonell KB, Chmiel JS, Poggensee L, Wu S, Phair JP. Predicting progression to AIDS: combined usefulness of CD4 lymphocyte counts and p24 antigenemia. Am J Med 1990;89:706–712.

27. Paul DA, Falk LA, Kessler HA, et al. Correlation of serum HIV antigen and antibody with clinical status in HIV-infected patients. J Med Virol 1987;22:357–363.

28. Jacobsen MA, Abrams DI, Volberding PA, et al. Serum beta-2 microglobulin decreases in patients with AIDS or ARC treated with azidothymidine. J Infect Dis 1989;159:1029–1036.

29. Schwartlander B, Bek B, Skarabis H, Koch J, Burkowitz J, Koch MA. Improvement of the predictive value of CD4+ lymphocyte count by ß-2 microglobulin, immunoglobulin A, and erythrocyte sedimentation rate. AIDS 1993;7:813–821.

30. Munfeldt-Manson L, Bottiger B, Nilsson B, von Stedingk L. Clinical signs and laboratory markers in predicting progression to AIDS in HIV-1 infected patients. Scand J Infect Dis 1991;23:443–449.

31. Lefrere J-J, Salmon D, Doinel C, et al. Sedimentation rate as a predictive marker in HIV infection. AIDS 1988;2:63–64.

32. Huber C, Batchelor JR, Fuchs D, et al. Immune response-associated production of neopterin: release from macrophages primarily under control of interferon-gamma. J Exp Med 1984;160:310–316.

33. Fuchs D, Hausen A, Reibnegger G, Werner ER, Dierich MP, Wachter H. Neopterin as a marker for activated cell-mediated immunity: application in HIV infection. Immunol Today 1988;9:150–155.

34. Jacobsen MA, Bacchetti P, Kolokathis A, et al. Surrogate markers for survival in patients with AIDS and AIDS related complex treated with zidovudine. Brit Med J 1991;302:73–78.

35. Kaslow RA, Phair JP, Friedman HB, et al. Infection with the human immunodeficiency virus: clinical manifestations and their relationship to immune deficiency. Ann Intern Med 1987;107:474–480.

36. Jost J, Tauber MG, Luthy R, Siegenthaler W. HIV-assoziierte thrombozytopenie. Schweiz Med Wochenschr 1988;118:206–212.

37. Ratner L. Human immunodeficiency virus-associated autoimmune thrombocytopenic purpura: a review. Am J Med 1989;86:194–198.

38. Murphy MF, Metcalfe P, Waters AH, et al. Incidence and mechanism of neutropenia and thrombocytopenia in patients with human immunodeficiency virus infection. Br J Haematol 1987;66:337–340.

39. Karpatkin S, Nardi M. Cross-reactive anti-idiotype antibody vs anti-HIVgp 120 in HIV-1-thrombocytopenia: correlation with thrombocytopenia (abstract). Blood 1989;74(suppl 1):128.

40. Stricker RB, Abrams DI, Corash L, Shuman MA. Target platelet antigen in homosexual men with immune thrombocytopenia. N Engl J Med 1985:313:1375–1380.

41. Walsh C, Krigel R, Lennette E, Karpatkin S. Thrombocytopenia in homosexual patients: prognosis, response to therapy, and prevalence of antibody to the retrovirus associated with the acquired immunodeficiency syndrome. Ann Intern Med 1985;103:542–545.

42. Ballem PJ, Belzberg A, Devine DV, et al. Kinetic studies of the mechanism of thrombocytopenia in patients with human immunodeficiency virus infection. N Engl J Med 1992:327:1779–1784.

43. Schimpff SS. Overview of empiric antibiotic therapy for the febrile neutropenic patient. Rev Infect Dis 1985;7:734–740.

44. Zon L, Groopman JE. Hematologic manifestations of the human immunodeficiency virus. Semin Hematol 1988;25:208–218.

45. Van der Lelie J, Lange JMA, Vos JJE, van Dalen CM, Danner SA, von der Borne AE. Autoimmunity against blood cells in human immunodeficiency virus infection. Br J Haematol 1987;67:109–114.

46. Stella CC, Ganser A, Hoelzer D. Defective in vitro growth of the hematopoietic progenitor cells in the acquired immunodeficiency syndrome. J Clin Invest 1987;80:286.

47. Folks TM, Kessler SW, Orenstein JM, Justement JS, Jaffe ES, Fauci AS. Infection and replication of HIV-1 in purified progenitor cells of normal human bone marrow. Science 1988;242:919–922.

48. Richman DD, Fischl MA, Grieco MH, et al. The toxicity of azidothymidine (AZT) in the treatment of patients with AIDS and AIDS-related complex: a double-blind, placebo-controlled trial. N Engl J Med 1987;317:192–197.

49. Volberding P, Lagakos SW, Koch MA, et al. Zidovudine in asymptomatic human immunodeficiency virus infection. A controlled trial in persons with fewer than 500 CD4-positive cells per cubic millimeter. N Engl J Med 1990;322:941–949.

50. Fischl MA, Richman DD, Hansen N, et al. The safety and efficacy of zidovudine (AZT) in the treatment of subjects with mildly symptomatic human immunodeficiency virus type 1 (HIV-1) infection. Ann Intern Med 1990;112:727–737.

51. Shaunak S, Bartlett JA. Zidovudine-induced neutropenia: are we too cautious? Lancet 1989;1:91–92.

52. Jacobson MA, O'Donnell JJ, Porteous D, Brodie HR, Feigal D, Mills J. Retinal and gastrointestinal disease due to cytomegalovirus in patients with acquired immunodeficiency syndrome: prevalence, natural history, and response to ganciclovir therapy. Q J Med 1988;254:473–486.

53. Gordin FM, Simon GL, Wofsy CB, Mills J. Adverse reactions to trimethoprim-sulfamethoxazole in patients with acquired immunodeficiency syndrome. Ann Intern Med 1984;100:495–499.

54. Sattler FR, Cowan R, Nielsen DM, Ruskin J. Trimethoprim-sulfamethoxazole compared with pentamidine for treatment of *Pneumocystis carinii* pneumonia in the acquired immunodeficiency syndrome. Ann Intern Med 1988;109:280–287.

55. Glatt AE, Chirgwin K, Landesman H. Current concepts: treatment of infections associated with human immunodeficiency virus. N Engl J Med 1988;318:1439–1448.

56. Mitsuyasu R, Levine J, Miles SA, et al. Effect of long-term subcutaneous (SC) administration of recombinant granulocyte-macrophage colony-stimulating factor (GM-CSF) in patients with HIV-related leukopenia (abstract). Blood 1988;72:357.

57. Frontiera M, Myers A. Peripheral and blood abnormalities in the acquired immunodeficiency syndrome. West J Med 1987;147:157–160.

58. Spivak JL, Barnes DC, Fuchs E, Quinn TC. Serum immunoreactive erythropoietin in HIV infected patients. JAMA 1989;261:3104–3107.

59. Zon LL, Arkin C, Groopman J. Hematologic manifestations of the human immune deficiency virus (HIV). Br J Haematol 1987;66:251–256.

60. Namiki TS, Boone DC, Meyer PR. A comparison of bone marrow findings in patients with acquired immunodeficiency syndrome (AIDS) and AIDS related complex. Hematol Oncol 1987;5:99–106.

61. Weber JN, Walker D, Engelkins H, Bain B, Harris JR. The value of hematologic screening for AIDS in an at-risk population. Genitourin Med 1985;61:325–329.

62. Bogner JR, Gathof B, Heinrich A, et al. Erythrocyte antibodies in AIDS are associated with mycobacteriosis and hypergammaglobulinemia. Klin Wochenschr 1990;68:1050–1053.

63. Jacobson MA, Peiperl L, Volberding PA, Porteous D, Toy PT, Feigal D. Red blood cell transfusion therapy for anemia in patients with AIDS and ARC: incidence, associated factors, and outcome. Transfusion 1990;30:133–137.

64. Burkes RL, Cohen H, Krailo M, Sinow RM, Carmel R. Low serum cobalamin levels occur frequently in the acquired immunodeficiency syndrome and related disorders. Eur J Haematol 1987;38:141–147.

65. Harriman GR, Smith PD, McDonald K, et al. Vitamin B_{12} malabsorption in patients with acquired immunodeficiency syndrome. Arch Intern Med 1989;149:2039–2041.

66. Erythropoietin Epo Study Group, Rudnick SA. Human recombinant erythropoietin (rHuEpo): a double blind, placebo-controlled study in acquired immunodeficiency syndrome (AIDS) patients with anemia induced by disease and AZT (abstract). Proc Am Soc Clin Oncol 1989;8:2.

67. Bloom EJ, Abrams DI, Rodgers GM. Lupus anticoagulant in the acquired immunodeficiency syndrome. JAMA 1986;256:491–493.

68. Cohen AJ, Phillips TM, Kessler CM. Circulating coagulation inhibitors in the acquired immunodeficiency syndrome. Ann Intern Med 1986;104:175–180.

69. Gold JE, Haubenstock A, Zalusky R. Lupus anticoagulant and AIDS. N Engl J Med 1986;314:1252–1253.

70. LeFrere JJ, Gozin D, Modai J, Vittecoq D. Circulating anticoagulant in the acquired immunodeficiency syndrome. Ann Intern Med 1987;107:429–430.

12

Medical Assessment of HIV-Infected Dental Patients

Michael Glick

Successful treatment of HIV-infected patients depends on proper medical assessment. The main concerns for the dental practitioner are bleeding, infections, and drug interactions. However, to formulate a suitable treatment plan, the patient's prognosis and survival must also be considered. An appropriate medical assessment will help prevent complications from dental therapy, as well as aid the diagnosis of oral lesions (Table 12-1).

Some information about patients with HIV disease might prove uncomfortable to elicit for dental practitioners. This chapter presents background for obtaining such information and shows how these data help dental health-care workers to better understand the medical relevance of such facts. This chapter also provides an overview of how dental practitioners can interpret medical information to evaluate the medical status of HIV-infected patients. Such information will help dental health-care workers differentiate oral pathologic conditions, reduce complications, and safely provide dental care. Since some oral manifestations may indicate disease progression, this chapter will also discuss why the dental provider should be familiar with appropriate HIV support groups and patients' individual support networks.

Table 12-1. Categories to Consider When Assessing Patients with HIV for Dental Treatment

- Transmission category
    - Homosexual or bisexual men
        - High incidence of particular oral manifestations
        - High incidence of HBV
    - Injection drug users
        - High risk for SBE
        - Avoid using narcotics
    - Hemophiliacs
        - High risk for increased bleeding tendencies
        - High incidence of HBV, HBC, HDV
- Date of initial HIV infection or HIV test
    - Will help to assess disease progression
- History of sexually transmitted diseases
    - Frequent episodes of STDs are associated with increased disease progression
    - Infections with syphilis may result in neurosyphilis and cardiomyopathies
- Past and present infectious diseases
    - Exposure to HBV, HCV, and HDV may result in liver disease
    - Exposure to TB and time period on medication may indicate infectious status
    - Noncompliance with anti-TB medications may result in multiple drug resistant–TB
- Past and present HIV-related opportunistic infections
    - Indicates immune status, disease progression, and medications
    - Indicates gastrointestinal and neurologic conditions
- Medications
    - Indicates past and present HIV-related conditions, immune status, disease progression
    - Indicates possible hematologic abnormalities

- Allergies
    - Increased incidence of drug allergies during disease progression
- Tobacco and alcohol use
    - Alcohol use may enhance HIV replication
    - Habitual injection drug users need to be referred for counseling
- Social support network
    - Dentists need to access support networks since oral findings may indicate disease progression*
- Laboratory values
    - High incidence of anemia, granolucytopenia, and thrombocytopenia
    - Evaluation of immune status
- Review of systems
    - Head and neck
        - Lymphadenopathy
        - Sinusitis
    - Gastrointestinal
        - Wasting syndrome
        - Hepatitis
        - Splenectomies
    - Pulmonary
        - TB
    - Neurologic manifestations
        - Cognitive and motor impairments
        - Neuropathies
- Examination
    - Extraoral
    - Intraoral

*Eliciting patients' transmission category enables referrals to appropriate support groups for counseling and support.

Transmission Category

It is helpful to ascertain how a patient acquired HIV infection since modes of transmission have been associated with specific oral lesions. Furthermore, prescription of medications, risk of carrying, as well as developing, certain infections, as well as being prone to hematologic abnormalities are particular for different transmission categories. These transmission categories includes homosexual or bisexual men, injection drug users, hemophiliacs, recipients of blood products, and those who acquired HIV through heterosexual contact.

Oral lesions, such as Kaposi's sarcoma, necrotizing ulcerative periodontitis, and oral hairy leukoplakia, occur more commonly among homosexual or bisexual men. Thus, a bluish macular area on the hard palate of an African-American woman who is an intravenous drug user is most probably due to physiologic pigmentation, and not HIV. In this case, the patient must be followed up to ensure that the affected area does not change in size and appearance. The same manifestation in a homosexual or bisexual man, however, may necessitate a biopsy to rule out Kaposi's sarcoma.

Patients acquiring HIV by intravenous drug use present with different concerns. Such patients are at high risk for subacute bacterial endocarditis (SBE), and many of these individuals have already experienced bouts with SBE. As with all patients with a history of SBE, antibiotic prophylaxis must be instituted prior to dental therapy. The antibiotic prophylactic protocol of the American Heart Association is adequate for patients with HIV. Narcotic analgesics should not be prescribed for patients with a history of drug abuse unless no other choices are available.

Patients with hemophilia must be assessed prior to procedures that produce bleeding. The level of factor deficiency determines appropriate therapy. Patients with hemophilia who received blood products prior to 1985 have an estimated 5% to 10% hepatitis B surface antigen positivity;[1] 25% to 50% are hepatitis non-A, non-B carriers;[2] 50% have been exposed to hepatitis delta virus (HDV);[3] 60% to 90% have HIV antibody;[4] and 88% have been exposed to parvovirus.[5] In a recent study of patients with hemophilia A and B, 53% had HIV and over 99% of these individuals had been exposed to hepatitis B virus (HBV), hepatitis C virus (HCV), or hepatitis delta virus (HDV).[6] Only 12% had evidence of active HBV infection, while 98% were anti-HCV positive.

Patients who acquire HIV from infected needles or sexual contacts, both heterosexual and homosexual, need counseling. They need to be made aware that the continuation of high-risk behavior may affect their own disease progression and put other individuals at risk. Many individuals with HIV have not connected with support networks, and the dental healthcare worker should be able to refer patients to an appropriate group or organization (see Appendix C).

Date of Initial Infection and HIV Test

The date of initial infection is very hard to ascertain in most patients, except for infections that are acquired congenitally or through blood transfusions. The time of infection is the best predictor for disease progression. Long-term asymptomatic patients have an excellent prognosis compared to individuals experiencing opportunistic infections shortly after initial HIV infection. To approximate the time of initial infection, it is advantageous to obtain the date of a patient's first positive HIV test result and the reason the patient was tested. Many individuals are asymptomatic but want to know their HIV status because they believe they are at risk for being infected. Others seek testing when they start to experience signs and symptoms of HIV disease. Others are encouraged to seek testing at drug treatment centers, which provide counseling to their clients. It is also important to try to elicit information on the patient's CD4+ cell count at the time of testing. This is another useful parameter for assessing progression of the patient's HIV disease.

History of Sexually Transmitted Diseases

Patients with HIV and a history of multiple sexually transmitted diseases (STD) show a faster progression of HIV disease. Herpes simplex virus infections, gonorrhea, and syphilis are the most common STDs reported among this group of patients. If successfully treated, these diseases do not directly effect dental therapy. However, oral lesions in patients with active disease are highly contagious and can be transmitted to a dental practitioner by direct contact. A history of syphilis may result in neurosyphilis or cardiac myopathies. Neurosyphilis is particularly worrisome, since it may cause a wide variety of symptoms including dementia, manic-depressive behavior, and a higher incidence of cardiovascular accidents, but it is rare.[7] The prevalence of neurosyphilis in HIV-positive individuals appears to be less than 2%.[8] While this complication of syphilis has little direct impact on dentistry, syphilitic involvement of the heart can include aortic valvular insufficiency.[9] As with other patients with organic valvular regurgitation, antibiotic prophylaxis must be instituted prior to dental therapy.

History of Infectious Diseases

Concurrent infections with HBV and HIV may occur in over 90% of HIV-infected individuals.[10] Studies from the United States indicate that prior to the onset of the HIV epidemic, an estimated 60% of homosexual men had been exposed to HBV infection and approximately 5% were chronic carriers.[11] However, liver damage in patients with concurrent chronic HBV infection and AIDS appears to be less severe than that in patients without HIV infection,[12] despite the fact that a higher incidence of HBeAg expression is noted among homosexual men with HIV compared to homosexual men without HIV.[13] Consequently, HBV infection in homosexual men with HIV may indicate a more contagious state but cause less liver damage.

Hepatic manifestations in HIV disease are usually associated with drug toxicity, hepatitis C virus, or hepatitis D virus infections.[14-16] Active hepatitis B infections are relatively rare, probably because of the high incidence of previous infections in this cohort. However, reports have suggested that reactivation of prior hepatitis B virus infection may occur during HIV disease progression.[17] Furthermore, a previous exposure to HBV increases the incidence of subsequent HIV seroconversion.[18] Transmission of HBV is similar to that of HIV; therefore, it is not surprising to find a high prevalence of HBV among individuals with HIV. However, the relationship between HBV and HIV infection is more than just an epidemiologic occurrence. The presence of previous infection with HBV is associated with a more rapid progression of HIV disease.[19] Furthermore, HBV infection in individuals with prior HIV infection will increase the incidence of a carrier state threefold.[20] This is probably due to the decreased clearance of HBV infection as a result of the impaired T-lymphocyte function in HIV-infected individuals.

The incidence of HCV infection in HIV-infected patients is estimated to be approximately 7%.[21] However, this prevalence depends on the number of patients with hemophilia included in such a study. Hepatitis C virus infection is a severe form of hepatitis and has been associated with a carrier state of 50%. Approximately 20% of chronic carriers develop liver disease from HCV. The incidence among the general population in the United States is estimated to be 0.5% to 1.5%, but dental providers are reported to have a prevalence rate of approximately 10%. This is not a surprising finding since HCV is present in saliva and may be transmitted by exposure to it.[22] Although individuals with HIV appear to have a higher incidence of HCV infection than the general population, the sexual transmission of HCV seems to be inefficient.[23] Hepatitis C virus infections in injection drug users is very common, corresponding to an incidence of approximately 65%.[24]

Patients with active hepatitis may present with hematologic abnormalities affecting dental therapy. Even if liver disease is not present, coagulation abnormalities have been reported. One study indicated that in a group of patients presumably without HIV but with infectious hepatitis and without liver failure, 41% presented with an increased prothrombin time (PT; mean, 16.5 seconds; range, 13 to 60 seconds; normal, 12 to 15 seconds) and 16% presented with thrombocytopenia (mean, 230,000 cells/mm^3; range, 60,000 to 500,000 cells/mm^3; normal, 150,000 to 450,000 cells/mm^3).[25] In patients with liver failure, 100% of patients presented with an elevated PT (mean, 44 seconds; range, 23 to 60 seconds; normal, 12 to 15 seconds). Thrombocytopenia was present in 52% of patients with liver failure

Table 12-2. Interpretation of PPD Skin Tests*

- A reaction ≥ 5 mm is classified as positive in

  Persons with HIV infection or at risk for HIV infection with unknown HIV status

  Persons who have had recent close contact[†] with persons with TB

  Persons who have abnormal chest radiographs consistent with previous TB episode

- A reaction of ≥ 10 mm is classified as positive in all persons who do not meet any of the criteria above but who have other risk factors for TB, including

  High-risk groups:

  Intravenous drug users known to be HIV seropositive

  Persons with other medical conditions that have been reported to increase the risk of progressing from latent TB infection to active TB, including silicosis, gastrectomy, jejuno-ileal bypass surgery; being ≥ 10% below ideal body weight; chronic renal failure; diabetes mellitus; high-dose corticosteroids and other immune suppressive therapy; some hematologic disorders (eg, leukemias and lymphomas), and other malignancies

  High-prevalence groups:

  Foreign-born persons from high-prevalence countries in Asia, Africa, and Latin America

  Persons from medically underserved, low-income populations

  Residents of long-term care facilities (eg, correctional institutions, nursing homes)

  Persons from high-risk populations in their communities, as determined by local public health authorities

- Induration ≥ 15 mm is classified as positive for persons who do not meet any of the above criteria

- Recent converts are defined on the basis of both induration and age:

  ≥ 10 mm increase within a 2-year period is classified as positive for persons < 35 years of age

  ≥ 15 mm increase within a 2-year period is classified as positive for persons ≥ 35 years of age

  ≥ 5 mm increases under certain circumstances

*From CDC. Federal Register. 1993;195(58):52830. Used with permission.
[†]Recent close contact implies household contact or unprotected occupational exposure similar in intensity and duration to household contact.

(mean, 139,000 cells/mm^3; range, 40,000 to 255,000 cells/mm^3; normal, 150,000 to 450,000 cells/mm^3).

Tuberculosis (TB) is the only major opportunistic infection that may be contagious to immune-competent health-care workers. Patients with active TB infections should not undergo elective dental procedures. Dental providers need to recognize the typical signs and symptoms associated with TB. These include productive cough, cough with blood in the sputum, chest pain, fever, night sweats, weight loss, and malaise. Patients may also report the result of their purified protein derivative (PPD) skin test (Table 12-2). It is important to remember that TB skin test results may be negative due to anergy in severely immunosuppressed individuals. Over 70% of HIV-infected individuals with

CD4+ cell counts below 200 cells/mm[3] may be anergic and only 1% may show tuberculin reactivity.[26] The risk for developing active TB may be similar for individuals with a positive PPD test result and in anergic patients with low CD4+ cell counts.[27] Many patients with HIV are treated prophylactically for TB infections. Treatment and prophylaxis for TB last between 6 and 18 months. As a rule of thumb, patients taking anti-TB medications are not considered contagious after 3 weeks of complying with medication regimen. It is important to learn if the patient has been compliant with taking anti-TB medications. Noncompliance is the most common cause for the development of multiple drug resistant–TB (see Chapter 6).

Past and Present HIV-Related Opportunistic Infections

Past and present HIV-related opportunistic infections (Table 12-3) may indicate what type of medications the patient is taking, as well as HIV status and staging, and immune status. This information will indicate proper treatment planning and suggest if precautionary measures are required prior to providing dental therapy.

Medications

A patient's HIV-associated medications usually indicate past and/or present infections and suggest possible hematologic abnormalities and sometimes immune status.

Antiretroviral drugs, such as zidovudine, ddI, and ddC, are usually not used in individuals with CD4+ cell counts above 500 cells/mm[3]. Furthermore, these drugs are used solely in patients with HIV. Side effects from some of these drugs, particularly zidovudine, include thrombocytopenia, neutropenia, and anemia. In severe cases, patients require blood transfusions to replenish missing cellular components. These patients must be assessed for increased bleeding tendencies, by evaluating platelet counts, and for increased susceptibility to infections, by evaluating neutrophil counts. An increased incidence of neutropenia is noticed in patients taking zidovudine together with trimethoprim-sulfamethoxazole, pyrimethamine and sulfadiazine, or ganciclovir. *Pneumocystis carinii* pneumonitis (PCP) prophylaxis is instituted for individuals with CD4+ cell counts below 200 cells/mm[3] or for patients with prior episodes of PCP. Since some of the medications used for this purpose, such as trimethoprim-sulfamethoxazole, are associated with a high incidence of allergic reactions, this information needs to be documented. Patients with histories of drug allergies tend to have a high incidence of allergic reactions toward more than one medication.

Prophylactic medications for *Mycobacterium avium-intracellulare* complex (MAC) and toxoplasmosis are usually instituted in patients with CD4+ cell counts below 100 cells/mm[3]. Some medications are administered through indwelling catheters. Although there are no indications that dental therapy

Table 12-3. HIV-Related Opportunistic Infections

- Central nervous system

  *Toxoplasma gondii** (AIDS diagnosis; severe immune deterioration)

  *Cryptococcus neoformans** (AIDS diagnosis; severe immune deterioration)

  Lymphoma (AIDS diagnosis; severe immune deterioration)

  Progressive multifocal leuko-encephalopathy (stable mental status; AIDS diagnosis; severe immune deterioration)

  HIV-associated dementia (can occur during all stages of HIV disease)

  Cytomegalovirus encephalitis (AIDS diagnosis; severe immune deterioration)

- Pulmonary

  Bacterial infections (if recurrent is considered an AIDS diagnosis and is associated with severe immune deterioration)

  *Hemophilus influenzae**

  *Streptococcus pneumoniae**

  Mycobacteria (AIDS diagnosis; severe immune deterioration)

  Mycobacterium avium-intracellulare

  Mycobacterium tuberculosis†

  Multiple drug resistant–TB

  Fungi (AIDS diagnosis; severe immune deterioration)

  Cryptococcus neoformans

  Histoplasma capsulatum†

  Viruses

  Cytomegalovirus (AIDS diagnosis; severe immune deterioration)

  Influenza

  Parasites

  Pneumocystis carinii pneumonia* (AIDS diagnosis; severe immune deterioration)

  Neoplasms

  Kaposi's sarcoma (AIDS diagnosis; severe immune deterioration)

  Miscellaneous

  Lymphoid interstitial pneumonia: more common among children

- Gastrointestinal

  Diarrhea—if associated with HIV wasting syndrome is considered an AIDS diagnosis

  Bacteria

  Clostridium difficile

  Clostridium jejuni

  *Salmonella**

  Shigella

  Mycobacterial

  *Mycobacterium avium-intracellulare**

  Fungi

  *Candida albicans**

  Parasites

  *Cryptosporidium parvum**

  Giardia lambia

  Isospora belli†

  Microsporidium

  Viruses

  CMV*

  HIV*

  Idiopathic*

*More common, †common.

results in dissemination of bacteria that may cause catheter failure, some physicians still prefer antibiotic prophylaxis prior to dental treatment for these patients.

The administration of medications ordinarily used for oral infections in patients without HIV is usually not contraindicated for patients with HIV. However, there are some exceptions. Patients with reduced salivary flow should not be given troches that are dissolved in the mouth. Furthermore, most medications that are dissolved in the mouth contain cariogenic carbohydrates, which increase the risk for odontogenic infections.

Patients with reduced gastric secretion should not be given medications that are activated by gastric acid, such as ketoconazole or dapsone. Furthermore, patients with severe diarrhea and wasting syndrome will not be able to efficiently absorb oral medications.

Broad spectrum antibiotics have been associated with an increased incidence of oral candidiasis. This phenomenon is noticed even more in patients with an impaired immune response.

Overall, medications should be administered only if there is a clear medical indication. An increased number of medications may cause unanticipated adverse drug interactions as well as increase the patient's financial burden.

Allergies

During the progression of HIV disease, patients show an increased susceptibility to developing drug allergies. This is a curious occurrence since drug reactions are usually associated with an intact T-lymphocyte response. Therefore, reduced allergic reaction would be expected in individuals with advanced HIV disease. However, it has been proposed that T-lymphocyte depletion and dysfunction enables allergens to directly induce histamine release.

Tobacco and Alcohol Use

Tobacco smoking has not been associated with immune impairment in individuals with HIV. Instead, an increased white blood cell count has been documented in smokers during the earliest stages of HIV disease.[28] However, heavy smokers may be at higher risk for developing opportunistic pneumonias such as PCP.[29]

The consumption of alcohol in amounts similar to those in social drinking increases and may augment HIV replication.[30] Furthermore, the risk of acquiring HIV infection after alcohol intake may increase due to the body's decreased resistance and impaired immune response caused by the alcohol. Chronic alcoholism has also been associated with profound depression of T-suppressor lymphocyte function.[31] As mentioned previously, these cells may play an important role in the initial elimination of HIV and subsequent reduction in HIV replication.

Patients who continue to use injection drugs need to be counseled. This habit will enhance HIV disease progression in the drug user and may put other persons at risk.

Social Support System

Many oral manifestations are early signs of HIV disease and AIDS. Therefore, a dentist may have to inform a patient that he or she has clinical indications of HIV disease. At other times, a patient's progression from HIV disease to AIDS may first manifest in the oral cavity. It is essential that the dental provider refer the patient to appropriate support networks in the patient's geographical area. This support group may comprise individuals belonging to the same transmission category or ethnic or religious background (see Appendix C). The patient should be given all options to choose what is most suitable for him or her.

It is also pertinent to inquire about a patient's personal support system. These people usually offer the most valuable support to the patient, but only if the patient is accepted by them.

Laboratory Values

Laboratory values indicate hemostasis and risk of infection, two of the most common concerns affecting the provision of dental care. However, with HIV-infected patients, the dental provider also needs to pay special attention to the patient's overall immune status. Platelet counts below normal levels of 150,000 cells/mm^3

are not automatically associated with bleeding abnormalities. For general dentistry procedures, including dental hygiene procedures, endodontics, and simple extractions, a platelet count of 60,000 cells/mm^3 is sufficient. When the platelet counts drops below 20,000 to 25,000 cells/mm^3, spontaneous gingival bleeding can occur. In cases of HIV-related immune thrombocytopenia (ITP), a bleeding time will appropriately assess bleeding tendencies (see Chapter 11). The red blood cell count is important when performing procedures associated with significant blood loss. However, these types of procedures are usually not performed on an outpatient basis. On the other hand, patients with severe anemia should not be given medications associated with respiratory depression. Thus, some medications, such as narcotics, should not be administered to patients with hemoglobin levels below 9 to 10 g/dL.

Patients with absolute neutrophil counts below 500 cells/mm^3 should receive antibiotic prophylaxis prior to dental therapy. Bactericidal antibiotics are the most appropriate agents since bacteriestatic antibiotics given to patients with low white blood cell counts may result in enhanced bacteremia. Although the number of other white blood cells does not indicate prophylactic interventions, it is appropriate to administer postoperative antibiotics after major surgical procedures in leukopenic patients (absolute white blood cell counts below 4,500 cells/mm^3).

A progressive decrease in CD4+ cell counts is the hallmark of HIV disease.

Indications of a patient's prognosis are usually based on absolute CD4+ cell counts or CD4%. However, these numbers give only a very limited view of the disease progression. A more appropriate measure is to follow CD4+ cell counts over a longer period and assess the trend of these values. A declining trend is a poorer prognosis than a stable or even a gradually increased CD4+ cell count. According to the National Institutes of Health Consensus Panel 1990,[32] and U.S. Public Health Service Task Force,[33] patients with CD4+ cell counts of 300 to 500 cells/mm³ should be re-evaluated every 6 months. Patients with CD4+ cell counts between 200 and 300 cells/mm³ should have a test every 3 months, while patients with counts below 200 cells/mm³ do not need further CD4+ cell counts, since below this level therapeutic interventions will not change. However, many physicians continue to check CD4+ cell counts well below 100 cells/mm³, since many of the major fatal opportunistic infections occur at this CD4+ cell count and prophylactic medications for toxoplasmosis and MAC are sometimes initiated at this level.

After initial HIV infection, the CD4+ cell count usually stabilizes at a level of 500 to 700 cells/mm³ (median normal CD4+ cell count, 935 cells/mm³), followed by a median annual reduction of 60 cells/mm³.[34] It is important to realize that these figures cannot be applied to all patients. Tremendous variations are present. Some patients have stable CD4+ cell counts for up to 10 years, while others exhibit a rapid decline. The prognosis of individuals exhibiting CD4+ cell counts below 50 cells/mm³ is very poor, with a median survival of approximately 12 months.[35,36] In dentistry, the CD4+ cell count helps with differential diagnosis of oral lesions; indicates prognosis of survival; and when it is below 50 to 100 cells/mm³, it also suggests possible platelet and white blood cell count deficiencies.

Review of Systems

The dissemination of HIV within different body systems, as well as the associated immune deterioration, create specific manifestations throughout the body.

Head and Neck

Sinusitis appears to be a common complication of HIV disease. In one study, over 60% of individuals with HIV were reported to have sinusitis.[37] Thirty-two percent of affected individuals presented with nasal congestion, and 25% needed decongestants or antihistamines. The incidence and severity of sinusitis increased with progression of HIV disease. With disease progression, multiple sinuses become involved and respond poorly to antibiotic therapy.[38] The high incidence of dry mouth in patients with HIV may be partially explained by mouth breathing and xerostomia-inducing medications associated with chronic sinusitis.

Past and present episodes of epistaxis indicate possible bleeding abnormalities. If this is a frequent occurrence, the patient needs hematologic evaluation prior to undergoing dental procedures that result in bleeding.

Persistent generalized lymphadenopathy (PGL) occurs commonly in the cervical lymph nodes of individuals with HIV and is characterized by lymph nodes approximately 10 mm in diameter, rubbery to hard, and usually freely moveable. This type of lymphadenopathy appears during the earliest stages of HIV disease and close to the time of an AIDS diagnosis. The HIV-related lymphadenopathy phenomenon probably represents a period of increased viral replication within the lymph nodes, which increase in size. Cervical lymphadenopathy can also be caused by Kaposi's sarcoma or lymphoma as well as infections by TB, syphilis and cytomegalovirus.

Gastrointestinal Tract

Diarrhea and malabsorption both play an important part in the development of wasting syndrome in HIV-infected individuals. This syndrome can be caused by a variety of infectious diseases and pathogens, such as cryptosporidiosis, isosporiasis, microsporidiosis, MAC, bacterial overgrowth, cytomegalovirus colitis, *Shigella, Salmonella, Campylobacter, Clostridium difficile* toxin, fungal infections, and HIV.[39] Wasting syndrome may occur in up to 80% of patients with AIDS. The pathogens causing diarrhea can usually be found in patients with AIDS,

while unexplained diarrhea is more common in patients with HIV but without AIDS. A progressive loss of lean body mass (LBM) can be seen in patients with AIDS and, if not halted, will result in death. More than 40% loss of lean body mass is not compatible with life.

Nutritional deficiencies will also impair the immune response. Reduction of T lymphocytes, impaired cell-mediated immune response, reduced natural killer cell activity, and altered phagocytic functions have all been associated with nutritional deficiencies.[40–43]

Vitamin B_{12} malabsorption is not uncommon in patients with HIV[43] and may initially present as an oral manifestation. Oral intake of nutrition and medications may not be the desired route in patients with wasting syndrome since absorption in the gastrointestinal tract is impaired.

Severe malabsorption may eradicate vitamin K–producing bacteria in the gut, causing coagulopathy. The lack of vitamin K prevents the formation of prothrombin. This deficiency can be detected by performing a prothrombin time assay.

Patients with HIV may have undergone splenectomies as treatment for immune thrombocytopenia purpura.[44] In such instances the dental-care provider needs to be aware of potential complications associated with dental therapy. Asplenic patients have an increased susceptibility to bacterial infections and may develop bacterial sepsis without identification of a primary site of infection. It is recommended that asplenic patients receive microbial antibiotics prior to dental therapy.[45]

Coagulation abnormalities due to HBV are rare in patients with HIV, as HIV infection may ameliorate chronic HBV disease.[12] This may be due to HIV infection of HBV-infected hepatocytes and their subsequent destruction. Furthermore, the immune reaction to HBV disease is the cause of the liver destruction seen in HBV carriers. Thus, in immune-suppressed individuals, decreased liver involvement is to be expected.

Cardiac System

The true incidence of cardiac involvement in HIV disease is not clear. Cardiomyopathy can be caused by a wide variety of opportunistic infections associated with HIV infection. One study of 101 patients with HIV found more frequent cardiac abnormalities in the group with HIV compared to healthy control subjects, but most abnormalities were of no clinical significance. Fourteen percent of the patients with AIDS and 6.6% of the other symptomatic and asymptomatic subjects with AIDS presented with valvular regurgitation. This is surprising since this phenomenon is more common in women and the study included 96 men and only 5 women.[46]

Pulmonary System

Pneumocystis carinii pneumonia is by far the most common type of pulmonary disease in patients with AIDS.

P. carinii pneumonitis is an AIDS diagnosis in HIV-infected individuals and is usually only found in patients with severe immune suppression. Furthermore, patients with a history of PCP will take prophylactic medications to prevent relapse of the disease, including trimethoprim-sulfamethoxazole, dapsone, a combination of the two, atovaquone, or aerosolized pentamidine. The transmission of PCP to healthy health-care workers has not been documented, but there are reports of nosocomial infections between patients.[47,48]

The emergence of TB has justifiably caused great concern among health-care providers. Since dentists are constantly in contact with aerosolized particles, they are exposed to pathogens present in the sputum and saliva. *Mycobacterium tuberculosis* has been transmitted from infected patients to healthy health-care providers.[49,50] Identification of patients with TB becomes essential to treat the patient with appropriate precautions and facilitate referrals for medical treatment. A diagnosis of TB should be considered in a patient with a persistent cough for more than 2 weeks, bloody sputum, night sweats, weight loss, lack of appetite, or fever.[51] The risk of active TB increases in patients with these signs and symptoms, particularly among those living in correctional institutions, homeless shelters, long-term care facilities for the elderly, or drug treatment centers. The result of a purified protein derivative (PPD) skin test may be relayed to the dental-care provider who needs to interpret the result (see Table 12-2).

Patients with active TB should not be treated for elective dental procedures. All treatment should be deferred to a later date when patients are no longer contagious. Patients are considered noninfectious after 3 weeks on antituberculosis medications. A definitive confirmation of a noninfectious state is three consecutive daily negative sputum samples.

Neurologic Manifestations

Patients with AIDS may exhibit signs of HIV encephalopathy (AIDS dementia), which is associated with decreased motor and cognitive abilities. This type of patient may have difficulties performing normal oral hygiene procedures, forget appointments, and have an unstable mental status. Progressive multifocal leukoencephalopathy may present with symptoms of personality changes, memory deficits, and severe cerebral dysfunction. Dental treatment for such patients should be symptomatic until there is improvement in the patient's neurologic deficiency.

Examination

Extraoral examinations can reveal lymphadenopathies, cutaneous manifestations, and central as well as peripheral neuropathies. Asymptomatic, soft-to-hard and freely moveable enlarged cervical lymph nodes, greater than 10 mm in diameter, may be present in over 50% of individuals with HIV. This phenomenon usually represents active HIV replication and is more common during the earlier stages of HIV disease as well as surrounding the time of an AIDS diagnosis. This type of lymphadenopathy may also be caused by other complications such as neoplastic growth, TB, cytomegalovirus infection, or syphilis.

An overview of cutaneous manifestations can be found in Chapter 7. However, attention should be paid to purplish, bluish lesions on the skin that resemble hematomas. Such lesions may be the first sign of Kaposi's sarcoma or signs of increased bleeding tendencies.

Neuropathies in HIV disease may be associated with acute and subacute encephalitis; caused by HIV directly; a function of an autoimmune response; neoplastic infiltration of nerve tissue; viral, bacterial, protozoal, and fungal infections; or secondary to chemotherapeutic interventions. Peripheral neuropathy can present as painful manifestations as well as motor deficiencies. Cytomegalovirus infections have been implicated in severe painful neuropathies but occur usually only in patients with CD4+ cell counts below 100 cells/mm^3.

An intraoral examination will reveal changes in the oral mucosa, decreased salivary flow, and the status of the periodontium and teeth. The significance and interpretation of oral findings in HIV-infected patients is described in Chapter 8. However, most oral as well as cutaneous lesions are early signs of immune suppression and disease progression.

The importance of a medical assessment of all dental patients cannot be overstated, but it is of particular importance for HIV-infected patients. For them, an updated medical evaluation needs to be performed at each dental visit, since changes in their medical condition occur rapidly and sometimes unpredictably.

References

1. Gomperts ED, Lazerson J, Berg D, Lockhart D, Sergis-Deavenport E. Hepatocellular enzyme patterns and hepatitis B virus exposure in multiple transfused young and very young hemophilia patients. Am J Hematol 1981;11:55–59.

2. Dienstag JL, Alter HJ. Non-A, non-B hepatitis: evolving epidemiologic and clinical perspective. Semin Liver Dis 1986;6:67–81.

3. Rizzetto M, Morello C, Mannucci PM, et al. Delta infection and liver disease in hemophilic carriers of the hepatitis B surface antigen. J Infect Dis 1982;145:18–22.

4. Evatt BL, Gomperts ED, McDougal JS, Ramsey RB. Coincidental appearance of LAV/HTLV III antibodies in hemophiliacs and the onset of the AIDS epidemic. N Engl J Med 1985;312:483–486.

5. Mortimer P, Luban N, Kelleher J, Cohen B. Transmission of serum parvovirus-like virus by clotting factor concentrates. Lancet 1983;2:482–484.

6. Troisi CL, Hollinger B, Hoots WK, et al. A multicenter study of viral hepatitis in a United States hemophilic population. Blood 1993;81:412–418.

7. Talbot MD, Morton RS. Neurosyphilis: the most common things are most common. Genitourin Med 1985;61:95–98.

8. Berger JR. Neurosyphilis in human immunodeficiency virus type-1 seropositive individuals. Arch Neurol 1991;48:700–702.

9. Grabau W, Emanuel R, Ross D, Parker J, Hedge M. Syphilitic aortic regurgitation: an appraisal of surgical treatment. Br J Vener Dis 1976;52:366–373.

10. Lebovics E, Dworkin BM, Heier SK, Rosenthal WS. The hepatobiliary manifestations of human immunodeficiency virus infection. Am J Gastroenterol 1988;83:1–7.

11. Szmuness W, Stevens CE, Harley EJ, et al. Hepatitis B vaccine: demonstration of efficacy in a controlled clinical trial in a high-risk population in the United States. N Engl J Med 1980;303:833–841.

12. Rustgi VK, Hoofnagle JH, Gerin JL, et al. B virus infection in the acquired immunodeficiency syndrome. Ann Intern Med 1984;101:795–797.

13. Bodsworth N, Donovan B, Nightingale BN. The effect of concurrent human immunodeficiency virus infection on chronic hepatitis B: a study of 150 homosexual men. J Infect Dis 1989;160:577–582.

14. Kotler DP. Intestinal and hepatic manifestations of AIDS. Adv Intern Med 1989;34:43–71.

15. Martin P, DiBisceglie AM, Kassianides C, Lisker-Melman M, Hoofnagle JH. Rapidly progressive non-A non-B hepatitis in patients with human immunodeficiency virus infection. Gastroenterology 1989;97:1559–1561.

16. Solomon RE, Kaslow RA, Phair JP, et al. Human immunodeficiency virus and hepatitis delta virus in homosexual men: a study of four cohorts. Ann Intern Med 1988:108:51–54.

17. Lazizi Y, Grangeot-Keros L, Delfraissy J-F, et al. Reappearance of hepatitis B virus in immune patients infected with human immunodeficiency virus type-1. J Infect Dis 1988;158:666–667.

18. Twu SJ, Detels R, Nelson K, et al. Relationship of hepatitis B virus infection to human immunodeficiency virus type 1 infection. J Infect Dis 1993;167:299–304.

19. Eskild A, Magnus P, Petersen G, et al. Hepatitis B antibodies in HIV-infected homosexual men are associated with more rapid progression to AIDS. AIDS 1992;6:571–574.

20. Hadler SC, Judson FN, O'Malley PM, et al. Outcome of hepatitis B virus infection in homosexual men and its relation to prior human immunodeficiency virus infection. J Infect Dis 1991;163:454–459.

21. Hayashi PH, Flynn N, McCurdy SA, Kuramoto IK, Holland PV, Zeldis JB. Prevalence of hepatitis C virus antibodies among patients infected with human immunodeficiency virus. J Med Virol 1991;33:177–180.

22. Young K-C, Chang T-T, Liou T-C, Wu H-L. Detection of hepatitis C virus RNA in peripheral blood mononuclear cells and in saliva. J Med Virol 1993;41:55–60.

23. Hallam NF, Fletcher ML, Read SJ, Majid AM, Kurtz JB, Rizza CR. Low risk of sexual transmission of hepatitis C virus. J Med Virol 1993;40:251–253.

24. Osmond DH, Padian NS, Sheppard HW, Glass S, Shiboski SC, Reingold A. Risk factors for hepatitis C virus seropositivity in heterosexual couples. JAMA 1993;269:361–365.

25. Gallus AS, Lucas CR, Hirsh J. Coagulation studies in patients with acute infectious hepatitis. Br J Haematol 1972;22:761–771.

26. Markowitz N, Hansen NI, Wilcosky TC, et al. Tuberculin and anergy testing in HIV-seropositive and HIV sero-negative persons. Ann Intern Med 1993;119:185–193.

27. Moreno S, Baraia-Etxaburu J, Bonza E, et al. Risk for developing tuberculosis among anergic patients infected with HIV. Ann Intern Med 1993;119:194–198.

28. Park LP, Margolick JB, Giorgi JV, et al. Influence of HIV-1 infection and cigarette smoking on leukocyte profiles in homosexual men. J Acquired Immune Deficiency Syndrome 1992;5:1124–1130.

29. Nieman RB, Fleming J, Coker RJ, Harris JRW, Mitchell DM. The effect of cigarette smoking on the development of AIDS in individuals infected with HIV-1. AIDS 1993;7:705–710.

30. Bagasra O, Kajdacsy-Balla A, Lischner HW, Pomeranz RJ. Alcohol intake increases human immunodeficiency virus type 1 replication in human peripheral blood mononuclear cells. J Infect Dis 1993;167:789–797.

31. Bagasra O, Howeedy A, Dorio R, Kajdacsy-Balla A. Functional analysis of T-cell subsets in chronic alcoholism. Immunology 1987;61:63–69.

32. National Institute of Allergy and Infectious Diseases, NIH. State-of-the-art conference on azidothymidine therapy for early HIV infection. Am J Med 1990;89:335–344.

33. CDC. Recommendations for prophylaxis against *Pneumocystis carinii* pneumonia for adults and adolescents infected with human immunodeficiency virus. MMWR 1992;41:1–11.

34. Lang W, Perkins H, Anderson RE, Royce R, Jewell N, Winkelstein W Jr. Patterns of T-lymphocyte changes with human immunodeficiency virus infection: from seroconversion to the development of AIDS. J Acquired Immune Deficiency Syndrome 1989;2:63–69.

35. Yarchoan R, Venzon DJ, Pluda JM, et al. CD4 count and the risk of death in patients infected with human immunodeficiency virus receiving antiretroviral therapy. Ann Intern Med 1991;115:184–189.

36. Mills GD, Jones PD. Relationship between CD4 lymphocyte count and AIDS mortality, 1986–91. AIDS 1993;7:1383–1386.

37. Zurlo JJ, Feuerstein IM, Lebovics R, Lane HC. Sinusitis in HIV-1 infection. Am J Med 1992;93:157–162.

38. Godofsky EW, Zinreich J, Armstrong M, Leslie JM, Weikel CS. Sinusitis in HIV-infected patients: a clinical and radiographic review. Am J Med 1992;93:163–170.

39. Smith PD. Gastrointestinal infections in AIDS. Ann Intern Med 1992;116:63-77.

40. Kotler DP, Tierney AR, Wang J, Pierson RN Jr. Magnitude of body cell-mass depletion and timing of death from wasting in AIDS. Am J Clin Nutr 1989;55:444–447.

41. Keusch CT, Orrutia JJ, Fernandez R. Humoral and cellular aspects of intracellular bacteria killing in Guatemalan children with protein-calorie malnutrition. In Suskind RM (ed): Malnutrition and The Immune Response. New York: Raven Press; 1977.

42. Chandra RK. Mucosal immune responses in malnutrition. Ann NY Acad Sci 1983;409:345–352.

43. Harriman GR, Smith PD, Horne MK, et al. Vitamin B_{12} malabsorption in patients with the acquired immunodeficiency syndrome. Arch Intern Med 1989;149:2039–2041.

44. Ravikumar TS, Allen JD, Bothe A Jr, Steele G Jr. Splenectomy. The treatment of choice for human immunodeficiency virus–related immune thrombocytopenia? Arch Surg 1989;124:625–628.

45. Terezhalmy GT, Hall EH. The asplenic patient: a consideration for antimicrobial prophylaxis. Oral Surg Oral Med Oral Pathol 1984;57:114–117.

46. Fong IW, Howard R, Elzawi A, Simbul M, Chiasson D. Cardiac involvement in human immunodeficiency virus–infected patients. J Acquired Immune Deficiency Syndrome 1993;6:380–385.

47. Bensousan T, Garo B, Islam S, Bourbigot B, Cledes J, Garre M. Possible transmission of *Pneumocystis carinii* between kidney transplant recipients (letter; comment). Lancet 1990;336:1066–1067.

48. Francioli P, Prod'hom G, Poloni C. Progress and problems in hospital infections: exemplified by pneumonia. Schweiz Med Wochenschr 1991;121:1423–1428.

49. Pearson ML, Jereb JA, Frieden TR, et al. Nosocomial transmission of multidrug-resistant *Mycobacterium tuberculosis:* a risk to patients and health care workers. Ann Intern Med 1992;117:191–196.

50. Iseman MD. Treatment of multidrug-resistant tuberculosis. N Engl J Med 1993;329:784–791.

51. CDC. Draft guidelines for preventing the transmission of tuberculosis in health-care facilities, ed 2. Federal Register 1993;195 (58):52810–52854.

13

Modifications of Dental Care

Michael Glick

For dental practitioners, the medical evaluation of patients with HIV is three-tiered. They need to anticipate: complications that may arise during dental therapy secondary to a patient's immunologic, hemostatic, and pharmacotherapeutic status; medical conditions that may directly interfere with provision of dental procedures (since a patient's physical well-being determines his or her ability to endure dental treatment and schedule and maintain appointments); and a patient's prognosis for survival, which influences the formulation of an appropriate treatment plan.

Overall, the provision of dental care for HIV-infected individuals is similar to that of noninfectious patients. Stud-ies have indicated that the overall complication rate secondary to dental procedures, even with severely immunosuppressed individuals with CD4+ cell counts below 200 cells/mm^3, is the same or even lower than that among patients without HIV. In one study, 2,477 dental procedures were performed on 331 patients who had an average CD4+ cell count of 70.6 cells/mm^3.[1] Procedures included oral examinations, periodontal therapy (scaling, curettage, root planing, and surgery), restorative procedures with different types of materials, prosthodontic procedures including both fixed and removable appliances, endodontic therapy for single and multiple canals and apicoectomies, simple and surgical extractions, and soft tissue biopsies. More than 1,800 procedures were defined as invasive, ie, when breakage of intact mucosa or other oral tissues occurs and only 17 complications—including dry sockets, slow healing after extractions, an oroantral fistula and a bone sequestrum after extractions, and one case of prolonged bleeding after a periodontal procedure—were documented. These results indicated an overall complication rate for invasive procedures of only 0.9%. All complications were treated by the attending dentist on an outpatient basis. The low complication rate was credited to proper medical evaluation of the patients and, when indicated, the modification of provision of dental care.

Treatment Planning

Treatment planning for patients with HIV is similar to that of other medically complex patients with potentially fatal disorders. Four parameters need to be considered when formulating an appropriate treatment plan for these patients.

1. A patient's medical condition determines his or her ability to endure dental visits, ie, long or short appointments as well as the frequency of dental visits, which will influence what types of procedures can be performed. Patients with severe weight loss may not be able to sit comfortably in a dental chair for more than 20 minutes without pillows, and even this may not alleviate the pain caused by pressure from the dental chair. Some patients with wasting syndrome suffer from incontinence, nausea, or vomiting, which limits the amount of time they can continuously sit for a dental appointment. The ability of patients to physically show up for a dental appointment may also change during the course of the disease. This not only depends on a patient's physical condition but also on his or her mental status.

2. It is essential to restore masticatory function in patients with an impaired ability to process oral nutrition. Due to a patient's deteriorating condition, such interventions do not always follow the standard progression of a dental treatment protocol.

3. A patient's prognosis for survival also influences the choice of dental procedures. One such example is the placement of dental implants. Although dental implants have successfully been placed in HIV-infected patients, this type of prosthetic rehabilitation may not be a viable solution for patients with advanced HIV disease and a poor prognosis for survival.[2]

4. Finally, as for other patients, financial resources determine the type of dental restorations and sometimes even a patient's ability to return for dental appointments.

Thus, treatment planning for patients with HIV is determined by a patient's changing medical condition, mental condition, and financial resources. It must be regarded as an evolving process that, despite its ever-changing nature, must address the same functions as with other patients—the alleviation of pain, the restoration of dental function, and esthetic considerations.

Antibiotic Prophylaxis

Antibiotic prophylaxis prior to dental procedures should be approached judiciously. Patients with HIV have demonstrated a higher propensity for developing allergic reactions to antibiotics during the more advanced stages of the disease; therefore, antibiotics should not be used without a clear medical indication.

According to the Council on Dental Therapeutics of the American Dental Association and the guidelines of the American Heart Association (AHA),[3] patients who are at risk for developing subacute bacterial endocarditis (SBE) need antibiotic prophylaxis prior to dental therapy, regardless of HIV status. The regimen for patients with HIV does not differ from that in patients without HIV. The highest risk for developing SBE is found in individuals with previous episodes of SBE. Thus, patients with a history of intravenous drug use, where SBE is not uncommon, may need prophylactic antibiotics more often than patients in other high-risk groups.

Patients with severe neutropenia, below 500 cells/mm^3, are highly susceptible to bacterial infections. For such patients, a prophylactic antibiotic regimen must be instituted.

The regimen for prophylaxis follows the AHA guidelines, but the type of antibiotic must be chosen carefully. Since a patient with severe neutropenia has a diminished ability to kill invading bacteria, only bactericidal antibiotics should be used, such as penicillin, amoxicillin, or cephalosporin. Bacteriostatic antibiotics, such as erythromycin, clindamycin, or tetracyline, may contribute to an increased bacterial load after withdrawal of the antibiotic.

Antibiotic medications should not be instituted based solely on a patient's CD4+ cell count, CD8+ cell count, p24 antigenemia, or HIV status. However, severe neutropenia is more common in two groups of patients: patients with CD4+ cell counts below 100 cells/mm^3; and patients who have experienced side effects from certain medications, such as long-term users of zidovudine in advanced stages of HIV disease, or individuals receiving zidovudine and who are concomitantly taking other neutropenia-inducing drugs such as trimethoprim-sulfamethoxazole, pyrimethamine and sulfadiazine, or ganciclovir. In each case, obtaining preoperative neutrophil counts may be pertinent. However, many patients with advanced stages of HIV disease are already taking antibiotics that may protect them from the dissemination of oral bacteria.

Many patients are being treated

with intravenous medications on an outpatient basis. Such individuals will have indwelling catheters to facilitate administration of the necessary drug. The more common medications delivered by this route are ganciclovir and amphotericin B. There are no clear indications in the literature for the use of antibiotic prophylaxis prior to dental therapy in patients with Hickman's or other indwelling catheters. Most indwelling catheters fail due to skin-associated bacterial infection and not from bacteria commonly found in the oral cavity. However, a patient's physician may still recommend prophylactic antibiotics prior to dental therapy.

Modification of Dental Procedures

In general, there is no justification to modify dental treatment based solely on patient's HIV status. Treatment plans for asymptomatic patients with HIV follow the same guidelines as those for all other patients. However, during the more advanced stages of HIV disease, the patient's illnesses may directly interfere with or require modification of dental procedures.

Before initiating any dental procedure, it is prudent to give the patient an antibacterial mouthrinse, such as chlorhexidine gluconate. This lowers the bacterial load inside the oral cavity and may reduce the incidence of bacterial dissemination during treatment.

For patients with a history of increased bleeding tendencies, hemorrhagic-prone procedures should be approached conservatively. Bleeding should not be induced in inaccessible areas or at multiple sites before assessing hemostasis in such patients.

Local Anesthetics

The delivery of local anesthetics is not associated with the dissemination of intraoral opportunistic infections, even in patients with oral candidiasis. However, deep block injections should be avoided in patients with a recent history of poor hemostasis. In such cases, local infiltration or intraligamentary injections can be used.

Preventive Oral Health Care

Many of the oral pathologic conditions associated with HIV disease are first discovered by alert dental health-care providers. Other changes in the oral cavity, such as xerostomia, become more common during progression of the disease. Therefore, patients at risk for developing oral manifestations associated with HIV disease should be seen at shorter intervals than regular patients.

Patients without any indication for disease progression, or with CD4+ cell counts above 200 cells/mm^3, or without previous oral manifestations associated with HIV disease should be placed on a regular 6-month recall. Patients with indications for disease progression, or with CD4+ cell counts below 200 cells/mm^3, or with a history of oral pathologic conditions, and patients with reduced salivary flow, especially patients taking multiple medications as oral suspensions (not uncommon among children with HIV), need to be seen at least every 3 months.

The institution of daily antibacterial mouthrinses should be considered for patients with poor oral hygiene, patients with periodontal disease not responding to conventional therapy, and patients with a history of necrotizing ulcerative periodontitis or linear gingival erythema.

Decreased salivary flow has been associated with HIV disease and with medications used in HIV disease (see Chapters 8 and 9). Patients exhibiting reduced flow rates should be given fluoride supplements in the form of topically applied gels, fluoride mouthrinses, and high-fluoride concentrated toothpastes.

Periodontal Therapy

Scaling, curettage, and root planing cause iatrogenic bacteremia but have not been associated with a higher incidence of systemic signs and symptoms, such as fevers and chills, in patients with HIV. This was borne out in a study evaluating complications caused by bacteremia after scaling and curettage in a cohort of 22 HIV-infected patients.[4] Due to the limited number of patients in this study, it may not be possible to draw any general conclusions: the results, however, indicated that antibiotic prophylaxis was not necessary prior to performing these types of procedures.

Periodontal conditions may worsen secondary to gingival lesions, such as those in Kaposi's sarcoma.[5] These lesions will also be affected and may become inflamed, further compromising the periodontium. To achieve periodontal health, treatment of the periodontal condition must be accompanied by treatment of the lesion.

Periodontal infections may have unusual appearances due to other underlying pathologic conditions, such as lymphomas and cytomegalovirus infections; on the other hand, lesions may mimic periodontal pathosis.[6–8] Dental providers need to be aware of such occurrences to differentiate oral manifestations in patients with HIV. They should not institute therapy that can exacerbate other pathologic conditions. Periodontal surgery can safely be performed even in patients with low CD4+ cell counts.[1] However, surgery should only be performed after evaluating the patient's overall medical condition. Patients with CD4+ cell counts below 100 cells/mm^3 need to be evaluated for neutropenia. If the neutrophil count is below 500 cells/mm^3, preoperative and postoperative antibiotics must be administered and the patient alerted to the signs and symptoms of infection in the area. However, a typical inflammatory response may not be present because of the patient's immune status.

Restorative and Prosthetic Procedures

Restorative procedures should be performed with an unabridged standard of care. All treatment options available to the patient should be fully explained prior to starting therapy, including the advantages and disadvantages of each option based on a patient's medical condition. The choice of restoration is governed by the patient's ability to withstand the length of dental appointments and to return for continuous therapy, the urgency to restore masticatory functions, and financial resources.

Full coverage prosthetic restoration is advantageous for long-term use, but such a procedure requires lengthy appointments, multiple visits, and is usually costly. For single posterior teeth, amalgam pin buildups are a viable solution for patients who can withstand only short appointments, are not able to immediately return for follow-up appointments, or cannot afford expensive dental therapy. Amalgam pin buildups, however, do have a shorter life expectancy compared to full prosthetic coverage. For restorations of single anterior teeth, glass ionomers or composite restorations are appropriate alternatives to complete coverage.

Intact masticatory function is essential for many patients with HIV disease to maintain adequate oral nutritional intake. Vitallium removable dentures provide long-lasting functional dentition for patients with several missing teeth. However, to fit such appliances, multiple visits may be required to restore existing dentition prior to fabrication of the dentures. Furthermore, they are more expensive than alternative acrylic treatment partial dentures with wrought iron clasps. For patients with limited financial resources or an urgent need to restore masticatory functions, acrylic treatment partial dentures with wrought iron clasps are a viable solution. In medical conditions such as rapid weight loss due primarily to an inability to chew, this type of denture can be placed in a patient's mouth to temporarily or permanently restore masticatory function without necessarily having to restore the existing dentition.

Patients who can withstand only very short dental appointments, and who do not know when they may be able to return for continuous treatment, may need longer-lasting temporary fillings. This can be accomplished with glass-ionomer restorations. These types of restorations require minimal tooth preparation and can even be placed on the occlusal surfaces of posterior teeth without the risk of immediately losing vertical dimension.

Endodontic Therapy

The incidence of endodontic interappointment flare-ups in a general population is estimated to be 3.2%.[9] In one retrospective study previously mentioned,[1] endodontic therapy in patients with severe immune deterioration was not associated with a higher incidence of postoperative flare-ups compared to that of the general dental patients. However, due to the limited number of endodontic procedures (76) it may not be possible to use the results from this study to establish a definitive protocol. When interappointment flare-ups occur, they are usually not more severe than those in patients without HIV and can be managed with nonsteroidal anti-inflammatory drugs and antibiotics. Meticulous instrumentation, avoiding passing the apex, may further reduce the incidence of postoperative flare-ups.

Long-term follow-up of endodontically treated teeth with periapical radiolucencies in HIV-infected patients shows that the success rate during all stages of the disease does not differ from that in patients without HIV (Glick M, unpublished data). At least two case reports in the dental literature support this finding.[10,11] However, an additional study indicated that periapical lesions in an immunodeficient individual with HIV contained polyclonal immunoglobulin-producing plasma cells and lacked CD4+ T lymphocytes. Furthermore, these lesions did not resolve after conventional endodontic therapy.[12] There is no indication for preoperative administration of antibiotics or antiinflammatory medications prior to endodontic therapy.

As for other invasive procedures, patients with CD4+ cell counts below 100 cells/mm³ require evaluation of their neutrophil count, and if it is below 500 cells/mm³, preoperative and postoperative antibiotics should be administered when apicoectomies are performed.

Oral Surgical Procedures

Surgical procedures are associated with bleeding and risk of infection. All such procedures must be performed in a manner that minimizes the risk of excessive bleeding and invasion of pathogens from the oral cavity to deeper facial planes and spaces.

Hemostasis

Patients with a history of bleeding tendencies must be evaluated prior to surgical procedures. However, even if hemostasis appears normal, excessive bleeding can occur due to unforeseen circumstances, such as HIV-associated immune thrombocytopenia[13] (see Chapter 11). In such instances, the surgical team needs to be able to stop the hemorrhage with local or systemic measures. Also, extraction of teeth in hemophiliac patients may result in patients with excessive bleeding if a proper medical evaluation has not been performed preoperatively.[14]

Extractions

Scaling prior to extractions and gingival flap procedures decreases the potential for dissemination of pathogens. This should always be performed on teeth that have a heavy accumulation of calculus.

One of the more common complications associated with extractions are dry sockets, occurring in approximately 3.0% to 4.0% of all such procedures among the general population.[15] This complication rate is similar to that found among patients with HIV. A large study of dry sockets among 86 men with HIV reported an incidence of 3.0%.[16] Since no data on the patients' immune status were available in this study, at least patients' HIV status did not appear to alter complication rates after dental procedures. Another study of postextraction complications in 38 individuals with HIV reported a similar incidence of 3.7% for dry sockets.[14]

In a study of patients with CD4+ cell counts below 200 cells/mm^3,[1] 16 (4.9%) of 326 extractions were accompanied by complications: four cases of slow healing, nine cases of dry sockets, one case of prolonged bleeding, one case of bone sequestration, and one case of an oroantral fistula. A total of 292 simple extractions were associated with a complication rate of 4.1% while 34 surgical extractions were associated with a complication rate of 11.8%. Because of the limited number of surgical extractions, it was not possible to ascertain if this type of procedure is more prone to complications when compared to simple extractions. However, all complications were treated by the attending dentist on an outpatient basis.

As all oral surgery procedures are highly invasive, patients with CD4+ cell counts below 100 cells/mm^3 should be evaluated for neutropenia. If the neutrophil count is below 500 cells/mm^3, patients should receive preoperative and postoperative antibiotics.

Extensive Surgical Interventions

Screening tests for bleeding tendencies, anemia, and leukopenia are appropriate prior to extensive surgical interventions. Consultation with a patient's primary physician is recommended.

Orthodontic Procedures

Nonsurgical orthodontic procedures can be safely performed on HIV-positive patients. One case involving orthodontic treatment of a patient with HIV reported no complications due to the patient's HIV status.[17]

Tissue Healing

A major concern when performing any type of procedure that results in tissue manipulation is the patient's healing ability. In surgical procedures as wide-ranging as biopsies, surgical extractions, periodontal surgery, apicoectomies, and placement of dental implants, no significant impaired healing or significant increased incidence of dry sockets has been documented in patients during all stages of HIV disease. However, in cases of impaired healing after extractions, underlying infections may be responsible and should be treated accordingly.[18]

References

1. Glick M, Abel SN, Muzyka BC, DiLorenzo M. Dental complications after dental treatment of patients with AIDS. J Am Dent Assoc 1994;125(3):296-301.

2. Glick M, Abel SN. Dental implants and HIV disease (editorial). Implant Dent 1993;2:149–150.

3. Council on Dental Therapeutics, American Heart Association. Preventing bacterial endocarditis: a statement for dental professionals. J Am Dent Assoc 1992;122: 87–92.

4. Lucatorto FM, Franker CK, Maza J. Postscaling bacteremia in HIV-associated gingivitis and periodontitis. Oral Surg Oral Med Oral Pathol 1992;73:550–554.

5. Shiboski CH, Winkler JR. Gingival Kaposi's sarcoma and periodontitis. A case report and suggested treatment approach to the combined lesions. Oral Surg Oral Med Oral Pathol 1993;76:49–53.

6. Vallejo GH, Garcia MD, Lopez A, Mendieta C, Moskow BS. Unusual periodontal findings in an AIDS patient with Burkitt's lymphoma. J Periodontol 1989;60:723–727.

7. Dodd CL, Winkler JR, Heinic GS, Daniels TE, Yee K, Greenspan D. Cytomegalovirus infection presenting as acute periodontal infection in a patient infected with the human immunodeficiency virus. J Clin Periodontol 1993;20:282–285.

8. Glick M, Cleveland DB, Salkin LM, Alfaro-Miranda M, Fielding AF. Intraoral cytomegalovirus lesion and HIV-associated periodontitis in a patient with acquired immunodeficiency syndrome. Oral Surg Oral Med Oral Pathol 1991;72:716–720.

9. Walton R, Fouad A. Endodontic inter-appointment flare-ups: a prospective study of incidence and related factors. J Endodontics 1992;18:172–177.

10. Hillman D. Combination treatment for a patient with AIDS-related complex and a chronic periapical lesion. J Conn State Dent Assoc 1986;60:165–170.

11. Goodis HE, King T. Endodontic treatment of HIV infected patients. J Calif Dent Assoc 1989;17:23–25.

12. Gerner NW, Hurlen B, Dobloug J, Brandtzaeg P. Endodontic treatment and immunopathology of periapical granuloma in an AIDS patient. Endodont Dent Traumatol 1988;4:127–131.

13. Maron G, Helmy E, Bays R. Immune thrombocytopenia in AIDS patients: a case report. J Oral Maxillofac Surg 1989; 47:1093-1095.

14. Porter SR, Scully C, Luker J. Complications of dental surgery in persons with HIV disease. Oral Surg Oral Med Oral Pathol 1993;75:165–167.

15. Field EA, Speechley JA, Rotter E, Scott J. Dry socket incidence compared after a 12 year interval. Br J Oral Maxillofac Surg 1985;23:419–427.

16. Robinson PG, Cooper H, Hatt J. Healing after dental extractions in men with HIV infection. Oral Surg Oral Med Oral Pathol 1992;74:426–430.

17. Williams BJ. Modified orthodontic treatment goals in a patient with multiple complicating factors. Special Care Dent 1992; 12:251–254.

18. Watkins KV, Richmond AS, Langstein IM. Nonhealing extraction site due to *Actinomyces naeslundii* in patient with AIDS. Oral Surg Oral Med Oral Pathol 1991;71:675–677.

14

Infection Control

Milton E. Schaefer

Infection control in a dental setting is twofold. First, it involves the prevention of the passage of infectious disease from the patient to health-care providers and other patients who may be subsequently treated in the same area. Second, it involves the prevention of transmission of any additional infectious disease to the already compromised patient, such as HIV-infected patients.

Preventing the transmission of infectious disease from patient to health-care worker has always been a concern. It became of major importance with the rising numbers of persons in the general population who became infected with hepatitis B virus, genital herpes viruses, and HIV. The Occupational Health and Safety Administration (OSHA) created a standard for health-care workers to follow to prevent the transmission of blood-borne pathogens in the health-care setting.[1,2] The American Dental Association (ADA),[3,4] the Centers for Disease Control and Prevention (CDC),[5] and the Office Sterilization and Asepsis Procedures Research Foundation (OSAP)[6] have all issued guidelines pertaining to infection control in the dental office.

Dental offices in the United States have incorporated elements of these standards and guidelines into their everyday practices. The concern for the health and safety of the patients and the treating personnel has fueled this effort. The infection control program for the special patient is strict adherence to these currently promulgated standards and guidelines, called *universal precautions*. They are called universal because they are to be applied to *all* patients and *all* treatment procedures. These infection control guidelines include appropriate procedures to protect all dental patients, as well as all dental-care providers, from the hazard of infectious disease transmission in the dental office. It is incumbent on all dental-care providers to recognize these guidelines to render safe dental care to their patients.

Immunization Against Hepatitis B Virus

All personnel in the dental office, including the receptionist, should be antibody-positive for the hepatitis B virus. The employer must provide the vaccine at no cost to the employee as required by OSHA. Each vaccine recipient should be tested 2 or 3 months after the series of injections is complete. The health-care worker is protected when the test is positive for the antibody to hepatitis B.

Barrier Techniques

The proper use of barrier techniques as part of universal precautions is extremely important. The wearing of gloves, masks, protective eyewear, and clinic attire by all personnel who have direct patient contact is required for all treatment sessions, regardless of their nature. There are no exceptions to this rule.

Gloving and Handwashing

Hands must be washed carefully with an antiseptic lotion soap that has persistent antibacterial activity, each time gloves are donned or removed, to remove the bacterial buildup that occurs in the warm, moist environment beneath the gloves. Hands should be dried thoroughly and a lotion applied to help maintain healthy skin. Petroleum-based lotions are avoided since they may degrade the latex in the gloves. Gloves are changed for each patient, when they are damaged or torn, or if the procedure extends longer than 1 hour. Gloves should be changed or covered with an overglove if it becomes necessary to temporarily leave the immediate field of operation.

To avoid cross-contamination, special care should be taken to avoid touching items with the gloved hands that are not directly in the field of operation, including the face mask, protective eyewear, the patient care record, progress slips, pencils, computer keyboards, radiographs, and amalgamators.

Masks

Masks should have at least 95% filtration efficiency for particles 3.0 to

5.0 μm in diameter, and they should be changed for each patient. When dealing with a patient with TB, a mask with greater filtration capabilities should be worn. A chin-length face shield may be worn in addition to the mask for greater protection against particulate splatter.

Protective Eyewear

This third member of the barrier technique group must be worn by the dental team at all times—when treating a patient, when proportioning dental materials, and when cleaning up following treatment. Side shields on eyeglasses are required by OSHA (Fig 14-1).

Chin-length face shields are now available that offer protection considered equal to protective eyewear when worn with a mask. The choice is a personal one.

Clinic Attire

Appropriate clinic attire provides protective covering for street clothing and exposed skin. This is especially important for individuals who participate directly in patient treatment to avoid contamination by infectious aerosols and splatter. Gowns that have been worn during treatment of patients should be removed before leaving the office or while eating. The clinic clothing should be laundered in hot water, with bleach if the fabric allows it. According to OSHA regulations, clinic personnel may not take these gar-

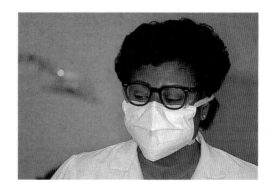

Fig 14-1. A mask and safety glasses with OSHA required solid side shields are to be worn for every visit with a patient where splatter may be reasonably anticipated.

ments home to launder. They may be laundered in the office if the machines are there, or they may be taken to a commercial laundromat properly bagged for proper compliance with the OSHA regulations.

Hair Control

All personnel involved in direct patient care should take steps to assure that hair does not come into contact with equipment or supplies used in patient care or intrude into the treatment field. Aerosols and splatter commonly contaminate the hair as well as the equipment and surfaces in the dental operatory. Disposable caps are available at dental or medical supply houses and may be worn for routine patient care if desired. Bearded persons should consider routine use of the chin-length face shield.

Sterilization

Sterilization refers to the complete destruction of all microbial life. Disinfection refers to the destruction of most vegetative bacteria, but not their spores. Therefore, these terms are not synonymous.

Each office must properly clean, disinfect, and sterilize all instruments and equipment used in the treatment of one patient before it is used with another patient. The current standards put forth by the ADA and CDC state clearly that any instrument or other article used in the mouth of one patient must be heat sterilized before being used in the mouth of another patient. This clearly limits the use of other modes of sterilization, such as liquid chemical solutions.

Cleaning of Instruments

The removal of gross organic soil (bioburden), ie, saliva, blood, and residues of dental restorative materials, before attempting a sterilization process is extremely important. The idea that the soil will become sterile is not necessarily true. If the amount or thickness of soil is sufficient, living bacteria may remain on the instrument underneath the layer of soil.[7]

The simplest and safest method for accomplishing this cleaning process is with an ultrasonic cleaner. Instruments are rinsed free of gross debris in the operatory, but scrubbing with a brush is neither necessary nor desirable, since this could result in injury to the health-care worker. The machine is able to do the work when used properly, and it saves time.

A presoak solution prevents the bioburden from drying on the instruments and allows the cleaning process to remove it easily. The liquid may be water, an enzyme solution, or a disinfectant.

Heat Sterilization

It is wise to review your armamentarium and replace those items that have poor plating, or are otherwise in poor condition and will deteriorate further. Replacements should be chosen for their ability to withstand the temperatures required for heat sterilization.

Steam autoclave. The steam autoclave is the instrument of choice for sterilization if there are many cloth- or paper-wrapped packs to deal with, such as those found in the offices of periodontists and oral surgeons. Steam penetrates multiple layers of wrapping material best.

Chemiclave® A. Chemiclave works well with single- or double-layer wraps, such as the mylar and paper tubing or pouches. It has the added advantage of operating below the threshold of rust, 12% water vapor, when operated according to the manufacturer's directions.

Dry heat. Conventional dry heat sterilizers are the least desirable of the accepted methods because of the extended time required to kill all pathogens and their spores, the high temperature used, the difficulty in biologic testing, and the fact that some instruments may be harmed by the process.

There are two forms of monitoring of sterilizers: process indicators and biologic testing.

Process indicators. These take the form of colored printing on the wrap, or a striped piece of tape on the package. If a color change takes place, it indicates that the package was processed in the sterilizer. This does not guarantee that the contents are sterile, only that the bundle was processed.

Biologic testing. To ascertain that each load run through the sterilizer is subjected to all three parameters of the sterilization process (proper temperature, proper pressure, and correct amount of time) the sterilizer is checked by performing a biologic test with spore strips. This test may be performed daily or weekly in-house, and the results should be carefully recorded in a log. A spore test should also be performed and sent to an outside laboratory service at least once a month to gain third-party assurance that the sterilizer is functioning properly. The test results should be carefully noted when received and then placed in a special file for this purpose. If one elects not to do in-house monitoring, the sterilizer should be monitored by a third-party service weekly.

Disinfection

Disinfection is a chemical process whereby the total numbers of microbes are reduced in number, but may not be totally eliminated. This level of kill is impossible to monitor. The process of chemical disinfection is used in the dental office for the decontamination of environmental surfaces and other items touched or splashed while treating a patient but too large to be placed in the sterilizer. Alcohol, either ethyl or isopropyl, has been used for many years in the dental office for this purpose. Since 1978, the Council on Dental Therapeutics of the American Dental Association has not accepted alcohol for use as a surface disinfectant, in part because the alcohol evaporates before a sufficient exposure time to kill the organisms has elapsed.

The chemical solution chosen for surface disinfection must be tuberculocidal, that is, capable of destroying the bacillus that causes tuberculosis. Microbiologists consider this pathogen to be the most difficult to kill. Therefore, any chemical that can eradicate Mycobacterium tuberculosis is considered to be an effective disinfectant.

Proper disinfection requires that the surfaces be cleaned first, and then wetted with the disinfectant solution for the length of time specified by the manufacturer for tuberculocidal activity, usually 10 minutes. Therefore, if only one solution is to be used, that chemical solution must be a detergent as well as a disinfectant.

The surfaces to be cleaned and disinfected should be sprayed until they glisten and then thoroughly wiped with a paper towel moistened with the disinfectant to remove the gross contamination. The solution should be sprayed a second time and allowed to remain on the surface for the recommended time.

Items that were properly covered with foil, plastic, or impervious paper to prevent contamination during treatment do not need to be disinfected after each patient but should be chemically disinfected at the end of the working day. Covers are advantageous in that they are 100% effective in preventing contamination, where disinfecting may be less than 80% effective in removing or inactivating contaminating organisms.

Chemicals that are acceptable for disinfection of environmental surfaces include aqueous iodophor solutions, combined synthetic phenolics, phenol-alcohol sprays, and sodium hypochlorite solutions diluted 1:5 to 1:100.

Operatory Management[8]

The Removal of Extraneous Items

The removal of extraneous items from treatment rooms is important because of the fallout of bacterial aerosols and gross splash and splatter that constantly occur. Removing the bulk storage containers and substituting "unit dose" amounts of each item in small packets is simple. In place of the cotton roll dispenser, four or five cotton rolls may be placed in a small envelope, stapled if a steam autoclave will be used to sterilize them, or simply sealed if a Chemiclave is the preferred method of sterilization. Several dozen of these should be made up and sterilized as backup for the cotton rolls

placed in each setup. The same goes for the cotton pellet dispenser, and for cotton-tipped swabs and 2 × 2 gauze squares. The basic starting amount, or "unit dose," of all these disposables should be included in the setup. Should the need arise for more, tearing open an envelope will deliver an additional supply of sterile material. Because they may be easily contaminated, products from a bulk dispenser are no longer appropriate (Fig 14-2).

Restorative materials should not be kept in cardboard boxes out on open counters in the operatories. They should be brought from the central supply area as needed, in procedure tubs, with all the necessary materials and supplies for a specific dental treatment, and handled with freshly washed hands or gloves. In a busy office, this is an excellent use of a third pair of hands.

Bur blocks, as well as other forms of bulk dispensers, no longer remain on the unit tray. The burs required for each treatment are packaged and sterilized in the instrument setup, on a small bur block, or the new single-use disposable burs are used. Should a need arise for an additional bur, the assistant can obtain it from a backup bur block in the cabinet. (Use backup cotton pliers or overgloves to enter storage areas.) When treatment is completed, the extra bur can be processed with the setup or wrapped separately for return to the backup bur block. Should a bur become dull, it should be discarded and a new one obtained from the cabinet to take its place in the setup, using overgloves or the second uncontaminated forceps.

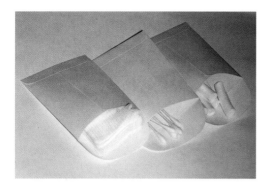

Fig 14-2a. Unit dose amounts of 2 x 2 gauze, cotton-tipped applicators, and cotton rolls are packaged in small envelopes to replace bulk dispensers for these items.

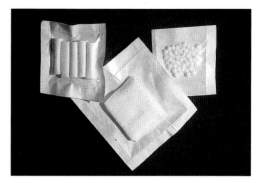

Fig 14-2b. Unit dose amounts of cotton pellets, 2 x 2 gauze, and cotton rolls may be packaged in heat-sealed packets to replace bulk dispensers for these items.

Between Patient Appointments

These activities can be divided into: removal, cleaning and disinfection, and resetting. Each section is completed before the next is begun.

Removal

1. Remove the drape from the patient and use it to cover the instruments on the setup tray. Dental workers should remove gloves, wash hands, make the next appointment, and dismiss the patient.
2. Don utility gloves (Fig 14-3).
3. Remove the handpieces from the unit and put them on the tray with the contaminated instruments for removal to the central sterilization area, so that they may be properly cleaned and wrapped for sterilization.
4. Remove the headrest cover, disposable saliva ejector, high velocity evacuator, and three-way syringe tips and place them in the trash bag on the cabinet.

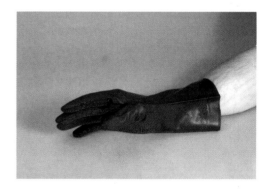

Fig 14-3. Utility gloves should be worn for all cleaning procedures where contact with contaminated instruments or surfaces could occur (photo courtesy of Health Sonics Corp).

5. Place in the trash bag attached to the mobile cabinet any other patient-contaminated waste remaining on the cabinet top, as well as the used patient towel, which has been used to cover the instruments during dismissal.
6. Remove the trash bag from the cabinet, twist it tightly to enclose the debris, cycle it through the heat sterilizer if required in one's area,

and dispose of it in the properly marked waste receptacle.

Cleaning and disinfection

1. Wash the utility-gloved hands, properly disinfect any items remaining on the cabinet top with the spray, wipe, and spray technique (those that cannot be heat sterilized), and return them to their proper place in the cabinet drawers.

2. Heat sterilize the handpieces. The usual pattern is to clean the exterior of gross soil first. Then a cleaner is introduced into the drive air line and the handpiece is activated, expelling the cleaner into a paper towel or other form of absorbent material. The handpiece is packaged and processed through the sterilizer. A lubricant is sprayed into the drive air line before the handpiece is connected to the air line. The excess lubricant is expelled in the same manner as the cleaner, into a paper towel, or the bag in which it was wrapped. It is important to follow the specific recommendations of the manufacturer of the handpiece for cleaning and lubrication, especially if fiber optics are involved.

3. If the unit reaches to the sink, run a large volume of water through each evacuator and saliva ejector hose by passing the handles back and forth through a stream of running water. Otherwise, use a container to bring rinse water to the unit. At the end of the day, use a container filled with the cleaning product suggested by the manufacturer of the vacuum unit.

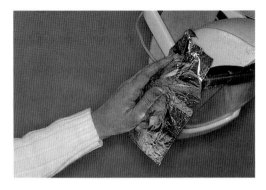

Fig 14-4. Aluminum foil light handle covers will prevent contamination of the handle and make frequent disinfection unnecessary.

4. Spray with disinfectant and wipe the cabinet top, drawer handles, light handles, chair switch buttons, top of unit, three-way syringe, and evacuator handles and handpiece hoses. Respray. The three-way syringe tip is removed and discarded if disposable, or placed in a small envelope and sterilized for each patient. Clean the plastic light shield as required. (Covering the light handles, chair switches and unit top will make this job easier. The covers should be waterproof to prevent contamination. Aluminum foil, plastic wrap, or plastic-backed towels are examples. Preventing of contamination is better than attempting to wipe it away after it occurs.) (Fig 14-4.)

5. Rinse dental impressions immediately on removal from the mouth to remove all blood and saliva. Then immerse them in an acceptable disinfectant solution and take them to the laboratory for casting. The earlier the disinfection process occurs in the procedure, the fewer the areas that will be contaminated.

The operatory and dental equipment should now be free from contamination by blood and saliva and ready to set up for the next patient. Place a fresh headrest cover.

Seating the patient and resetting the operatory

1. Seat the patient. Dental workers should adjust their mask and protective eyewear, wash their hands with the antibacterial lotion soap, and put on fresh gloves. Place a disposable saliva ejector tip and high-velocity evacuator tip. Run the water through the three-way syringe handle for 30 seconds before placing the sterilized tip or disposable tip. Open the sealed pouch containing the sterilized handpiece, partially remove it, and lubricate it as recommended by the manufacturer. Step on the controller and run water through the handpiece hose for 30 seconds before connecting the handpiece. Run the handpiece dry into the partially removed sterilizing bag to expel any excess lubricant. Patients appreciate when dental workers take the time to explain what they are doing as they do it.

2. Ask the patient to rinse their mouth with an antibacterial mouthwash prior to the procedure. This lowers the number of bacteria present in the mouth and may help to prevent their spread to uncontaminated areas by splatters and aerosols during treatment.

3. Attach the trash bag to a convenient location on the edge of back

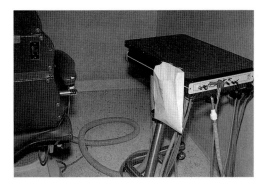

Fig 14-5. A trash bag affixed to side of mobile dental cart will make it convenient to dispose of waste generated during a treatment session.

or side bar, or edge of cart (Fig 14-5).

4. From the procedure tub or tubs brought from the central sterilization area, assemble the required armamentaria on the covered tray or mobile cabinet top.

5. Dental workers should try to anticipate all their needs for that particular treatment. Should you need to go back to a storage container during the course of the appointment, it is essential to wash the gloved hands first, or use overgloves, before selecting additional materials or instruments from clean storage areas, so that contamination is not spread. If it becomes necessary to leave the treatment area for any reason, put on overgloves or remove the gloves for the same reason. When returning, reglove or remove the overgloves prior to resuming treatment.

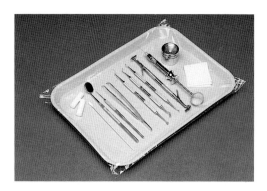

Fig 14-6. A plastic tray cover completely covers the tray, preventing contamination (photo courtesy of Pinnacle Products, Inc).

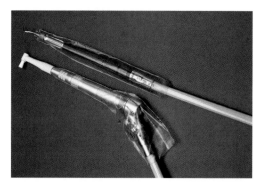

Fig 14-7. Disposable sleeves on slow speed handpiece and ultrasonic scaler handpiece will provide good protection from contamination by oral fluids (photo courtesy of Pinnacle Products, Inc).

Covers and Disposables

It is easier to prevent contamination with the proper use of covers than it is to decontaminate a soiled surface. It is safer to prevent contamination than to try to eliminate it after it has occurred. And it is more certain to prevent contamination than to assume that the disinfection process will totally kill any organisms that have accumulated on the uncovered surface. A good cover has the following attributes: low in cost, waterproof, and large enough to cover completely the area to be protected. It does little good to cover part of a surface and then go through the effort of disinfecting that surface.

The common practice of placing a stack of paper covers on a unit tray is a poor practice. They are not waterproof, and material spilled on the top sheet will often soak down several layers. Additionally, they are not large enough to cover the entire tray; therefore, the edge or lip of the tray will be

contaminated and must be disinfected. Third, many instruments, because of their design, will hang over the edge of the paper stack and contaminate that area. Therefore, if tray covers are the method of choice, they should be used singly and the tray should be disinfected after each use. More correctly, a waterproof cover larger than the tray should be used and discarded after each patient. Another version of cover for this particular application is a plastic bag pulled over the tray. When treatment is complete, the plastic bag may be removed by turning it inside out, and used to collect the other disposables. It may then be tied tightly to contain the waste (Fig 14-6).

Other uses of covers could include the newly introduced finger cots for slow-speed handpieces and ultrasonic scaler handles (Fig 14-7). Yet another type of cover is the aluminum foil square crimped over the lamp handle. It can be easily placed and removed, and it does away with the need for disinfecting the handle after each patient since it prevents contamination (see Fig 14-4). There are many other possibilities for the use of covers, limited only by the imagination of the user.

Products that are purchased for single use are not intended to be sterilized and reused. They are often plastic and will not tolerate the heat required for sterilization. It is not safe to try to clean and disinfect these items for reuse. The time required to do so can make it uneconomical. Therefore, use and then dispose of all single-use items.

Properly cleaning, lubricating, and sterilizing by heat a prophy angle after each use can consume a considerable amount of time. The new disposable angles are an answer to this problem. They can be obtained individually packaged, sterile, with a rubber-cup fitted. Showing the patient that a brand new, never-used-before article of equipment is going to be used in treating them, and then discarded, is another excellent way to let them know what is being done is for their protection (Fig 14-8).

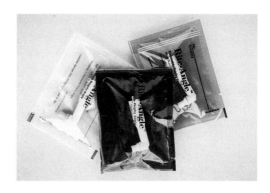

Fig 14-8. Sterilized disposable prophy angles sealed in individual wraps (photo courtesy of Ash/Dentsply) demonstrate to the patient your concern for their protection against the transfer of infectious disease.

Central Sterilization Area

It is recommended that the processes of cleaning and sterilizing dental instruments be carried out in an area devoted to that sole purpose. In the past, the instrument management was often carried out in the operatory, or in another room. Since we now know that there are a great number of bacteria and other infectious organisms present on soiled dental instruments, it makes sense to perform the cleaning and sterilization of these items in an area where the chance of contamination of instruments or persons is more remote. The movement of instruments should be in a flow pattern that does not require clean materials and contaminated items to cross paths.

Cleaning of Instruments

Thorough cleaning of recyclable instruments must precede any efforts at sterilization. Bioburden must be removed. The safest way to perform this cleaning is a two-step process. A container should be on or near the field of operation in the treatment room, and it should contain either a disinfectant or a detergent solution. When an instrument has been used for the last time in the procedure, simply place it in the liquid in the container. When the patient is dismissed, the container, along with all the other contaminated articles, may be removed from the treatment room to the central sterilization area for handling. The instruments in the container will be kept moist by the solution and the blood, saliva, etc, will not dry and become difficult to remove. When it is time to clean the instruments, the liquid should be poured into the sink and the instruments placed into the ultrasonic cleaner.

Manual scrubbing of instruments is no longer considered acceptable. Utility gloves are always worn when handling contaminated instruments. At the end of the day, the utility gloves are pulled off inside out and sprayed with the disinfectant, or run through the sterilizer with the last load (see Fig 14-3).

Following this protocol results in minimum contact with contaminated instruments throughout the process and prevents the possibility of a puncture wound from these sharp instruments.

Instrument Setups and Packaging

Historically, dental instruments were purchased, placed in a cabinet drawer in a treatment room and circulated between the drawer, the instrument tray, the sink, the dish of disinfectant, the sink, and the drawer again. Practice management people realized the folly of this, and began urging the use of setups, that is, all the instruments needed for a specific procedure packaged together, thus saving the time it took to assemble them the next time they were needed.

With the present requirement that all items that have been used in the mouth of one patient be sterilized by heat before being used with another patient, it makes even more sense to use setups, since they can be packaged together with the disposable materials needed for the restoration, sterilized together, and then kept that way until ready to be used again.

Methods for Cleaning, Packaging, and Sterilization of Dental Hand Instruments

1. Clean all instruments ultrasonically before wrapping and sterilization.
2. Place the instruments on a paper towel and dry them with another paper towel.
3. Separate the instruments into the appropriate groups or setups. Placing rubber bands around individual setups before cleaning makes this easier.
   a. Place a small envelope over each end of a group of instruments and tack together with a piece of tape. This prevents the sharp points from penetrating the sterilizing bag. Slide the entire group into a sterilizing bag (Fig 14-9).
   b. Arrange the instruments on their appropriate setup trays, if this is the preferred method in one's office.
4. Add a unit dose of 2×2 gauze, cotton rolls, and cotton pellets for the

intended procedure to the setup tray or bagged setup.

Note: Backup packages of 2 × 2s, cotton rolls, cotton pellets, and other disposable goods can be conveniently made by placing the amount that will be sufficient for one treatment session into individual small envelopes, available at stationery stores. Mark the contents with a soft lead pencil and sterilize. These are distributed among the operatories in a convenient location. Should the operator use all the cotton rolls that were included in the setup, the assistant may use an uncontaminated cotton forceps or put on overgloves, open a drawer, retrieve one of the coin envelopes containing cotton rolls, tear off the top and spill them out on the work space (see Fig 14-2a).

5. The packages are wrapped in such a way that the sterility of the contents may be maintained for a reasonable length of time.
   a. Fold the opening of the sterilizing bag over two times and fasten with a length of indicator tape long enough to go completely around the folded edge to seal it. Write the setup type and the date clearly on the bottom border of the bag with a soft lead pencil. If other types of markers that contain ink are used to write the number on bags that will be processed in a Chemiclave, the ink will be dissolved by the chemical vapor and deposited on all the instru-

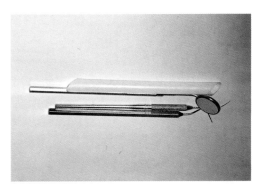

Fig 14-9a. The instrument setup for examination has been ultrasonically cleaned and is ready to be wrapped for sterilization.

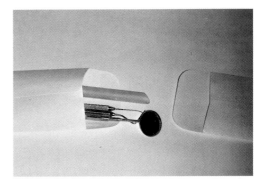

Fig 14-9b. Instruments are placed in a small envelope and a second envelope will be placed on other ends to prevent tearing through the sterilization bag.

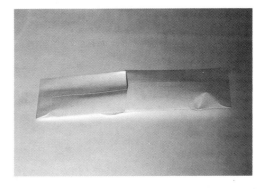

Fig 14-9c. Instruments covered with both small envelopes are ready to be placed in larger wrap.

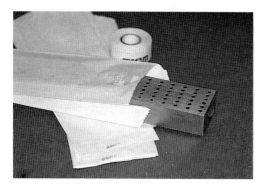

Fig 14-10. A perforated setup tray is partially inserted into a sterilization bag to maintain sterility when the process is completed.

ments and the chamber walls, creating a cleaning problem.

b. The solid setup tray is closed and a strip of indicator tape is placed over the edge. The setup type and date may be written on the tape with a soft lead pencil. If a perforated setup tray is used, it must be placed in a bag or wrapped, and marked. (Fig 14-10).

6. Sterilize in the autoclave or Chemiclave, and store in the central sterilizing area.

Wrapping Techniques for Other Articles

Burs and Mounted Stones. Clean in the ultrasonic unit and blot dry on a paper towel. Place in a coin envelope and seal. With a soft lead pencil, identify the contents on the envelope. These may be placed in a larger sterilizer bag with other smaller items to be sterilized. If sterilization will be by steam autoclave, use of an anticorro-

sion spray on the burs will minimize damage by the water vapor.

Sharpening Stones and Contraangles. Wipe off any excess oil or grease and bag separately in the smaller sterilization bags. Place in the larger bag with any other small wrapped articles. Be sure to identify the article enclosed in the small bag as before. Contraangles must be lubricated after sterilization according to manufacturers' directions.

Handpieces: High and Low Speed. Most handpieces manufactured after 1980 are sterilizable by steam autoclave or chemical vapor sterilizers or can be retrofitted to make this possible. Follow the manufacturer's instructions carefully for cleaning and lubrication before and after sterilization. This is extremely important to prolong the life of the turbine.

Sterilization bags or tubing that can be made into bags are available in several sizes and materials. One of the most convenient is the combination of clear mylar film and paper. Instruments placed in these bags can be processed in the autoclave or Chemiclave, and stored in drawers or on shelves. A glance is all that is necessary to identify the contents (Fig 14-11).

Packaged instruments should be stored so that the contents can be easily identified, either by looking through the clear material or reading the markings on the bag, and then removed without major movement of the other packages. The paper that makes up the sterilizing bags becomes brittle when exposed to sterilizing conditions and may crack when handled excessively.

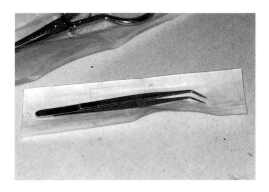

Fig 14-11. The cotton forceps can be easily identified in a sterilization bag of paper and mylar film.

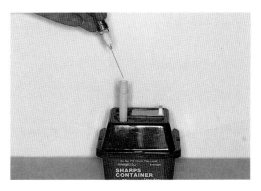

Fig 14-12. A sharps container with a needle cap held for one-hand recapping of the needle complies with OSHA guidelines.

Of utmost importance is letting the patient see these efforts at patient protection. Dental workers should make a point of telling the patient as they open the bag or tray that these instruments have all been sterilized since they were used.

Waste Control

To comply with CDC, ADA, and OSHA guidelines, needles and other sharps must be disposed of in a hard-walled, puncture-proof container as close to the point of use as possible. This means a sharps container in each operatory (Fig 14-12).

Guidelines from the CDC state that we should not bend or break needles but dispose of them in sharps containers that allow the removal of the needle without the hazard of recapping by hand. If recapping must be done, the cap may be placed in a holder (see Fig 14-12) or held in a hemostat, or use the one-handed swoop technique to put the point of the needle in the cap, then raise the syringe to a vertical position and allow the cap to settle down over the needle. The cap is then pushed to place (Fig 14-13).

Cotton rolls, 2 × 2 gauze, patient towels, and other items that have absorbed patient secretions during treatment may be considered contaminated or infectious waste, depending on the area in which one's practice is located. Dental practitioners must contact their local dental organization to find out the status of patient-contaminated waste in their particular locale.

If this patient-contaminated waste must be handled differently from common trash, it can be handled easily if a small bag is attached to the cabinet or unit for each patient (see Fig 14-5). Place all the patient-contaminated waste into this bag as it is generated. At the conclusion of treatment, close the bag securely and heat sterilize it. It may then be disposed of as

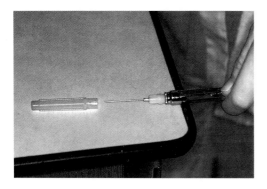

Fig 14-13a. The needle cover is placed on the surface of the cabinet and the syringe is ready for a one-hand recapping procedure.

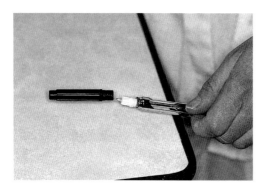

Fig 14-13b. The tip of the needle is placed in the cover.

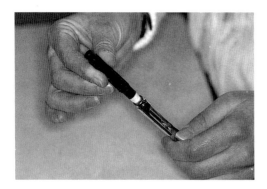

Fig 14-13c. The syringe is raised to allow the cover to slide down and cover the entire needle, making the removal safe.

common trash, if allowed by local health department rules. There should be some indication on the bag that it has been exposed to sterilizing conditions, such as a printed process indicator, or a piece of indicator tape.

The other alternative is to collect all the contaminated waste separately from your towel waste and other non-patient waste, and pay a disposal service a monthly fee to pick it up and incinerate it. It would be wise to do business with a firm that has been in the business for a number of years, and where required, licensed by the state or local community. If dentists are using this option, then OSHA mandates that they have the proper biohazard label on all containers in their office that will be used for the storage of this contaminated waste (Fig 14-14).

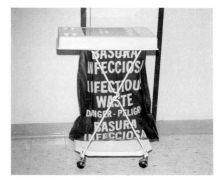

Fig 14-14. This container for patient contaminated waste will be removed by an outside agency when full.

Prosthetic Considerations

Disinfecting Impressions

The commonly used impression materials such as alginates, reversible hydrocolloids, polysulfides, polyethers, and vinyl polysiloxanes have all been subjected to spraying with, or immersion in, the various disinfectants and for the most part have been found to undergo no significant dimensional stability changes. To be absolutely sure that no problem arises, it would be wise to consult the manufacturer of the particular brand or brands of impression material used in one's office for their recommendation of a disinfectant.

Regardless of the chemical disinfectant used, the impression must be removed from the mouth and taken directly to the sink and thoroughly rinsed to remove all blood, saliva, and other contaminants. In following the 1991 ADA guidelines,[9] it is then immersed in a fresh solution of the disinfectant for the time recommended by the manufacturer of the product for it to destroy TB-causing Mycobacterium (Table). It is taken to the laboratory and after the prescribed soaking time, preferably under 30 minutes, it is rinsed thoroughly. The model is then poured. The disinfectant is discarded, and the container cleaned well and set aside until its next use. Reuse of the disinfectant in the container is not acceptable.

This technique disinfects the tray and the impression material so no contamination is brought into the laboratory area. This is the same technique used for denture try-ins, sore spot removals, and any other procedure that requires an item to be placed in the mouth of a patient.

Remember, the closer to the source of contamination (oral cavity) that one begins infection control practices, the less chance there is of carrying disease-causing microorganisms into the laboratory or other parts of the dental office.

If the impression is to be sent to the commercial laboratory for casting, the same routine is advisable. It should be removed from the mouth, thoroughly rinsed at the sink, and then soaked for the required length of time. It is then rinsed and dried and placed in a Zip loc bag before being packed in the laboratory box. The laboratory should understand what procedure for disinfection has been followed so that it does not repeat it.

Other prosthetic devices such as the fox plane, face bow, and the wrench used to tighten it, and any other items that were touched by saliva-contaminated hands during the prosthodontic procedure, may be taken to the central sterilization area, placed in the sink, and thoroughly washed with an iodophor scrub. They are rinsed, dried, and placed in a clean environment until required again.

The dental office that understands and carefully follows the guidelines set forth by the ADA, the CDC, and OSHA can be certain that it has taken every precaution to ensure that no infectious disease is spread from patient to health-care worker, or health-care worker to patient. These guidelines apply regardless of the infection potential of the patient.

Table. Guide for Selection of Disinfectant Solutions

Type of Material	Disinfectant Solutions*			
	Glutaraldehydes†	Iodophores‡	Chlorine Compounds§	Complex Phenolics†
Impressions				
Alginate	–	+	+	–
Polysulfide	+	+	+	+
Silicone	+	+	+	+
Polyether	±	±	+	±
ZOE impression paste	+	+	–	?
Reversible hydrocolloid	–	+	+	?
Compound	–	+	+	–
Prostheses/appliances¶				
Fixed (metal/porcelain)	+	–	–	?
Removable (metal/porcelain)	–	+	+	–
Removable (metal/acrylic)	–	+#	+#	–
Appliances (all metal)	+	–	–	?

Impressions/prostheses should be rinsed under running tap water and then immersed for the time recommended for TB disinfection with selected product. Thorough rinsing of impressions and prostheses under running tap water following disinfection is necessary to remove any residual disinfectant.

*+ = recommended method; – = not recommended; ± = Use with caution. Consult manufacturer's recommendations; ? = data not available or conclusive.
†Prepared according to the manufacturer's instructions for disinfection.
‡1:213 dilution.
§1:10 dilution of commercial bleach or prepared according to the manufacturer's instruction for disinfection.

¶May also be ethylene oxide sterilized; prostheses or appliances that have been worn by patients must be thoroughly cleaned prior to disinfection.
#Use minimal exposure time (10 min) to avoid damage to metal.
Table courtesy of Virginia A. Merchant, MS, DMD.

References

1. US Department of Labor, OSHA. Occupational exposure to bloodborne pathogens: Final rule. 29 Federal Register CFR Part 1910.1030, Vol. 54 No. 235 (December 6): 64175–64182, 1991.

2. US Department of Labor, OSHA. Controlling occupational exposure to bloodborne pathogens in dentistry. OSHA 1992; 3129.

3. ADA. OSHA's bloodborne pathogens standard: questions and answers. J Am Dent Assoc 1992; Supplement.

4. ADA. OSHA compliance checklist for the dental office. L200. 1993.

5. CDC. Recommended infection control practices for dentistry. Recommendations and reports series. MMWR 1993; 42(No. RR-8):1–12.

6. Infection Control in Dentistry Guidelines. Denver: Office Sterilization and Asepsis Procedures Research Foundation; 1993.

7. Miller CH, Palenik CJ. Infection control in dentistry. In Block S (ed): Sterilization, Disinfection, Preservation and Sanitation, ed 4. Philadelphia: Lea and Febiger; 1991.

8. Schaefer ME. The Manual for Infection Control. Pleasanton, CA: Health Sonics Corp; 1989, 1992.

9. ADA Council on Dental Materials, Instruments and Equipment. Disinfection of impressions. J Am Dent Assoc 1991;122:110.

15

Management of Occupational Exposures to Blood-borne Pathogens

David K. Henderson and Susan E. Beekmann

Dental-care providers are at risk for occupational infections with blood-borne viruses, including hepatitis B virus (HBV), hepatitis C virus (HCV), and human immunodeficiency virus (HIV). Although current concern for infection is focused on the risk of HIV infection, the magnitude of risk associated with a parenteral occupational exposure to HIV is lower than that associated with either HBV or HCV.[1–11] Perhaps more than any other group of health-care professionals, dental providers have applied universal precautions in their practices. The impact of these changes in the practice of dentistry is just now beginning to be appreciated.[12–14] Behavior modification in the practice of dentistry should serve as a model for other health-care disciplines.

Management Immediately After Exposure

Although the efficacy of first aid for occupational exposures to blood-borne pathogens remains to be established definitively, many centers routinely recommend that puncture wounds and other cutaneous injuries be rinsed thoroughly with water or saline and then washed with soap and water.[15,16] Mucosal exposures involving the mouth and nose should be flushed vigorously with water. Eyes should be irrigated with clean water, saline, or sterile eye irrigants. Although no evidence documents the efficacy of disinfectants used for decontaminating wounds contaminated with blood from patients known to be infected with blood-borne pathogens, their use in this setting seems intuitively rational.[15,16]

An important component of post-exposure management is assuring that all occupational exposures to blood-borne pathogens are documented by and reported to appropriate occupational medicine professionals. Both institution-based dental practices as well as private dental offices should develop plans for managing occupational exposures to blood-borne pathogens. Employees should be made aware of the appropriate procedures to follow, and information about post-exposure management should be readily available in the work site. Ideally, reporting systems should both allow prompt access to expert consultants and also protect the confidentiality of the exposed worker. If an emergency department or employee health service is used for post-exposure management, staff in these departments responsible for providing post-exposure care should be familiar with treatment protocols and knowledgeable about the importance of maintaining the exposed worker's medical privacy.

The exposed worker should provide accurate information about the type of exposure experienced (eg, puncture, laceration, mucous membrane splash), the mechanism of exposure, the device causing the exposure, the severity of the exposure, the source of the exposure, and the type of body fluid to which the worker was exposed (eg, blood, bloody saliva, other body fluids or tissues, or inflammatory exudates). Exposure to all body fluids, tissues, and laboratory specimens, regardless of HIV risk, should be reported and evaluated to assess the risk of transmission of blood-borne pathogens and to determine the need for post-exposure care.

In addition, the worker should report whether gloves, eye protection, and masks were in use at the time of exposure. These latter data may help evaluate the risk for infection (eg, in experimental studies, a needle puncture though a glove reduces the blood inoculum by approximately 50%[17,18]) and may assist in the identification of procedures and techniques toward which infection control educational efforts should be aimed.

Serologic Evaluation of Source Patients

When the source patient for an exposure is identifiable, these patients should be evaluated clinically and epidemiologically for evidence of infection with HIV, HBV, HCV, and other blood-borne pathogens. Although state laws vary somewhat, testing for hepatitis B usually does not require informed consent if serum is already available from the source patient. Serum from source patients should be evaluated for hepatitis B surface antigen (HBsAg), and, if positive, for hepatitis B e antigen (HBeAg) as well.

Some practitioners also evaluate for antibody to surface antigen (anti-HBs) and/or antibody to hepatitis B core antigen (anti-HBc) to determine prior exposure to this blood-borne pathogen.[2]

Dental practitioners often will not have ready access to serum; thus, obtaining consent and blood samples may be the most practical way to evaluate risk in a timely manner. Testing for HCV is not readily available in all locations and is not yet routinely recommended.[15] If the source patient is identified as being at high risk for HCV infection (eg, a source patient who has a history of intravenous drug use, hemodialysis, or a history of either HCV infection or non-A, non-B hepatitis), the source patient should be tested for HCV antibodies (preferably using a second-generation assay) to identify workers at risk for occupational infection. Neither the nosocomial epidemiology of HCV infection nor the magnitude of risk for infection with HCV following an occupational exposure to HCV have been fully characterized.[2,15] Furthermore, unlike the setting of an occupational exposure to HBV, to date no safe and effective chemoprophylactic regimen has been established for HCV exposure.

Unless the clinical and epidemiologic assessment suggests that HIV infection of the source patient is highly improbable, the source patient should be offered HIV testing. Some states permit mandatory testing of source patients; others do not.[19] Knowledge of testing limitations imposed by state and local laws is crucial. We advocate using an informed consent document for HIV testing of source patients. At the Clinical Center, National Institutes of Health (NIH), most source patients agree to testing with this voluntary process. Results of source patient testing must be held confidentially. Dental practitioners should align source patient testing protocols with state and local laws.

Managing Occupational Exposures to HIV

The occupational risk for HIV infection associated with parenteral exposures to blood from source patients with HIV is approximately 0.3% per exposure.[3,6,19,20] The risk associated with mucosal exposures and exposures of nonintact skin to blood from such patient exposure is below the level of detection in clinical studies performed to date.[20] Combining the data from 15 longitudinal studies attempting to measure the risk for occupational infection following a mucous membrane exposure, the 95% confidence interval for the risk for transmission associated with a single such exposure is 0 to 0.36 per exposure.[20] Finally, the risk for intact skin exposures appears to be even smaller.[21] The overwhelming likelihood is that this latter risk is so small that it will never be measured with precision.

Health-care providers occupationally exposed to HIV should be counseled and tested for HIV antibody as soon as possible after the exposure. Staff sustaining occupational exposures should be counseled extensively about the risks of infection and about the early manifestations of HIV infection. The need for such counseling should not be underestimated. Strong psychological reactions to occupational HIV exposures are not uncommon; supervisors and occupational medicine personnel are likely to encounter anger, sadness, depression, fear, anxiety, and denial. Curiously, these exposures often result in the surfacing of pre-existing related problems (eg, interpersonal problems, understaffing, other workplace issues), so the counselor and the workplace supervisor need to be prepared to manage these types of issues as well. Finally, the needs of sexual partners, family members, friends, and coworkers of the exposed employee should not be minimized or overlooked. The counselor may be asked to intervene with family or friends or to provide additional information about the exposure, the risks, and risk management strategies. Counseling employees is perhaps the single most critical component of post-exposure management.[15,16]

Equally important in post-exposure management is accurate, timely serologic testing. Should transmission occur, having the employee's baseline seronegativity documented is an important protection for the employee. An alternative approach is to draw and save a serum sample to permit retrospective baseline testing if post-exposure infection ultimately is documented. Post-exposure follow-up HIV testing should be performed 6 weeks, 3 months, and 6 months after exposure.[22] Delayed seroconversion following an occupational exposure has, to our knowledge, not yet been documented; thus, additional testing (after 6 months) may be unnecessary. Staff should be counseled to return for re-evaluation if symptoms consistent with the acute retroviral infection develop.[15,16] Antibody tests for HIV are somewhat unreliable in the interval immediately surrounding seroconversion. Although ancillary and research-based tests, such as antigen testing, viral cultures, and gene amplification (polymerase chain reaction [PCR] studies) have no place in the routine management of occupational exposures to HIV, these tests may be useful in the clinical setting in which seroconversion is suspected.

The issue of whether to offer post-exposure chemoprophylaxis with an antiretroviral agent (eg, zidovudine) to health-care workers who sustain occupational exposure to HIV is complex and controversial. Because of the relatively low risk for infection following an exposure, a clinical efficacy trial is not feasible.[23] Despite its use in this setting for several years, neither the efficacy nor the safety of zidovudine for use as a post-exposure chemoprophylactic agent following occupational exposure to HIV has been established. A thorough discussion of rationale for offering or not offering post-exposure nucleoside analog chemoprophylaxis following occupational exposures to HIV in the health-care workplace is beyond the scope of this chapter; however, this subject has been reviewed in detail elsewhere.[15,24–29]

Primarily because of the formidable

population requirements for such studies,[23] placebo-controlled efficacy trials of nucleoside analogs administered as post-exposure prophylaxis are not currently practical. Employers must develop rational interim positions regarding the use of these agents in this setting.[27] Sentient arguments can be made for and against offering these agents to workers who sustain occupational exposures to HIV.[25,27,28] In our opinion, at this time, available data are inadequate to provide support for a clear mandate—either to provide these agents in this setting or to advise against their provision.

At the Clinical Center, NIH, we have elected to offer zidovudine to health-care workers who have been occupationally exposed to HIV. In collaboration with Gerberding and coworkers at San Francisco General Hospital, this program has now been incorporated into a multicenter clinical trial that is attempting to evaluate the safety of zidovudine administered in this setting.[30] This decision represents our interim strategy and should not be construed either as a recommendation or as a statement of the standard of care. We await definitive data about the safety and efficacy of these agents for this indication.

Managing Occupational Exposures to HBV and HCV

The risks for occupational infection associated with percutaneous exposure to blood from patients known to be infected with HBV or HCV are much larger than for those known to be infected with HIV. For HBV this risk is between 5% (for sources who are HBeAg negative) to as high as 43% (for sources known to be HBeAg positive).[7,9,31] Post-exposure management strategies for HBV begin with prevention and immunization. Dental-care providers who are at risk for blood exposure in the workplace should be immunized with the hepatitis B vaccine, unless already immune or unless contraindications to immunization exist. The Occupational Safety and Health Administration Blood-borne Pathogen Standard requires immunization of all providers at risk for blood exposure.[32]

Health-care workers who sustain occupational exposure to blood and other materials posing a HBV transmission risk should be evaluated for immunity to HBV. The Clinical Center, NIH, evaluates the anti-HBs status of any health-care workers reporting occupational HBV exposures whose anti-HBs antibody titers have not been evaluated within the preceding year. It routinely offers booster doses of HBV vaccine to those whose titers have fallen below the cutoff level; depending on the exposure, such individuals may also be candidates for a single dose of hepatitis B immune globulin (HBIG).[2,16] For susceptible employees, in instances in which the source patient is known to be HBsAg positive, in addition to beginning the HBV immunization series, one dose of HBIG (0.06 mL/kg) should be administered to provide passive protection until vaccine-induced antibody develops. Passive immunoprophylaxis with

HBIG should be given as soon as possible after exposure and within 24 hours, if possible (its utility beyond 7 days after exposure is undocumented). If the worker refuses to, or cannot, be immunized, a second dose of HBIG should be administered 1 month following the occupational exposure. Follow-up should include serologic evaluation for HBsAg, anti-HBs, anti-HBc and hepatic enzymes 6 months from the time of exposure (at the time of the third dose of vaccine).

Management of situations in which the source patient's hepatitis status is unknown is less straightforward. Since employees reporting occupational exposures represent a captive audience, the Clinical Center, NIH, administers hepatitis B vaccine to all susceptible employees after any exposure incident, irrespective of the source patient's hepatitis B status. A more detailed discussion of management of occupational exposures to HBV can be found elsewhere.[2]

In some dental offices and clinics, post-exposure management for HBV may be somewhat more complicated because expeditious HBV testing of patients and exposed workers is not available. In such settings, the empiric use of HBIG immunoprophylaxis for staff sustaining occupational exposures is likely to be effective, albeit expensive. A better alternative may be to establish a protocol for testing that ensures rapid results.

As previously noted, the nosocomial epidemiology of HCV infection and occupational risks for infection with HCV for health-care providers are incompletely understood. Several anecdotal cases of occupational infections in health-care workers (usually following documented parenteral exposures) have been reported in the medical literature,[33–36] and a number of prevalence studies have demonstrated health-care providers to be at only slightly elevated risk for HCV infection compared with first-time blood donors.[10,11,37–44] Combining the results from 14 such studies evaluating more than 6,700 at-risk health-care workers, the overall seroprevalence of HCV infection was 2.75%.[45] Eight of these 14 studies included some sort of control group, and in seven of those eight studies the health-care worker population had a slightly higher seroprevalence than did the control group.[45] Using the first-generation anti-c100-3 (nonstructural-region-antigen-based assay), Kiyosawa et al observed hepatitis in four of 110 exposed health-care workers and observed anti-HCV seroconversion in three of these four workers.[11] In a second study that used first- and second-generation assays, Hernandez and coworkers found no seroconversions among 81 workers who had experienced documented parenteral exposures to blood from patients known to have HCV. In this study, the exposed health-care workers were evaluated for HCV infection 3, 6, and 12 months following exposure.[38] In a third study, Mitsui and colleagues used a combination of three detection techniques: anti-c100-3; an assay for HCV-core-derived antibodies; and a PCR assay for HCV RNA to detect evidence of HCV infection in seven of 68 health-care workers (10.3%) who had sustained needle-stick exposures to blood from patients with HCV.[10] In this latter study, the presence of high-titer anti-core antibodies (anti-cp10) in the source patient's blood correlated with an increased risk for HCV transmission from a needle-stick, but did not correlate with detectable HCV RNA in the source patient's blood.[10]

Based on the experience with hepatitis B, many centers (including our own) have elected to offer standard immune serum globulin (ISG) prophylaxis (2 mL per dose) to health-care workers who have sustained occupational exposures to HCV. The efficacy of ISG as post-exposure immunoprophylaxis for HCV exposures is unproven; and, to our knowledge, none of the early studies of ISG efficacy in non-A, non-B hepatitis has been repeated with HCV serologies. No effective prophylaxis strategies have, as yet, been identified. Some investigators have presented theoretical arguments against the use of ISG, including: 1) neutralizing antibodies for HCV have as yet not yet been identified and may not exist; 2) donors who contribute blood from which standard ISG is prepared are now screened for antibody to HCV and are eliminated from the donor pool if they are found to be anti-HCV positive; thus, any efficacy of ISG present in older ISG preparations may progressively decrease as such anti-HCV-positive donors are excluded by the screening process; and 3) use of ISG is associated with a theoretical risk for disease transmission[46] (although with the broad experience in the use of ISG for a variety of indications, transmis-sion of HCV seems extremely unlikely in this setting and has not yet, to our knowledge, been documented with the intramuscular immunoglobulin preparation).

Some investigators have suggested alternative approaches to HCV prophylaxis. Preliminary data suggest that some anti-HCV-envelope antibodies may be somewhat protective. If so, hyperimmune globulin preparations (ie, those enriched for such anti-envelope antibodies) might be useful as immunoprophylaxis. Furthermore, if these initial studies are confirmed, the development of an envelope-containing vaccine, analogous to the HBV vaccine, that could be used as active immunoprophylaxis may become possible.

No solid argument, either for or against, the post-exposure use of ISG (or any other agent) for HCV exposures can be made at this time. The Clinical Center, NIH, routinely offers baseline and follow-up HCV testing (including liver function tests) to health-care workers who sustain parenteral exposures to HCV. It also offers (but does not recommend) ISG post-exposure prophylaxis following HCV occupational exposures. With the new and improved HCV tests being more widely used, more information should be available to answer these questions in the future.

Based on currently available data, health-care workers who have HCV appear to be at very low risk of transmitting infection to sexual partners. The CDC has not yet recommended changes in sexual practices for individuals infected with HCV.[47] Until additional information becomes available to help guide decisions, health-care providers who are exposed to HCV should be reassured that sexual transmission is an infrequent event.[47]

Preventing HIV Transmission in Dental Practice

The systematic use of universal precautions[22] —wearing gloves and appropriate barriers to prevent mucous membrane exposure, using good work practices, modifying procedures to prevent occupational exposures, and using devices that have been engineered to make the dental workplace safer—represents the most effective strategy to reduce the risks for transmission of HIV in the dental practice setting. As previously noted, preliminary evidence suggests both that dentists and dental personnel are adhering to these recommendations and that the use of the precautions is contributing to a reduction in occupational exposures. Data collected from the annual survey conducted by the American Dental Association at its annual meeting demonstrate that dentists believe that they are experiencing fewer occupational exposures than in previous survey years.[12,14] Data collected annually from 1987 through 1991 demonstrate a stepwise, systematic decrease in self-reported parenteral exposures among dental personnel participating in the survey over these years. In 1987, survey participants reported an average of more than 11 parenteral exposures per year.

By 1991, this figure had fallen to 3.5. Dental surgeons reported the highest average rate of parenteral occupational exposure (4.6 injuries per year), while orthodontists reported the lowest rate among dental subspecialties (2.2 injuries per year). Participants reported that 58% of exposures occurred outside of the patient's mouth and more than 90% were hand injuries. More than 37% of the injuries resulted from bur exposures; 30% from needle sticks. Investigators found no clear association with years of practice experience.[12,14]

The dramatic decline in parenteral exposure among practicing dental personnel parallels the increase in the use of universal precautions by these professionals. The NIH's clinical experience parallels the dental experience with many fewer occupational exposures (reductions in both cutaneous[21] and percutaneous exposures observed following training staff in, and implementation of, universal precautions at the clinical center). The occurrence of a case cluster of HIV infections resulting from provider-to-patient transmission of HIV in a Florida dentist's practice[49-54] has produced a great deal of societal concern about the risk of transmission of HIV from infected providers to their patients. Numerous additional so-called "look-back" studies of more than 19,000 patients of infected providers have, as yet, failed to identify any additional iatrogenic infections.[51,52,55–57]

Despite the apparent low risk for provider-to-patient transmission of blood-borne pathogens, the CDC issued guidelines in 1991 in response to the anxiety generated by the documented cases of provider-to-patient transmission of HIV. These guidelines recommend that health-care workers who perform what the CDC termed exposure-prone invasive procedures know their hepatitis B and HIV serologic status.[58] According to these guidelines, providers who are either HBeAg positive or HIV positive are not to perform such procedures unless they have sought the counsel of an expert review panel that could advise these practitioners under what circumstances, if any, they could continue to perform the procedures.[58] According to the guidelines, such circumstances would include notifying the patient about the health-care provider's illness.[58] Subsequently a Federal Law was passed (PL. 102-141) requiring all states to adopt these (or equivalent) guidelines. As of April 1, 1993, only eight states or territories had certified that the CDC guidelines had been implemented; 26 noted that equivalent guidelines had been implemented, and 25 had asked for a 1-year extension (permissible by law).[13] Curiously, several of the states reporting that equivalent guidelines had been implemented have actually published guidelines that directly conflict with the CDC recommendations.

Estimates of the risk for infection associated with treatment by a dentist with HIV indicate that the risks are miniscule[12,14,59–62]; the far-reaching implications of restrictive policies for health-care providers infected with HIV or HBV have been discussed in detail elsewhere.[20,60–65] Almost all authorities agree that adherence to

sensible infection control procedures and the use of new, safer technologies represent the most effective prevention strategies and the best approaches to reducing this already small risk.[13,20,60,66]

An additional piece of evidence that strongly suggests both that dentists and dental personnel are following universal precautions and that the precautions are contributing to a reduction in transmission of blood-borne pathogens in dental practice comes from studies of provider-to-patient transmission of hepatitis B. Since universal precautions were recommended as a routine infection control strategy for dentists and dental professionals,[22] no instances of dental professional-to-patient transmission of hepatitis B have been detected.[13] Thus, the use of universal precautions, combined with education and retraining of dental staff regarding occupational risks and risk reduction strategies, the modification of procedures intrinsically associated with increased risk, modification of dental professional school curricula to focus on these risks and risk reduction strategies, the use of technological improvements in equipment, effective use of the hepatitis B vaccine, and the development of protocols for management of occupational exposures will make the dental office even safer from the risks associated with blood-borne pathogens for both providers and patients during the next decade.

References

1. Alter H, Seeff L, Kaplan P, et al. Type B hepatitis: the infectivity of blood positive for e antigen and DNA polymerase after accidental needlestick exposure. N Engl J Med 1976;295:909–913.

2. Beekmann SE, Henderson DK. Health care workers and hepatitis: risk for infection and management of exposures. Infect Dis Clin Pract 1992;1:424–428.

3. Gerberding JL, Bryant-LeBlanc C, Nelson K, et al. Risk of transmitting the human immunodeficiency virus, cytomegalovirus, and hepatitis B virus to health care workers exposed to patients with AIDS and AIDS-related conditions. J Infect Dis 1987; 156:1–8.

4. Gerberding JL, Brown A, Raniro N. Cumulative risk of HIV and hepatitis B among health care workers: longterm serologic followup and gene amplification for latent HIV infection (abstract 959). 30th Interscience Conference on Antimicrobial Agents and Chemotherapy, Atlanta; 1990.

5. Henderson DK, Fahey BJ, Willy M, et al. Risk for occupational transmission of human immunodeficiency virus type 1 (HIV-1) associated with clinical exposures: a prospective evaluation. Ann Intern Med 1990;113:740–746.

6. Marcus R, The Cooperative Needlestick Surveillance Group. Surveillance of health care workers exposed to blood from patients infected with the human immunodeficiency virus. N Engl J Med 1988;319: 1118–1123.

7. Seefe L, Wright E, Zimmerman H, Alter H, et al. Type B hepatitis after needlestick exposure: Prevention with hepatitis B immune globulin: final report of the Veterans' Administration Cooperative Study. Ann Intern Med 1978;88:285–293.

8. West D. The risk of hepatitis B infection among health professionals in the United States: a review. Am J Med Sci 1984;287: 26–33.

9. Werner B, Grady G. Accidental hepatitis-B-surface- antigen- positive inoculations: use of "e" antigen to estimate infectivity. Ann Intern Med 1982;97:367–369.

10. Mitsui T, Iwano K, Masuko K, et al. Hepatitis C virus infection in medical personnel after needlestick accident. Hepatology 1992;16:1109–1114.

11. Kiyosawa K, Sodeyama T, Tanaka E, et al. Hepatitis C in hospital employees with needlestick injuries. Ann Intern Med 1991; 115:367–369.

12. Gruninger SE, Siew C, Chang SB, et al. Human immunodeficiency virus type I. Infection among dentists. J Am Dent Assoc 1992;123:57–64.

13. Bell DM, Shapiro CN, Gooch BF. Preventing HIV transmission to patients during invasive procedures. J Public Health Dent 1993;53:170–173.

14. Siew C, Chang SB, Gruninger SE, Verrusio AC, Neidle EA. Self-reported percutaneous injuries in dentists: implications for HBV, HIV, transmission risk. J Am Dent Assoc 1992;123:36–44.

15. Gerberding JL, Henderson DK. Management of occupational exposures to bloodborne pathogens: hepatitis B virus, hepatitis C virus, and human immunodeficiency virus. Clin Infect Dis 1992;14:1179–1185.

16. Fahey BJ, Beekmann SE, Schmitt JM, Fedio JM, Henderson DK. Managing occupational exposures to HIV-1 in the healthcare workplace. Infect Control Hosp Epidemiol 1993;14:405–412.

17. Woolwine J, Mast S, Gerberding J. Factors influencing needlestick infectivity and decontamination efficacy: an ex vivo model (abstract 1188). 32nd Interscience Conference on Antimicrobial Agents and Chemotherapy. Anaheim, CA: American Society for Microbiology; 1992.

18. Mast S, Gerberding J. Factors predicting infectivity following needlestick exposure to HIV: an in vitro model. Clin Res 1991;39:58.

19. Beekmann SE, Fahey BJ, Gerberding JL, Henderson DK. Risky business: using necessarily imprecise casualty counts to estimate occupational risks for HIV-1 infection. Infect Control Hosp Epidemiol 1990; 11:371–379.

20. Henderson DK. Human Immunodeficiency virus in the health-care setting. In Mandell G, Bennett J, Dolin R (eds): Principles and Practice of Infectious Diseases, ed 4. New York: Churchill-Livingstone, in press.

21. Fahey BJ, Koziol DE, Banks SM, Henderson DK. Frequency of nonparenteral occupational exposures to blood and body fluids before and after universal precautions training. Am J Med 1991;90:145–153.

22. CDC. Recommendations for prevention of HIV transmission in health-care settings. MMWR 1987;36:1–19.

23. Beekmann SE, Henderson DK. The epidemiology of blood-borne infections in the health-care setting. In Sande M, Root R (eds): Contemporary Issues in Infectious Diseases. New York: Churchill-Livingstone, in press.

24. CDC. Public Health Service statement on management of occupational exposure to human immunodeficiency virus, including considerations regarding zidovudine postexposure use. MMWR 1990;39:1–14.

25. Henderson DK. Post-exposure chemoprophylaxis for occupational exposure to HIV-1: Current status and prospects for the future. Am J Med 1991;91:312–319.

26. Beekmann SE, Fahrner R, Koziol DE, Gerberding JL, Henderson DK. Safety of zidovudine (AZT) administered as post-exposure chemoprophylaxis to healthcare workers (HCW) sustaining occupational exposures (OE) to HIV (abstract 1121). 33rd Annual Meeting of the Infectious Diseases Society of America, New Orleans, LA; 1993.

27. Henderson DK, Gerberding JL. Prophylactic zidovudine after occupational exposure to the human immunodeficiency virus: an interim analysis. J Infect Dis 1989;160:321–327.

28. Henderson DK, Beekmann SE, Gerberding JL. Post-exposure antiviral chemoprophylaxis following occupational exposure to the human immunodeficiency virus. AIDS Updates 1990;3:1–8.

29. Gerberding JL. Is antiretroviral treatment after percutaneous HIV exposure justified? Ann Intern Med 1993;118:979–980.

30. Beekmann SE, Fahrner R, Koziol DE, Gerberding JL, Henderson DK. Safety of zidovudine (AZT) administered as post-exposure chemoprophylaxis to healthcare workers (HCW) sustaining occupational exposures (OE) to HIV (abstract). 30th Annual Meeting of the Infectious Diseases Society of America, Anaheim, CA; 1992.

31. Grady G, Lee V, Prince A, Gitnick G, et al. Hepatitis B immune globulin for accidental exposures among medical personnel: final report of a multicenter controlled trial. J Infect Dis 1978;138:625–638.

32. Department of Labor OSHA. Occupational exposure to blood-borne pathogens: final rule. Federal Register 1991;56:64175–64182.

33. Schlipkoter U, Roggendorf M, Cholmakow K, Weise A, Deinhardt F. Transmission of hepatitis C virus (HCV) from a haemodialysis patient to a medical staff member (letter). Scand J Infect Dis 1990;22:757–758.

34. Tsude K, Fujiyama S, Sato S, et al. Two cases of accidental transmission of hepatitis C to medical staff. Hepatogastroenterology 1992;39:73–75.

35. Sartori M, La Terra G, Aglietta M, Manzin A, Navino C, Verzetti G. Transmission of hepatitis C via blood splash into conjunctiva (letter). Scand J Infect Dis 1993;25:270–271.

36. Vaqlia A, Nicolin R, Puro V, Ippolito G, Bettini C, de Lalla F. Needlestick hepatitis C virus seroconversion in a surgeon (letter). Lancet 1990;336:1315–1316.

37. Perez TE, Cilla G, Alcorta M, Elosegui ME, Saenz DJ. Low risk of acquiring the hepatitis C virus for the health personnel. Med Clin (Barcelona) 1992;99:609–611.

38. Hernandez ME, Bruguera M, Puyuelo T, Barrera JM, Sanchez TJ, Rodhes J. Risk of needle-stick injuries in the transmission of hepatitis C virus in hospital personnel. J Hepatol 1992;16:56–58.

39. Thomas DL, Factor SH, Kelen GD, Washington AS, Taylor EJ, Quinn TC. Viral hepatitis in health care personnel at the Johns Hopkins Hospital. The seroprevalence of and risk factors for hepatitis B virus and hepatitis C virus infection. Arch Intern Med 1993;153:1705–1712.

40. Panlilio A, Chamberland M, Shapiro C, Schable C, Srivastava P, The Serostudy Group. Human immunodeficiency virus (HIV), hepatitis B virus, (HBV) and hepatitis C virus (HCV) serosurvey among hospital-based surgeons (abstract PO-C18-3024). 9th International Conference on AIDS, Berlin, 1993.

41. Wormser GP, Forseter G, Joline C, Tupper B, O'Brien TA. Hepatitis C infection in the health care setting. I. Low risk from parenteral exposure to blood of human immunodeficiency virus–infected patients. Am J Infect Control 1991;19:237–242.

42. Hayashi PH, Flynn N, McCurdy SA, Kuramoto IK, Holland PV, Zeldis JB. Prevalence of hepatitis C virus antibodies among patients infected with human immunodeficiency virus. J Med Virol 1991;33:177–180.

43. Cooper BW, Krusell A, Tilton RC, Goodwin R, Levitz RE. Seroprevalence of antibodies to hepatitis C virus in high-risk hospital personnel. Infect Control Hosp Epid 1992;13:82–85.

44. Kelen GD, Green GB, Purcell RH, et al. Hepatitis B and hepatitis C in emergency department patients. N Engl J Med 1992; 326:1399–1404.

45. Henderson DK. Prophylaxis for bloodborne infections. 31st Annual Meeting. New Orleans: Infectious Diseases Society of America; 1993:9.

46. Uemura Y, Yokoyama K, Nishida M, Suyama T. Immunoglobulin preparation: safe from virus transmission? Vox Sang 1989;57:1–3.

47. Alter MJ, Coleman PJ, Alexander WJ, et al. Importance of heterosexual activity in the transmission of hepatitis B and non-A, non-B hepatitis. JAMA 1989;62:1201–1205.

48. Beekmann SE, Vlahov D, Koziol DE, McShalley E, Schmitt J, Henderson DK. Implementation of universal precautions was temporally associated with a sustained, progressive decrease in percutaneous exposures to blood or body fluids. Clin Infect Dis 1994;181:562–569.

49. CDC. Update: Transmission of HIV infection during an invasive dental procedure — Florida. MMWR 1991;40:21–33.

50. CDC. Possible transmission of human immunodeficiency virus to a patient during an invasive dental procedure. MMWR 1990;39:489–493.

51. CDC. Update: investigations of patients who have been treated by HIV-infected health-care workers. MMWR 1992;41:344–346.

52. CDC. Update: Investigations of persons treated by HIV-infected health-care workers—United States. MMWR 1993;42:329–331,337.

53. Ciesielski C, Marianos D, Ou C-Y, et al. Transmission of human immunodeficiency virus in a dental practice. Ann Intern Med 1992;116:798–805.

54. Ou C-Y, Ciesielski CA, Myers G, et al. Molecular epidemiology of HIV transmission in a dental practice. Science 1992;256:1165–1171.

55. Danila RN, MacDonald KL, Rhame FS, et al. A look-back investigation of patients of an HIV-infected physician. N Engl J Med 1991;325:1406–1411.

56. Rogers AS, Froggatt JW III, Townsend T, et al. Investigation of potential HIV transmission to the patients of an HIV-infected surgeon. JAMA 1993;269:1795–1801.

57. Von Reyn CF, Gilbert TT, Shaw FE Jr, Parsonnet KC, Abramson JE, Smith MG. Absence of HIV transmission from an infected orthopedic surgeon: a 13-year look-back study. JAMA 1993;269:1807–1811.

58. CDC. Recommendations for preventing transmission of human immunodeficiency virus and hepatitis B virus to patients during exposure-prone invasive procedures. MMWR 1991;40:1–9.

59. Neidle E, American Dental Association. Estimates of the risk of endemic transmission of hepatitis B virus and human immunodeficiency virus to patients by the percutaneous route during invasive surgical and dental procedures. Open meeting on the risks of transmission of blood-borne pathogens to patients during invasive procedures. Atlanta: American Dental Association; 1991.

60. Henderson D. Management of health-care workers who are infected with the human immunodeficiency virus or other blood-borne pathogens. In DeVita V, Hellman S, Rosenberg S (eds). AIDS—Etiology, Diagnosis, Treatment, and Prevention, ed 3. Philadelphia: Lippincott Co; 1993.

61. Henderson DK. Human immunodeficiency virus infection in patients and providers. In Wenzel R (ed): Prevention and Control of Nosocomial Infections, ed 2. Baltimore, MD: Williams and Wilkins; 1992: 42–57.

62. Henderson D. The HIV- or HBV-infected healthcare provider and society's perception of risk: science, nonscience, and nonsense. Ann Allergy 1992;68:197–199.

63. Gostin L. HIV-infected physicians and the practice of seriously invasive procedures. Hastings Cent Rep 1989;19:32–39.

64. Feldblum C. Disability anti-discrimination laws and HIV testing of health-care providers. Courts Health Sci Law 1991;2: 136–142.

65. Feldblum C. A reply to Gostin. Law Med Health Care 1991;19:134–139.

66. Gerberding JL. Reducing occupational risk of HIV infection. Hosp Pract 1991;26: 103–110.

16

Staff Training

M. Ann Ricksecker and Susan R. Thompson

The dental team needs to be prepared to accept and treat HIV-positive patients. Assessment of the dental team's training needs and ways to involve members in planning the training are crucial for effective and safe treatment of HIV-infected patients. Supervisory issues and concerns about office practices or policies may not be effectively addressed or alleviated with staff training. It is therefore essential that the dental staff actively participates in the formulation of office policies.

Staff training is an important component in planning for the addition of any new protocol or service in the dental office. It includes preparing the team to accept patients with HIV as well as formal and informal educational opportunities designed to enhance knowledge, skills, and behavior. Office-wide agreement on procedures, regulations, and overall practice expectations is critical to the process of expanding a practice's services. This is certainly true with the treatment of patients with HIV. Concerns about HIV transmission in health-care settings, misconceptions about the disease, and a fear of adding a treatment component that involves patients who are immune-compromised are some of the issues, in addition to the actual treatment protocol, that must be addressed by the dental team to successfully integrate the treatment of patients with HIV.

The treatment of HIV-positive patients may pose professional and personal challenges for members of the dental team, who are affected by the HIV epidemic in various ways: as dental professionals who will be providing care for patients with HIV; as individuals personally confronted by the epidemic through infection or risk of infection outside of the dental office; and as dental professionals faced with patients who believe that dental personnel can transmit HIV to patients. Effective staff training considers the staff's professional and personal concerns, determines the knowledge and skills they already have, and uses learning tools most conducive to meeting the training goals defined by the team.

Preparing the Team to Accept Patients with HIV

To provide an accepting environment for patients with HIV as well as a comfortable workplace for the dental team, attention should be paid to the process of transition into providing treatment for people with HIV. Acceptance can be effectively fostered by encouraging staff involvement in planning training and activities that integrate HIV as a reality into their lives. For example, preparing the team to accept patients with HIV might begin with a look at how the AIDS epidemic has affected their lives. While it will be necessary to develop HIV-related policies and procedures for the workplace that define staff expectations and accountability, achieving acceptance from the team is best accomplished through fostering positive attitudes, gaining a strong knowledge base, acting as a model of acceptable behavior, and creating a work environment respectful of each team member's prior and current experience with the epidemic.

The Team Leader as Role Model

As you prepare the dental team to accept patients with HIV, be aware of the message that you convey through your behavior as the team leader. Your model of acceptance and acceptable behavior is one of your strongest training tools. Do you treat patients with HIV with respect for their confidentiality and appreciation for their right to quality care? Are you open to learning new techniques and treatments and discussing what you need to learn? Do you handle your misconceptions or fears by searching for opportunities to expand your experiences or knowledge? Do you greet patients with HIV in your practice with compassion and an eagerness to provide a model of care that is best for your patients and your team? "Practice what you preach" is a good adage as you build your team's capabilities through staff training.

Developing Staff Comfort with HIV Issues

It is important to provide experiences that help the team heighten HIV awareness and promote the comfort necessary to provide quality patient care. This is particularly important if HIV has not been a part of your staff's personal or professional lives to date.

There are a variety of ways to structure a learning experience that encourages team members to examine their attitudes regarding HIV in a non-threatening way. One way is to invite a person with HIV disease to your office to meet with your staff. While this seems like a simple and informal educational approach, it has served as a powerful tool in preparing clinical staff to treat people with HIV. However, to achieve your intended impact, this exercise requires preplanning.

1. Get good advice about how to find a speaker. Perhaps someone you know has heard a good speaker who can address HIV infection from personal experience. Or you can call a contact in your community for recommendations (see the resource section toward the end of chapter).

2. Talk with the speaker prior to the visit about the issues you believe your staff needs to address. For example, does your staff want help in understanding the emotional impact of receiving a diagnosis of HIV infection? Coach the speaker to discuss his or her own life experiences. For example, when the speaker was diagnosed with HIV, who was most helpful and why? What services and support did he or she need?

3. Be respectful of the speaker's time and the value of his or her contri-

bution by offering an honorarium or some token of your appreciation.

4. Allow ample time for the session. One hour is usually adequate for one speaker. You can begin by asking the speaker to spend the first 15 minutes talking about experiences relevant to the information your staff needs. The remaining 45 minutes can be spent in an informal discussion during which staff members ask questions and discuss concerns with the speaker. Be sure to talk with the speaker ahead of time to determine whether there are questions or issues he or she does not want to discuss.

Another effective technique to help develop staff comfort with HIV infection is arranging for the team to visit a dental service that is experienced and comfortable in providing treatment for people with HIV. Allow for discussion time between your staff and the staff at the site you are visiting so that your staff can ask questions and observe the level of comfort the experienced staff has achieved.

Setting Staff Development Goals

It is not difficult to develop a training plan that can meet your team's needs. Staff training and development should have goals that are broad and clearly stated so that your team understands the overall intentions. Generally, staff training goals include creating or enhancing a productive, comfortable work environment; showcasing optimum care, quality assurance, and consistency of practice; fostering team building and cooperation; and teaching or reinforcing professional behaviors you, as the manager, want to instill. Education for adults will be most successful if you include time for self-reflection and provide opportunities to integrate information into their life experience and values. It is also helpful to use a variety of teaching methods such as reading suggested articles, journals or books; attending lectures; self-learning tools; and skills practice. Since your training strives to foster a successful team approach to providing HIV treatment, it is important to recognize that presenting factual information alone will not meet the overall staff development goals.

Involving Staff in the Planning

An important component of the transition to providing treatment for patients with HIV is team involvement in planning for staff continuing education. If the staff is involved in the planning through a needs assessment process—a process that carefully identifies their educational needs—the training will be appropriate and useful. There are several ways to assess the educational needs of your staff:

1. *Informal involvement.*
   a) At a staff meeting, explain to your staff that you expect patients with HIV as part of the patient load and that you want to be sure the staff is prepared and comfortable in providing care for them. Ask them what training they want before this care begins. If this list is longer than is realistic in the available time, ask them to prioritize the needs so you can address them first.
   b) During this and other discussions with staff, listen for the types of questions they ask and how they react to the idea of treating an HIV-positive patient. The staff's questions and behavior can help guide you regarding what to include in the training. You may notice underlying myths, specific attitudes, or desired skills that need to be addressed.
   c) Group and individual discussions with staff as to their perceived HIV training needs are another informal way to assess their educational needs.
2. *Formal involvement.* A brief questionnaire with focused, directed questions completed by each staff member can serve as a guide for planning a training series.
3. *Determining what HIV training your staff needs.* As you review the information from the team regarding what training they want or need, focus on three categories:
   a) What knowledge do they need? What myths or misinformation seem to be common? Singling out the necessary knowledge and information will be helpful in determining effective training techniques. For example, lec-

tures, reading, and informational videos can be used to fulfill a need or desire for knowledge.

b) What skills do they need to learn? This is important to determine because skill-based learning is often best achieved through supervised practice instead of didactic presentation of information. For example, enhancing a staff member's skills in performing an office procedure could be achieved through first explaining the procedure, then demonstrating it, and finally asking them to practice it under your supervision.

c) What attitudes need to be addressed? During the needs assessment discussions or in the answers to the questionnaire, you may detect feelings of fear or prejudice that need to be addressed gradually throughout the training. For example, if you realize during the assessment that a staff member has a particular bias against a behavior that is known to transmit HIV, you could begin to address that by inviting speakers or guests to your office to talk to your staff.

Training the Dental Team

Knowledge and experience can reduce your team's fears or insecurities about adding this new service to your practice. After you and your team have assessed the training needed to begin effectively treating HIV-positive pa-

tients, set a short timeline—perhaps 6 months—for training activities. Set clear learning objectives that outline what you expect the team to be able to do better or differently at the conclusion of the training. Discuss accountability measures that will be used to evaluate staff and their role in the practice.

There is merit in incorporating a multifaceted approach to achieving the training objectives.

HIV-Related Conferences and Seminars

Selecting an appropriate conference or seminar is important. Inappropriate training wastes your staff's time or has a negative impact. Match the conference to the level of knowledge that is needed by your staff. Read the conference brochure or training announcement carefully to help determine its appropriateness. Consider the following:

1. Who is the intended audience?
2. What are the goals of the conference?
3. Who are the faculty and what is their expertise?
4. Who are the sponsors and cosponsors of the program?
5. Are continuing education credits offered?

If the conference literature does not clarify these questions, call the conference organizer to discuss your staff's specific educational needs. If this particular seminar is inappropriate, the conference organizer may know of other training organizations or conferences that will meet your needs. Finally, if there is a dental school or training program in your vicinity, consult them about other continuing education programs or seminars in this field.

After the conference, ask the staff who attended to present a summary of the information to the rest of the team. This provides teacher variety and gives the message to the team that they have something to teach as well as to learn.

Self-Teaching Tools

Often, videos can be previewed at no cost to determine whether they will meet your staff's needs. Depending on the topic, some videos on HIV are outdated within a year. Local health education agencies and other HIV education associations in your locale may have lending libraries that provide inexpensive access to updated videos, books, and programs.

In-Service Educational Sessions

An in-service educational series can increase the staff's HIV knowledge as well as encourage team-building. The sessions might be custom-designed for your dental team only. Alternatively, your team could elect to join forces with another practice that is addressing similar training and HIV practice goals and plan these educational sessions together.

Begin the planning process by agreeing as a group on the time and location of the series. For example, is it best to plan half-day sessions, twice a month during times when patients are not scheduled? Or might these be evening sessions over dinner? What schedule works best for everyone? Organizing an educational session or series entails setting educational objectives and designing a program with a realistic schedule. The chapters of this book can serve as a guideline for the type of information to be covered.

Do not attempt to accomplish more than time allows, and do not underestimate how much time is needed for discussion and questions. Consider inviting outside experts to join you in this training. For example, if one of the sessions is to be on HIV transmission, you might arrange for an infection control nurse from a local hospital to discuss the ways in which HIV is and is not transmitted. This session would probably require 45 minutes to cover factual information and an additional 30 minutes for discussion and questions. This could be followed by a discussion of infection control in the dental setting demonstrated by you or another dental teacher. In this segment, 30 minutes could be dedicated to lecture and discussion followed by 1 hour of demonstration of technique and supervised practice by your staff.

During all the sessions, listen for new questions or topics that need to be addressed. Proceed in planning other sessions based on both the original learning objectives and new topics that have surfaced.

Training tools to consider for an in-service educational series include:

1. Lecture by you or another expert. Always allow time for questions and discussion.
2. Video and discussion. Always preview the video before you show it and be prepared to discuss topics it will stimulate. Do not expect the video to do all the teaching for you.
3. Skill practice. This can be clinical or counseling practice, and usually includes demonstrating a technique or situation followed by others practicing in front of the group.

How will we make treatment decisions with a patient whose immune system and health are failing?

What if I see oral manifestations of HIV infection and I don't know if the person has been tested or has considered that he or she may have HIV?

As the team leader, be prepared for these kinds of questions. It is common for clinical providers to express anxiety or discomfort with issues such as these. Support your team, and continue to talk with them about what training they believe they need to resolve these questions.

Topics and Issues That May Arise During Training

Review the other chapters of this book to become familiar with topics regarding HIV care that could arise in a training session, and be prepared for questions during the process that may or may not be relevant to the particular topic being discussed. Below are examples of questions or issues that could arise during training:

Do you think Dr. Acer transmitted HIV to his patients?

What laws exist that prevent discrimination and how does it affect our practice on a daily basis?

At what point should we refer someone out of our setting, and what is our relationship with tertiary care?

Do I have a duty to warn partners or family members of an HIV-positive patient?

Training Tips

Paying attention to detail will enhance your team's potential to benefit from the educational program. An audience can develop resistance to learning if they are physically uncomfortable, are confused about the intention of the training, or believe their educational needs are not being met.

Always introduce the training by describing how it was planned, what is scheduled during the allotted time, and who will be involved.

Plan a break every 1½ hours. Be aware of people's attention spans.

Refreshments are always appreciated before or during a training. Nourishment will help keep people alert and comfortable.

Be aware of how comfortable the room is. Are the chairs comfortable? Is it a pleasant temperature? Is there a table for writing or taking notes, if appropriate? Does lighting allow for taking notes? Are there windows and adequate ventilation?

Enhance the educational session by providing the team with written materials if possible. Relevant articles and other materials reinforce what is being taught and can be used by staff to learn more on their own.

If audiovisual equipment is being used in the training, check the operation of the equipment well in advance.

Resources

There are many resources to help you develop an educational plan for your team (see Appendix C).

The federally funded regional AIDS education and training centers (ETCs) can be a good source of speakers, slides, videos, and written materials. Seventeen ETCs have been established through a cooperative agreement program of the Health Resources and Services Administration within the U.S. Public Health Service, Department of Health and Human Services. The ETCs are a national network of centers that have a responsibility for designated geographic areas in which they conduct targeted, multidisciplinary education and training programs for health-care providers. The goal of the ETCs is to increase the number of health-care providers who are effectively educated and motivated to counsel, treat, and manage individuals with HIV infection as well as diagnose disease. The ETCs can identify conferences and training opportunities, speakers, materials, and HIV care guidelines. For information about the ETC serving your area, call 301-443-6364.

The local county or state health department may have educators, nurses, physicians, or dentists on staff who have expertise in HIV disease.

The local AIDS service organization may have videos, articles, or a speakers bureau of people living with HIV who are able to speak to the dental team.

A local hospital infection control nurse may be a good resource for teaching or for directing you to other resources.

A local dental school may have faculty with expertise or may offer continuing education programs relevant to the team's HIV educational needs.

The Centers for Disease Control (CDC) has slides on HIV disease. Each slide set covers a topic such as AIDS epidemiology or oral manifestations. There is no charge for these slides, which can be ordered by calling the CDC at 404-639-2142.

Summary of the Training Process

Prepare the team to accept patients with HIV

- Consider how your behavior is a model for what you expect of the team
- Provide an experience that would help integrate HIV awareness into their lives
  - a) Invite a person with HIV to speak to the team
  - b) Arrange for a visit to a dental service experienced with HIV

Assess the team's educational needs and planning training

- Perform a needs assessment; ask team members what they want or need
  - a) Informally through meetings and discussions
  - b) Formally through questionnaires
- Plan the training
  - a) What knowledge needs did the needs assessment reveal?
  - b) What skills are needed?
  - c) What attitudes need to be addressed?
  - d) What expectations do you have of the team: what knowledge, skills, and behavior you expect as a result of the training and how will you evaluate this?

Train the dental team to treat patients with HIV

- Training methods
  - a) Send members of the team to conferences or seminars
    1. Select appropriate sessions
    2. Have staff present to team after the conference
  - b) Buy or rent videos or other self-learning instruments
  - c) Develop a series of sessions for the team
    1. You or an outside expert can lecture on a topic
    2. Show a video and then discuss it
    3. Small group discussions or assignments
    4. Skill practice
- Training tips
  - a) Allow time in the beginning to introduce and explain what will be covered
  - b) As you plan the session, be realistic with what can be covered in the time allowed
  - c) Allow plenty of discussion time
  - d) Plan for breaks at least every 1½ hours
  - e) Have refreshments
  - f) Check the comfort of the room
  - g) Supplement the session with written materials
- Evaluation
  - a) Ask the team how they liked the session and what they learned from it
  - b) Ask the team what else they need
  - c) As patients with HIV receive care in your practice, observe the team's practices to determine the effectiveness of training and further training requirements

Staff training is a critical activity for the dental team preparing to treat HIV-positive patients. There are many methods of providing training for the team. The impact of an educational experience can be evaluated through increased knowledge, enhanced skills, and appropriate behavior. If the training goals are clear, one can easily evaluate whether the desired change has occurred as a result of the education.

Laboratory Values

ß-2 microglobulin
(Normal, 250 nmol/L)

Increased values indicate active immune system stimulation and HIV disease progression.

Bleeding time
(Normal, 0–7 minutes)

Measures qualitative and quantitative platelet functions.

CD4%
(Normal, 32%–60%; median, 46%)

Measures the percent of CD4+ cells of total lymphocytes. The CD4% is less subject to variation on repeated measurements (see Table on next page).

CD4+ T-helper lymphocyte count
(Normal, 544–1663 cells/mm^3; median, 935 cells/mm^3)

Measures the number (cells/mm^3) of peripheral T4 (helper)-lymphocytes.

CD4+ cell counts will determine disease stage and thus influence appropriate treatment planning. It is also used for diagnostic differentiation of both medical and dental pathologic conditions. There is no need for prophylactic medication prior to dental therapy based solely on CD4+ cell status. CD4+ cell counts below 100 cells/mm^3 are associated with a higher incidence of neutropenia.

CD4+:CD8+ ratio
(Normal, 0.93–4.50; median, 1.72)

Low ratio indicates immune suppression. However, with very high CD8+ cell counts this ratio may be deceptive.

CD8+ T-cytotoxic/suppressor lymphocyte count
(Normal, 272–932 cells/mm^3; median, 519 cells/mm^3)

Measures the number (cells/mm^3) of peripheral CD8+ (suppressor/cytotoxic)-lymphocytes. These cells have been indicated in suppression of HIV. High stable numbers of CD8 cells may be suggestive of a better prognosis.

Differential white blood cell count
(Normal, neutrophils: 43%–77% or 2,500–7,000 cells/mm^3; lymphocytes: 21%–35% or 1,000–4,800 cells/mm^3;

CD4 (cells/mm³)	CD4%	Adults
> 600	32–50	Within normal limits.
< 500	< 29	Initial immune suppression. Prophylactic antiretroviral therapy is indicated.
< 400		Manifestations of early opportunistic infections such as oral candidiasis.
200–400	14–28	Constitutional symptoms and some major opportunistic infections. Oral lesions include oral hairy leukoplakia.
< 200	< 14	Severe immune suppression. Appearance of major opportunistic infections. AIDS diagnosis. HIV viremia is present. Prophylaxis against PCP is instituted. Oral lesions may include Kaposi's sarcoma, NUP, major aphthous ulcerations, necrotizing stomatitis.
< 100	< 7	Appearance of fatal opportunistic infections. Prophylaxis against MAC and toxoplasmosis may be instituted.

monocytes: 0%–9% or 0–800 cells/mm³)

Prophylactic bactericidal antibiotics need to be considered when the neutrophil count drops below 500 cells/mm³ (normal, 2,500–7,000 cells/mm³), but at this stage the patient is often already medicated with antibiotics due to frequent bacterial infections and as prophylaxis against opportunistic infections.

Neutropenia should be suspected in patients with advanced HIV disease (CD4+ cell count below 100 cells/mm³) taking zidovudine. Zidovudine together with trimethoprim-sulfamethoxazole, or pyrimethamine and sulfadizine, or ganciclovir may worsen neutropenia.

Erythrocyte sedimentation rate (ESR)
(Normal, men: 0–13 mm in 1 hour; women: 0–20 mm in 1 hour)

Increased ESR values in combination with low CD4+ cell counts and elevated ß-2 microglobulin levels are predictive of HIV progression. An ESR level greater than 35 mm/hr is a marker for the development of AIDS.

Hemoglobin
(Normal, men, 14–18 g/dL; women, 12–16 g/dL)

Many patients with HIV are anemic secondary to medications and as a direct result of the HIV infection. In many cases patients present with hemoglobin levels of 7.0 to 10.0 g/dL. It is important to establish a baseline value for each individual and correlate subsequent hemoglobin levels with the baseline value.

Patients taking zidovudine for long periods and are in more advanced stages of HIV disease have a higher incidence of anemia.

There are no contraindications for general dental procedures, including single extractions, for patients with normal bleeding time and coagulation values, and hemoglobin levels above 7.0 g/dL.

Avoid respiratory depressant drugs with hemoglobin levels below 10 g/dL.

HIV antibody

The presence of HIV antibodies, as detected by two enzyme-linked immunosorbent assays (ELISAs) and confirmed by one Western blot test, indicates HIV infection.

Neopterin

(Normal [serum]; 10 nmol/L)

Increased values indicate active immune system stimulation and HIV disease progression.

p24 antigen/antibody

The presence of p24 antigens (p24 antigenemia) indicates active viral replication and suggests disease progression. Presence of p24 antibody levels indicates a relative latent disease stage. This marker is usually only used for research purposes.

p24 status will determine disease stage and thus influence appropriate treatment planning. There is no need for prophylactic medication prior to dental therapy based solely on p24 status.

Platelet count

(Normal, 150,000–400,000 platelets/mm^3)

Thrombocytopenia (less than 150,000 platelets/mm^3) may be present in 50% to 60% of adults with AIDS.

Dental treatments, including extractions, can be safely performed in patients with platelet counts greater than 60,000 platelets/mm^3. ITP may be more common during early HIV disease.

Prothrombin time (PT) and partial thromboplastin time (PTT)

(Normal PT: less than 2 seconds deviation from control [usually 9–11 seconds]; Normal PTT: 28–38 seconds)

Normal values usually indicate absence of liver damage.

General dentistry, including extractions, can be safely performed with PT and PTT values of twice the normal levels and sufficient numbers of platelets.

Red blood cell count

(Normal, 4.0–5.5 million/mm^3)

Total white blood cell count

(Normal, 4,500–10,000 cells/mm^3. Leukopenia (below 4,500 cells/mm^3) is present in 40% to 60% of patients with AIDS. This is due mainly to a decreased lymphocyte cell count. Neutrophil cell count may be low during the more advanced stages of the disease.

Hepatitis serology

Serologic markers for hepatitis viral infections

HBsAg. Hepatitis B surface antigen (HBsAg) is an indicator of viral replication and can be present both during acute and chronic infections. Patients with HBsAg markers are considered infectious.

Anti-HBs. Antibody to hepatitis B surface antigen (HBsAg). Indicator of clinical recovery and subsequent immunity to HBV. Generally appears 1 to 4 months after onset of symptoms.

Can also be acquired by hepatitis B immune globulin (HBIG) or hepatitis B vaccine. Patients with anti-HBs markers are not considered infectious.

Anti-HBcIgM. Antibody (IgM) to hepatitis B core antigen (HBcAg). An early indicator of acute infection. Is prominent during the acute phase of infection and persists for 3 to 12 months. Will distinguish acute from chronic hepatitis B infection.

Anti-HBc. Total antibody (IgG and IgM) to hepatitis core antigen (HBcAg). A lifelong marker that represents past infection as well as active infection during the acute/chronic period. Some patients with anti-HBc markers are considered infectious; however, some patients are not infectious. These antibodies are not produced by HBV vaccination and can be used to establish past HBV infections.

HBeAg. Hepatitis B e antigen (HBeAg) is an indicator of the most infectious period during acute and chronic infection. Usually short-lived (3 to 6 weeks) but when present beyond 10 weeks, a progressive chronic state and probable chronic liver disease can be expected. Patients with HBeAg markers are considered highly infectious.

Anti-HBe. Antibody to HBeAg. Seroconversion from HBeAg to anti-HBe is prognostic for resolution of infection. Patients with anti-HBe markers are not considered infectious even in the presence of HBsAg.

Anti-HAVIgM. IgM antibody to hepatitis A antigen (HA Ag). This marker is detectable with the first symptoms of hepatitis A virus infection and persists for 3 to 12 months.

Anti-HAVIgG. IgG antibody to HA Ag. IgG antibodies appear within a week of the IgM response. This antibody has neutralizing activity and persists for life. Patients with anti-HAVIgG markers are not considered infectious.

Anti-HD. Total antibody (IgG and IgM) to hepatitis D virus. Indicator of exposure to hepatitis D virus. Anti-delta positive individuals may still transmit HDV infection. Patients with anti-HD markers are considered infectious.

Anti-HCV. Presence of antibody to hepatitis C virus (anti-HCV) may indicate infection with HCV. Anti-HCV seroconversion occurs 15 weeks to up to 1 year after infection and may disappear after resolution of the infection. Patients with anti-HCV markers are considered either infectious or noninfectious. Changes in anti-HCV titer together with changes in liver functions determine infectivity.

Appendix B

Abbreviations

Ab	antibody	**CNS**	central nervous system
ADC	AIDS dementia complex	**CT**	computed tomography
ADCC	antibody-dependent cellular cytotoxicity	**ddI**	dideoxyinosine
		ddC	dideoxycytodine
AIDS	acquired immunodeficiency syndrome	**EBV**	Epstein-Barr virus
Ag	antigen	**EI**	erythema infectiosum
anti-HBc	antibody to hepatitis B core antigen	**EIA**	enzyme immunoassay
		ELISA	enzyme-linked immunosorbent assay
anti-HBs	antibody to hepatitis B surface antigen	**FDA**	Food and Drug Administration
APC	antigen-presenting cells	**G-CSF**	granulocyte-colony stimulating factor
ARV	AIDS-associated retrovirus		
AZT	azidothymidine (Retrovir)	**GI**	gastrointestinal tract
BAL	bronchoalveolar lavage	**GM-CSF**	granulocyte-macrophage–colony stimulating factor
BEA	bacillary epithelioid angiomatosis		
CD	clusters of differentiation	**gp**	glycoprotein
CDC	Centers for Disease Control and Prevention	**HAV**	hepatitis A virus
CMV	cytomegalovirus	**HBeAg**	hepatitis B e antigen

HBIG	hepatitis B immune globulin		**ITP**	immune thrombocytopenic purpura
HBsAg	hepatitis B surface antigen		**IVDU**	intravenous drug user
HBV	hepatitis B virus		**kDa**	kiloDalton
HCV	hepatitis C virus		**KS**	Kaposi's sarcoma
HDV	hepatitis delta virus		**LAS**	lymphadenopathy syndrome
HCW	health-care workers		**LAV**	lymphadenopathy-associated virus
Hgb	hemoglobin			
HIV	human immunodeficiency virus		**LBM**	lean body mass
			LGE	linear gingival erythema
HIV-1	human immunodeficiency virus type 1		**MAC**	*Mycobacterium avium complex*
HIV-2	human immunodeficiency virus type 2		**MAI**	*Mycobacterium avium-intracellulare*
HIVD	human immunodeficiency virus disease		**MDR-TB**	multi-drug–resistant tuberculosis
HIV-G	human immunodeficiency virus-associated gingivitis		**MiAU**	minor aphthous ulcer
			MiRAU	minor recurrent aphthous ulcer
HIV-P	human immunodeficiency virus–associated periodontitis		**MjAU**	major aphthous ulcer
			MjRAU	major recurrent aphthous ulcer
HPV	human papilloma virus			
HSV	herpes simplex virus		**MRI**	magnetic resonance imaging
HSV-1	herpes simplex virus type 1		**MSM**	men having sex with men
HSV-2	herpes simplex virus type 2		**NDA**	new drug application
HTLV III	human T-cell lymphotropic virus type III		**NHL**	non-Hodgkin's lymphoma
			NIH	National Institutes of Health
IDU	injection drug user		**NK**	natural killer (cells)
IFA	immunofluorescence assay		**NS**	necrotizing stomatitis
IL	interleukin		**NUP**	necrotizing ulcerative periodontitis
IND	investigational new drug			
ISG	immune serum globulin			

OHL	oral hairy leukoplakia	**rCD4**	recombinant CD4
OSHA	Occupational Safety and Health Administration	**rHuEPO**	recombinant human erythropoietin
p	protein	**RT**	reverse transcriptase
PBMC	peripheral blood mononuclear cells	**SBE**	subacute bacterial endocarditis
PCP	*Pneumocystis carinii* pneumonia	**SCC**	squamous cell carcinoma
		SI	syncytia inducing
PCR	polymerase chain reaction (assay)	**STD**	sexually transmitted diseases
		TB	tuberculosis
PGL	persistent generalized lymphadenopathy	**TH1**	T-helper cell type 1 (response)
PML	progressive multifocal leukoencephalopathy	**TH2**	T-helper cell type 2 (response)
PPD	purified protein derivative	**VZV**	varicella zoster virus
PSN	predominantly sensory neuropathy	**WB**	Western blot
PT	prothrombin time	**WBC count**	white blood cell count
PTT	partial thromboplastin time	**WHO**	World Health Organization
PWA	people with AIDS	**ZDV**	zidovudine (Retrovir)

Resources

Hotlines (AIDS/Drugs/STD)

CDC National AIDS Hotline	1-800-342-AIDS
CDC Spanish AIDS Hotline	1-800-344-SIDA
CDC Hearing Impaired AIDS Hotline	1-800-243-7889
CDC National AIDS Clearing House	1-800-458-5231
CDC National AIDS Clearing House (Deaf access/TDD)	1-800-243-7012
CDC National Clearing House (International)	1-301-217-0023
AIDS Clinical Trials Information Service	1-800-TRIALS-A
Project Inform (HIV Treatment Hotline)	1-800-822-7422
National Indian AIDS Line	1-800-283-2437
Substance Abuse and Mental Health Service Administration (SAMHSA) Drug Abuse Information and Treatment Referrals Hotline	1-800-662-HELP

Center for Substance Abuse Prevention (CSAP) National Clearinghouse for Alcohol and Drug Information	1-800-729-6686
CDC National Sexually Transmitted Diseases Hotline	1-800-227-8922
National Herpes Hotline	1-919-361-8488

Recorded Information from the CDC

AIDS Statistical Information Line	1-404-332-4570
Fax Information Service Line	1-404-332-4565
General Information Including HIV/AIDS	1-404-332-4555

AIDS Hotlines by State
(Note: numbers subject to change)

Alabama	1-800-228-0469
Alaska	1-800-468-AIDS
Arizona	1-602-420-9396

Arkansas	1-800-445-7720	Nevada	1-800-842-AIDS
California (N)	1-800-367-AIDS	New Hampshire	1-800-752-2437
California (S)	1-213-876-AIDS	New Jersey	1-800-624-2377
Colorado	1-800-252-AIDS	New Mexico	1-800-545-AIDS
Connecticut	1-800-342-AIDS	New York	1-800-541-AIDS
Delaware	1-800-422-0429	North Carolina	1-800-342-AIDS
District of Columbia	1-202-332-AIDS	North Dakota	1-800-472-2180
Florida	1-800-352-AIDS	Ohio	1-800-332-AIDS
Georgia	1-800-551-2728	Oklahoma	1-800-535-AIDS
Hawaii	1-808-922-1313	Oregon	1-503-223-AIDS
Idaho	1-800-677-AIDS	Pennsylvania	1-800-662-6080
Illinois	1-800-243-AIDS	Puerto Rico	1-809-765-1010
Indiana	1-800-848-AIDS	Rhode Island	1-800-726-3010
Iowa	1-800-445-AIDS	South Carolina	1-800-322-AIDS
Kansas	1-800-232-0040	South Dakota	1-800-592-1861
Kentucky	1-800-654-AIDS	Tennessee	1-800-525-AIDS
Louisiana	1-800-992-4379	Texas	1-800-299-AIDS
Maine	1-800-851-AIDS	Utah	1-801-487-AIDS
Maryland	1-800-638-6252	Vermont	1-800-882-AIDS
Massachusetts	1-800-235-2331	Virgin Islands	1-809-773-AIDS
Michigan	1-800-872-AIDS	Virginia	1-800-533-4148
Minnesota	1-800-248-AIDS	Washington	1-800-272-AIDS
Mississippi	1-800-537-0851	West Virginia	1-800-642-8244
Missouri	1-800-533-AIDS	Wisconsin	1-800-334-AIDS
Montana	1-800-233-6668	Wyoming	1-800-327-3577
Nebraska	1-800-782-AIDS		

National Organizations

American Red Cross
1750 K St, NW, Suite 700
Washington, DC 20006
202-973-6025

HDI-National Hispanic Education and
    Communication Projects
1000 16th St, NW, Suite 504
Washington, DC 20036
202-452-0092

Health Resource and Service Administration
    (HRSA)
AIDS Program Office, Parklawn Building
5600 Fishers Lane
Rockville, MD 20857
301-443-4588

The NAMES Project AIDS Memorial Quilt
310 Townsend St, Suite 310
San Francisco, CA 94107
415-882-5500

The National Association of People with AIDS
    (NAPWA)
1413 K St, 10th Floor
Washington, DC 20005
202-898-0414

The National Coalition of Hispanic Health and
    Human Services Organizations
    (COSSMHO)
1501 16th St, NW
Washington, DC 20036-1401
202-387-5000

The National Gay and Lesbian Task Force
    (NGLTF)
1734 14th St, NW
Washington, DC 20009-4309
202-332-6483

The National Hemophilia Foundation (NHF)
The SOHO BLDG, 110 Greene St, Suite 303
New York, NY 10012
212-219-8180; 212-431-8541

National Pediatric HIV Resource Center
    (NPHRC)
Children's Hospital of New Jersey
15th S 9th St
Newark, NJ 07107
201-268-8251; 1-800-362-0071

National Minority AIDS Council (NMAC)
300 I St, NE, Suite 400
Washington, DC 20002-4389
202-544-1076

National Native American AIDS Prevention
    Center (NNAAPC)
3515 Grand Ave, Suite 100
Oakland, CA 94610
510-444-2051

Planned Parenthood Federation of America
    (PPFA)
810 7th Ave
New York, NY 10019
212-541-7800

Rural AIDS Network (RAN)
1915 Rosina
Santa Fe, NM 87501
505-986-8337

Substance Abuse and Mental Health Service
    Administration (SAMHSA)
Room 12C-10, 5600 Fishers Lane
Rockville, MD 20857
301-443-5305

*The above information has been adapted
    from Resource Booklet, American
    Association for World Health, 1129 20th St,
    NW, Suite 400, Washington, DC, 20036-
    3403.

Health Resource and Service Administration Funded AIDS Education and Training Centers

Serving New York and the Virgin Islands

New York/Virgin Islands AIDS ETC
Columbia University School of Public Health
600 W 168th St
New York, NY 10032
Cheryl Healton, Dr PH
212-305-3616, Fax 212-305-6832

Serving Washington, Alaska, Montana, Idaho, and Oregon

Northwest AIDS ETC
University of Washington
1001 Broadway, Suite 217 Mail Stop ZH-20
Seattle, WA 98122
Ann Downer, MS
206-720-4250, Fax 206-720-4218

Serving Ohio, Michigan, Kentucky, and Tennessee

East Central AIDS ETC
The Ohio State University
Department of Family Medicine
1314 Kinnear Rd, Area 300
Columbus, OH 43212
Lawrence L. Gabel, PhD
614-292-1400, Fax 614-292-4056

Serving Nevada, Arizona, Hawaii, and California (excluding six counties included in following entry)

Western AIDS ETC
University of California—Davis
5110 East Clinton Way, Suite 115
Fresno, CA 93727-2098
Michael Reyes, MD
209-252-2851, Fax 209-454-8012

Serving six counties in Southern California: Riverside, San Bernardino, Los Angeles, Orange, Ventura, and Santa Barbara

AIDS ETC for Southern California
University of Southern California
1420 San Pablo St, B207
Los Angeles, CA 90033
Jerry Gates, PhD
213-342-1846, Fax 213-942-2051

Serving Alabama, Georgia, North Carolina, and South Carolina

Emory AIDS Training Network
Emory University
735 Gatewood Rd, NE
Atlanta, GA 30322
Ira Schwartz, MD
404-729-2929, Fax 404-727-4562

Serving Arkansas, Louisiana, and Mississippi

Delta Region AIDS ETC
Louisiana State University
1542 Tulane Ave
New Orleans, LA 70112
William Brandon, MD, MPH
504-568-3855, Fax 504-568-7893

Serving North Dakota, South Dakota, Utah, Colorado, New Mexico, Nebraska, Kansas, and Wyoming

Mountain Plains Regional AIDS ETC
University of Colorado
4200 E Ninth Avenue, Box A-096
Denver, CO 80262
Donna Anderson, PhD, MPH
303-355-1301, Fax 303-355-1448

Serving Illinois, Indiana, Iowa, Minnesota, Missouri, and Wisconsin

Midwest AIDS Training Education Center
University of Illinois at Chicago
808 S Wood St (M/C 779)
Chicago, IL 60612
Nathan L. Linsk, PhD
312-996-1373, Fax 312-413-4184

Serving Delaware, Maryland, Virginia, and West Virginia

Mid-Atlantic AIDS ETC
Medical College of Virginia
P.O. Box 159, MCV Station
Richmond, VA 23298-0159
Lisa Kaplowitz, MD
804-371-2447, Fax 804-371-0495

Serving Connecticut, Maine, Massachusetts, New Hampshire, Rhode Island, and Vermont

New England AIDS ETC
University of Massachusetts
55 Lake Ave North
Worcester, MA 01655
Donna Gallagher, RN, MS, ANP
508-856-3255, Fax 508-856-6128

Serving Texas and Oklahoma

AIDS ETC for Texas and Oklahoma
The University of Texas
1200 Herman Pressler St
POB 20186
Houston, TX 77225
Richard Grimes, PhD
713-794-4075, Fax 713-794-4877

Serving Pennsylvania

Pennsylvania AIDS ETC
University of Pittsburgh
Graduate School of Public Health
130 DeSoto St, Room A425
Pittsburgh, PA 15201
Linda Frank, PhD, MSN, RN
412-624-1895, Fax 412-624-4767

Serving New Jersey

New Jersey AIDS ETC
University of Medicine and Dentistry of NJ
Office of Continuing Education
30 Bergen St, ADMC #710
Newark, NJ 07107-3000
Charles McKinney, EdD
201-982-3690, Fax 201-982-7128

Serving Florida

Florida AIDS ETC
University of Miami
P.O. Box 016960 (D-90)
Miami, FL 33101
Howard Anapol, MD
305-585-7836, Fax 305-324-4931

Serving Puerto Rico

Puerto Rico AIDS ETC
University of Puerto Rico
Medical Sciences Campus
GPO 36-5067 Room 745A
Rio Piedras, Puerto Rico 00936-5067
Angel Bravo, MPH
809-759-6528, Fax 809-764-2470

Serving metropolitan Washington DC

District of Columbia AIDS ETC
2112 Georgia Ave, NW
Washington, DC 20060
Eric Moolchan, MD
202-800-4002, Fax 202-806-4323

INDEX

Illustrations are indicated in *italics*.

Antidiscrimination laws, 28–32
  Americans with Disabilities Act of 1990, 30–31
  confidentiality issues, 32
  licensure laws, 31–32
  malpractice action, 32
  referral as discrimination, 25–27, 34–35
  Rehabilitation Act of 1973, 29–30
  tort law, 32
Antifungal medication, 197–198
Antigen/antibody, p24 Antigen/antibody, 219
Anti-HIV dementia medication, 199
Antimycobacterial medication, 195–197
Antineoplastic agents, 195
Antiparasitic agents, 198–199
Anti-retroviral therapy, 186–190
Antiviral medications, 195
Aphthous ulceration, intraoral manifestation of HIV, *172*, 172–173
  treatment, *173*
Aspergillus infection, as manifestation of AIDS, 101–102, 162
Attire, for infection control, 259

B

B19 parvovirus, as manifestation of AIDS, 102
Bacillary angiomatosis, cutaneous manifestations of HIV, 133–134
Bacillary epithelioid angiomatosis, intraoral manifestation of HIV, 165–166, *166*
Bacterial infection
  intraoral manifestation of HIV, 165–168
  pyogenic, localized, cutaneous manifestations of HIV, 132–134
Barrier techniques, for infection control, 258–259
  clinic attire, 259
  gloving, 258
  mask, 258–259
  protective eyewear, 259
Bisexual contact, HIV exposure, 50–52
Blame, of society, in response to epidemic, 16
Bleeding time, HIV, 221
Blood transfusion/products
  HIV exposure, 52–53
  HIV prevention, 61–62
  HIV transmission, 73–75
Blood-borne pathogen management
  exposure
    to HBC, 279–282
    to HIV, 277–279
    to HVC, 279–282
    immediately after, 275–276
  serologic evaluation of source patient, 276–277
Bubonic plague, impact of, 12–14

C

Calciphylaxis, cutaneous manifestations of HIV, 140
Candidiasis, intraoral manifestation of HIV, 102, 158–162, *159–161*
Cardiac system, review of, in medical assessment, 241
Casual contact, HIV transmission, 79–80
CD8+ cell count, HIV, 219
CD4+ T-Helper lymphocyte
  classification system, *118*
  HIV pathogenesis, 92
CD4+ T-lymphocyte cell count, HIV, 216–219
CD4+/CD8+ ratio, HIV, 219
Cellular infection, HIV, 88–90, *89*
Centers for Disease Control and Prevention
  Revised Classification System for HIV Infection, 116, *117*, 117–118, *118*
  surveillance for HIV/AIDS, 43–44
Characteristics, of persons reported with AIDS, *45*
Cholera, impact of, 14–15
Classification system
  CD4+ T-Helper lymphocyte, *118*
  Revised Classification System for HIV Infection, 116, *117*, 117–118, *118*
Cleaning of instruments, for infection control, 260
Clinic attire, for infection control, 259
Clinical manifestations, AIDS, 101–125
Coccidioides immitis infection, as manifestation of AIDS, 102–103
Confidentiality
  HIV test, 209
  issues, 32
Contact
  casual, HIV transmission, 79–80
  sexual, HIV transmission. *See* Sexual transmission
Corynebacterium diphtheriae, cutaneous manifestations of HIV, 133
Counseling, prevention, HIV, 209–210
Covers, infection control, 266, *266*
Cryptococcosis, intraoral manifestation of HIV, 162
Cryptococcus neoformans, cutaneous manifestations of HIV, 135
Cutaneous manifestations, HIV, 127–152, *128*
  bacillary angiomatosis, 133–134
  calciphylaxis, 140
  Corynebacterium diphtheriae, 133
  cryptococcus neoformans, 135
  cytomegalovirus, 129
  demodicidosis, 136–137
  ectoparasitic infestation, 136–137
  eosinophilic pustular folliculitis, 140, *140*
  erythema elevatum diutinum, 140
  exanthem, 128

fungal infection
  superficial, 134
  systemic, 134–136
Grover's disease, 142
hair disorder, 143
herpes simplex, 129–130, *130*
herpes zoster, 129–130, *130*
histoplasma capsulatum, 135–136
human papilloma virus infection, 131–132
infectious skin disease, 128–137
inflammatory dermatoses, 142
Kaposi's sarcoma, 143–145, *144*
localized pyogenic bacterial infection, 132–134
molluscum contagiosum, 130–131, *131*
morbilliform drug eruption, 139
mycobacterial infection, 133
neoplasm, 143
noninfectious skin condition, 137–142
nutritional disorder, 142
papular urticaria, 139–140
parasitic infection, 136–137
Penicillium, marneffei, 136
photodermatitis, 138–139
pigmentary disorders, 141, *141*
pityriasis rubra pilaris, 138
pruritus, 141–142
psoriasis, 137–138
scabies, 136
seborrheic dermatitis, 137–138, *138*
syphilis, 133
vascular abnormalities, 141
viral infection, 128–132
Cytokines, 199
Cytomegalovirus
  cutaneous manifestations of HIV, 129
  intraoral manifestation of HIV, 163, *163*
  as manifestation of AIDS, 103–104

D

Dementia, medication, 199
Demodicidosis, cutaneous manifestations of HIV, 136–137
Demographics
  AIDS, 44, *45, 46,* 47
  HIV, 47–50, *48–49*
Denial, of society, in response to epidemic, 15–16
Dental care, modifications of, 247–255
  antibiotic prophylaxis, 248–249
  endodontic therapy, 252–253
  extraction, 253–254
  hemostatis, in oral surgery, 253
  local anesthetics, 250
  oral surgery, 253–254

orthodontic procedures, 254
periodontal therapy, 251
preventive oral health care, 250–251
prosthetic procedures, 251–252
restorative procedures, 251–252
surgical intervention, extensive, 254
tissue healing from oral surgery, 254
treatment planning, 248–249
Dermatitis, seborrheic, cutaneous manifestations of HIV, 137–138, *138*
Discrimination
  against HIV-positive individual, 28–32
    Americans with Disabilities Act of 1990, 30–31
      sanctions, 31
    confidentiality issues, 32
    malpractice action, 32
    Rehabilitation Act of 1973, 29–30
      sanctions, 31
    tort law, 32
  licensure laws, 31–32
  referral as, 25–27, 34–35
Disinfection, for infection control, 261–262
Disposables, infection control, 266, *266–267*
Distribution, global, HIV, 56, *58,* 58–59
Drug approval process, 183–184
Duty to treat, 26–40

E

Ectoparasitic infestation, cutaneous manifestations of HIV, 136–137
Encephalopathy, as manifestation of AIDS, 109–110
Endodontic therapy, with HIV-infected patient, 252–253
Eosinophilic pustular folliculitis, cutaneous manifestations of HIV, 140, *140*
Epidemics
  impact of, 12–15
    Bubonic plague, 12–14
    cholera, 14–15
    smallpox, 14
  sexually transmitted disease, 17
  social response to, 15–16
Epidemiology
  AIDS, 17–19
    number of cases, 11, 41, *42, 45, 46*
  hepatitis B, 19
Erythema
  elevatum diutinum, cutaneous manifestations of HIV, 141
  gingival, linear, intraoral manifestation of HIV, 166–168, *168*
Erythrocyte sedimentation rate, HIV, 220
Ethical issues, 27–28

Plague, AIDS epidemic, compared, 19–20
Platelet count, HIV, 220–221
Pneumocystis carinii, 137
    pneumonia, 110
Pneumonia, *Pneumocystis carinii,* as manifestation
        of AIDS, 110
Positive result, HIV test, 210–211
Poverty, and AIDS, 20
Prevention, HIV, 59–62
    blood transfusion/products, 61–62
    counseling, 209–210
    in dental practice, 282–283
    in health-care setting, 62
    injection equipment, 61
    in oral health care, with HIV-infected patient,
        250–251
    perinatal infection, 62
    sexual transmission, 59–60
Progressive multifocal leukoencephalopathy, as
        manifestation of AIDS, 109–110
Prosthetic procedures
    with HIV-infected patient, 251–252
    infection control, impression disinfecting,
        273–274, *274*
Protective eyewear, for infection control, 259
Prothrombin time, HIV, 223–224
Pruritus, cutaneous manifestations of HIV, 141–142
Psoriasis, cutaneous manifestations of HIV,
        137–138
Pulmonary system, review of, in medical
        assessment, 241–242
Pyogenic bacterial infection, localized, cutaneous
        manifestations of HIV, 132–134

R

Referral, as discrimination, 25–27, 34–35
Refusal to treat, 26–40
Rehabilitation Act of 1973, 29–30
    sanctions, 31
Resources, HIV/AIDS, 306–309
Restorative procedures, with HIV-infected patient,
        251–252
Result, positive, HIV test, 210–211
Revised Classification System for HIV Infection,
        116, *117, 117*117–118, *118*

S

Saliva
    HIV testing, 212
    HIV transmission, 76–77
Scabies, cutaneous manifestations of HIV, 136

Seborrheic dermatitis, cutaneous manifestations of
        HIV, 137–138, *138*
Serologic testing, 206–207
    evaluation of source patient, for blood-borne
        pathogen management, 276–277
Sexual transmission
    AIDS/HIV, 72–73
        bisexual contact, 50–52
        homosexual male, 22
        prevention, 59–60
    epidemic, societal response, 17
    history of, in medical assessment, 232
Smallpox, impact of, 14
Social support system, 238
Sociological response
    AIDS, 20–21
    blame, in response to epidemic, 16
    denial, in response to epidemic, 15–16
    to epidemics, 15–16
    to sexually transmitted disease epidemic, 17
Squamous cell carcinoma, intraoral manifestation
        of HIV, 171
Staff training
    team preparation
        accepting patients with HIV, 290–291
        planning, staff involvement in, 292–293
        staff development goal-setting, 291–292
    team training, 293–296, *297*
Sterilization of instruments
    central area, 267–268
    for infection control, 260–261
        cleaning of instruments, 260
        heat sterilization, 260–261
Stomatitis, necrotizing, intraoral manifestation of
        HIV, 173–174, *174*
Surgery, oral, with HIV-infected patient, 253–254
Surveillance for HIV/AIDS, 43–44
Syphilis
    cutaneous manifestations of HIV, 133
    intraoral manifestation of HIV, 168
    as manifestation of AIDS, 111

T

Team preparation, HIV patient
    accepting patients with HIV, 290–291
    planning, staff involvement in, 292–293
    staff development goal-setting, 291–292
    staff training, 293–296, *297*
Tears, HIV transmission, 78
Testing, HIV, 205–213
    confidentiality, 209
    dentist's role in, 212
    indications for, 208–209